Library of Congress Cataloging-in-Publication Data
ISBN 0-8031-1895-3
ISSN 1071-720x
ASTM Publication Code Number (PCN) 04-01280-16

Peer Review Policy

Each paper published in this volume was evaluated by three peer reviewers. The authors addressed all of the reviewers' comments to the satisfaction of both the technical editor(s) and the ASTM Committee on Publications.

To make technical information available as quickly as possible, the peer-reviewed papers in this publication were printed "camera-ready" as submitted by the authors.

The quality of the papers in this publication reflects not only the obvious efforts of the authors and the technical editor(s), but also the work of these peer reviewers. The ASTM Committee on Publications acknowledges with appreciation their dedication and contribution to time and effort on behalf of ASTM.

Printed in Philadelphia, PA
February 1995

STP 1218

Environmental Toxicology and Risk Assessment: Third Volume

Jane Staveley Hughes, Gregory R. Biddinger, and Eugene Mones, Editors

ASTM Publication Code Number (PCN)
04-012180-16

ASTM
1916 Race Street
Philadelphia, PA 19103
Printed in the U.S.A.

Foreword

This publication, *Environmental Toxicology and Risk Assessment: Third Volume* contains papers presented at the symposium of the same name held in Atlanta, GA on 26–29 April 1993. The symposium was sponsored by ASTM Committee E-47 on Biological Effects and Environmental Fate. Jane S Hughes of Caroline Ecotox, Inc. in Durham, NC, Gregory R. Biddinger of Exxon Company USA in Benecia, CA, and Eugene Mones of Unilever Research U.S. in Edgewater, NJ presided as chairs, and are the editors of the resulting publications.

Contents

Overview ix

KEYNOTE ADDRESS

Critical Issues in Ecological Risk Assessment—S. M. BARTELL AND G. R. BIDDINGER 3

ECOTOXICOLOGY: PREDICTION AND ASSESSMENT

Bioassessment of Glovers Creed, West Union, Iowa, Using the USEPA's Rapid Bioassessment Protocol II—J. R. VIGNA, J. K. JOHNSON AND B. C. KROSS 29

Guidance for Performing Ecological Risk Assessments at Hazardous Waste Sites—J. M. DESESSO 44

A Framework for Field and Laboratory Studies for Ecological Risk Assessments in Wetland and Terrestrial Habitats: Two Case Studies—G. LINDER, M. BOLLMAN, G. GILLETT, R. KING, J. NWOSU, S. OTT, D. WILBORN, G. HENDERSON, T. PFLEEGER, T. DARROW AND D. LIGHTFOOT 61

Nonmetric Clustering and Association Analysis: Implications for the Evaluation of Multispecies Toxicity Tests and Field Monitoring—G. B. MATTHEWS, R. A. MATTHEWS AND W. G. LANDIS 79

MODELS IN ECOLOGICAL RISK ASSESSMENT

Conservative Uncertainty Propagation in Environmental Risk Assessment—S. FERSON AND T. F. LONG 97

Screening-Level Versus Refined Modeling Approaches to Estimating PCB Concentrations in Aquatic Food WEBS: A Case Study of Lake Ontario—P. K. SCOTT AND K. R. TROWBRIDGE 111

Non-linear Oscillations Detected by Multivariate Analysis in Microcosm Toxicity Tests: Implications for Risk Assessment and Biomonitoring—W. G. LANDIS, R. A. A. J. MARKIEWICZ AND G. B. MATTHEWS 133

Ecotoxicology of Predator-Prey Communities: An Individual-Based Modeling Approach—J. S. JAWORSKA, T. G. HALLAM, S. M. HENSON, W. R. MCKINNEY AND R. R. LASSITER 157

Volume Fraction Analyses for Selected Mechanisms of Toxic Action—T. W. SCHULTZ, J. S. JAWORSKA AND R. S. HUNTER 172

SEDIMENT TOXICOLOGY

Use of Vascular Aquatic Plants in Phytotoxicity Studies with Sediments—D. E. WEBER, G. E. WALSH AND M. A. MACGREGOR 187

A 28 Day Sediment Bioassay with the Marine Polychaete, NEREIS (NEANTHES) ARENACEODENTATA—T. M. DILLON, D. W. MOORE AND D. J. REISH 201

In-Situ Bioassays using Transplanted Mussels: I. Estimating Chemical Exposure and Bioeffects with Bioaccumulation and Growth—M. H. SALAZAR AND S. M. SALAZAR 216

In-Situ Bioassay using Transplanted Mussels: II. Assessing Contaminated Sediment at a Superfund Site in Puget Sound—M. H. SALAZAR, S. M. SALAZAR, P. B. DUNCAN AND K. A. ROSE 242

FATE AND EFFECTS OF CHEMICALS

Using Grass Shrimp Embryos to Determine the Effects of Sediment on the Toxicity and Persistence of Diflubenzuron in Laboratory Microcosms—J. E. H. WILSON, P. A. CUNNINGHAM, D. W. EVANS, AND J. D. COSTLOW, JR. 267

A Comparative Analysis of the Toxicity of Boron Compounds to Freshwater and Saltwater Species—P. S. HOVATTER AND R. H. ROSS 288

Net Photosynthesis and Respiration of Sago Pondweed (POTAMOGETON PECTINATUS) Exposed to Herbicides—W. J. FLEMING, M. S. AILSTOCK AND J. J. MOMOT 303

Development of a General QSAR for Predicting Octanol-Water Partition Coefficients and its Application to Surfactants—K. F. MOSCHNER AND A. CECE 318

Recent Developments in LCA and Critical Issues—D. POSTLETHWAITE 332

METHODS DEVELOPMENT

Probing the Routes, Rates, and Mechanisms of Xenobiotic Elimination by Rainbow Trout (ONCORHYNCHUS MYKISS) with a Physiological Chamber—M. C. BLACK, K. BJORKROTH AND A. OIKARI 351

Methods to Improve the Sensitivity of an Automated Biomonitoring by System—D. GRUBER AND C. FRAGO 365

Comparative Toxicities of Six Heavy Metals Using Root Elongation and Shoot Growth in Three Plant Species—J. W. GORSUCH, M. RITTER AND E. R. ANDERSON 377

A Modified ASTM Semi-Continuous Activated Sludge Test to Compare Nonionic Surfactant Biological Removal—A. M. NIELSEN, P. A. FILLER, J. E. HEINZE AND T. M. LACHOCKI 393

Author Index 409

Subject Index 411

Overview

The Third Symposium on Environmental Toxicology and Risk Assessment: Aquatic, Plant and Terrestrial was held in Atlanta, GA, during 26–29 April 1993. This symposium was actually the 17th consecutive annual ASTM symposium to address environmental toxicology and related issues. The symposium was sponsored by ASTM Committee E-47 on Biological Effects and Environmental Fate, and the platform and poster presentations were integrated over the four days with meetings of the various subcommittees that are actively engaged in developing the consensus standards for which ASTM is so well known.

A featured highlight of the symposium was a series of sessions on "The Exxon Valdez: Environmental Response and Assessment," in which the Exxon Valdez oil spill was examined as a "case study" in ecological risk assessment. The presentations from this portion of the symposium are published in a separate volume entitled *The Exxon Valdez Oil Spill: Fate and Effects in Alaskan Waters,* edited by Peter Wells, James Butler, and Jane Hughes (ASTM STP 1219).

The theme of the symposium was a review of "Critical Issues in Environmental Toxicology and Risk Assessment." It is a testament to the development of the field that we have come to the stage of refining those issues that are most critical to taking the next steps in advancing the science of estimating the fate and effects of chemicals in the environment. Across various matrices, over different levels of organization, from molecular to ecosystem, in the lab, in the field, and through models, we seek essentially the same types of information in order to improve the predictive value of our risk assessments.

The plenary session began with a presentation entitled "Critical Issues in Ecological Risk Assessment." This paper, by Bartell and Biddinger, reviews the current technical status of ecological risk assessment and offers suggestions for advancing the discipline. The prospects for standardization of procedures and methods for ecological risk analysis are discussed, and an argument is presented for adoption of environmental planning to minimize the future need to assess ecological risks.

The remaining 22 papers in this STP have been organized into 5 groups. However, it is indicative of the maturation of the field of environmental toxicology that most of the papers could be placed in a number of categories. Boundaries between traditional categories have become blurred, as we read about plants used to assess the toxicity of sediments, laboratory tests used to assess multiple environmental matrices, and field techniques integrating exposure and effects.

The papers in the first section, "Ecotoxicology: Prediction and Assessment," are concerned with the estimation and measurement of ecological effects. A protocol for rapid bioassessment, based upon the characterization of the macroinvertebrate community, was used to assess the biological condition of a stream by Vigna et al. DeSesso describes a three-phased approach to ecological risk assessment at hazardous waste sites including the determination of ecological quotients, assessment of biological diversity, and population studies. Linder et al. compare and contrast field and laboratory methods used for evaluating contaminant-impacted wetlands at two different sites. Matthews et al. present a tool for the analysis of multispecies data based upon an artificial intelligence technique known as nonmetric clustering, which characterizes a complex, multivariate system.

For the first time in this ASTM series, a significant number of papers are presented that address "Models in Ecological Risk Assessment." Ferson and Long compare the merits of dependency bounds analysis with Monte Carlo methods for yielding conservative risk estimates with realistic uncertainty. The use of a screening-level model is compared to the use of a more refined food web model for assessing bioaccumulation of Polychlorobenzene (PCBs) in Lake Ontario by Scott and Trowbridge. Based upon multivariate analysis of data from aquatic microcosms (a.k.a. "Wayne's Worms"), Landis et al. challenge the assumption that, after the initial stress, ecosystems recover to resemble the "unchaotic" control state. Physiologically structured models focusing on the individual were used to study the effects of nonpolar narcotic chemicals on two predator-prey systems by Jaworska et al. On the molecular scale, Schultz et al. describe the use of volume fraction analyses to distinguish different mechanisms of toxic action.

Continued interest in the topic, "Sediment Toxicology," is reflected in the next four papers. Weber et al. present procedures used to identify the effects of contaminated sediments on rooted aquatic plants through the use of laboratory toxicity tests involving natural and artificial sediments. Methods for conducting a 28-day sediment bioassay with a marine polychaete for use in the evaluation of dredged material are presented by Dillon et al. Salazar and Salazar measured bioaccumulation and growth to estimate chemical exposure and bioeffects for caged mussels. Transplanted mussels were also used by Salazar et al. to assess the extent and magnitude of contamination in water overlying the sediment at a Superfund site in Puget Sound.

Five papers examine the "Fate and Effects of Chemicals." Wilson et al. used grass shrimp embryos to determine the effects of estuarine sediment on the toxicity and persistence of diflubenzuron in two laboratory microcosm systems. Hovatter and Ross performed a comparative analysis of the toxicity of boron compounds to freshwater and saltwater fish and invertebrates. Fleming et al. examined net photosynthesis and respiration rates for sago pondweed exposed to various concentrations of 11 herbicides. An approach to develop a broad Quantitative Structure-Activity Relationships (QSAR), applicable to surfactants, to predict octanol-water partition coefficients based upon general molecular structural parameters is discussed by Moschner and Cece. This chapter concludes with a review of recent developments and critical issues in the growing field of Lifecycle Assessment by Postlethwaite.

Last, but certainly not least in the hearts and minds of die-hard ASTM members, are the papers addressing "Methods Development." The development and refinement of new methods to assess exposure and toxicity are crucial to progress in the field of risk assessment. Black et al. discuss the development and use of a special chamber to isolate the various xenobiotic elimination routes in fish. The design and use of an automated biomonitoring system using fish ventilatory response and activity as the detector of toxicity is the subject of the paper by Gruber and Frago. Gorsuch et al. discuss the use of vertically mounted seed pouches to assess the effects of heavy metals on the growth of terrestrial plants. Three different modifications to the ASTM Test Method for Biodegradability of Alkylbenzene Sulfonates (D 2667) for biodegradability were investigated by Nielsen et al.

We would like to thank the session chairs for their efforts in organizing the sessions and assistance in selecting manuscript reviewers: Ecological Risk Assessment: Models, Steve Bartell (SENES Oak Ridge, Inc., Oak Ridge, TN); Plants in Toxicity Assessments, Mike Lewis (U.S. EPA, Gulf Breeze, FL) and Nancy Lane (Westinghouse Hanford Co., Richland, WA); Sediment Toxicology, Chris Ingersoll (National Biological Survey, Columbia, MO); Ecological Risk Assessment at Contaminated Sites, Steve Friant (Battelle Pacific Northwest Laboratories, Richland, WA) and Suellen Pirages (Karch and Associates, Washington, DC); Environmental Neurotoxicology, Behrus Jahan-Parwar (NY State Department of Health, Albany, NY); Product Life-Cycle Assessment, Jim Fava (Roy F. Weston, Inc., West Chester,

PA); Research Trends in Ecological Risk Assessment, Greg Linder and Jerry Barker (Mantech Environmental Technology, Inc., Corvallis, OR); Aquatic Toxicology, Jerry Diamond (Tetra Tech, Inc., Owings Mills, MD) and Ian Hartwell (MD Department of Natural Resources, Annapolis, MD); and Poster Session, John Walker (U.S. EPA, Washington, DC). Our gratitude is also extended towards the ASTM staff members that assisted with planning the symposium and with the publication of this volume: Dorothy Savini (Symposium Planning); Kathy Dernoga, Therese Pravitz, and Shannon Wainwright (Acquisitions and Review); Susan Canning (Committee E-47 Staff Manager); and also Ken St. John (representative of Committee on Publications, University of Mississippi).

We would also like to express our appreciation to all of the people who volunteered to review the papers in this volume for their insights and constructive comments. Thanks are also due to the authors of the manuscripts for their patience and cooperation with the publication process.

Jane S. Hughes

Carolina Ecotox, Inc.
Durham, NC
symposium co-chairwoman and editor.

Gregory R. Biddinger

Exxon Company, USA
Benecia, CA
symposium chairman and editor.

Eugene Mones

Unilever Research U.S.
Edgewater, NJ
symposium co-chairman and editor.

Keynote Address

Steven M. Bartell[1] and Gregory R. Biddinger[2]

CRITICAL ISSUES IN ECOLOGICAL RISK ASSESSMENT

REFERENCE: Bartell, S. M., and Biddinger, G. R., **"Critical Issues in Ecological Risk Assessment,"** Environmental Toxicology and Risk Assessment - Third Volume, ASTM STP 1218, Jane S. Hughes, Gregory R. Biddinger, and Eugene Mones, Eds., American Society for Testing and Materials, Philadelphia, 1995.

ABSTRACT: Evaluation of current capabilities in assessing ecological risks suggests several avenues for advancing this dynamic and evolving discipline. Risk assessors should make every effort to incorporate state-of-the-art ecological understanding in identifying endpoints for assessments and in developing assessment tools. Efforts must increase in constructing, maintaining, and providing efficient access to electronic data bases for ecological and toxicological parameter values. Dose-response data for wildlife are often lacking, especially for chemicals other than pesticides. Innovative exposure-response assays directed at obtaining process-level data for extrapolations to field conditions are urgently needed. Critical assessment of current capabilities in ecological and environmental modeling can be used to effectively design the next generation of models for ecological risk analysis. A sequence of upwardly scaled models with additional emphasis on developing watershed or basin level risk estimation capabilities would advance the discipline. Linking geographic information systems with dynamic risk models will permit more effective site-specific assessment. Risk assessment should be developed in the context of formal decision theory. Most important, the difficult societal questions concerning population, resource demands, environmental quality, and sustainability must be addressed if ecological risk assessments are to have significant meaning.

KEYWORDS: ecological risk assessment, critical issues, data needs, modeling capabilities, environmental quality

[1] Vice-president and Director, SENES Oak Ridge, Inc.,Center for Risk Analysis, Oak Ridge, TN 37830

[2] Ecotoxicology Section Head, Exxon Biomedical Sciences ,Mettlers road East Millstone, NJ 08875-2350

INTRODUCTION

Ecological risk assessment (ERA), as currently practiced (e.g., Bartell et al. 1992, Suter 1992), uses methods of systems analysis to integrate aspects of ecology, environmental chemistry, environmental toxicology, hydrology, and other earth sciences to estimate conditional probabilities of the occurrence of undesired ecological events. In theory, ERA applies to both natural and human impacts on ecological resources. In practice, nearly all of the assessments address ecological impacts resulting from human activities.

The undesired ecological events represent an unbounded set of primarily negative impacts, ranging in theory across the entire spectrum of ecological measures. In a more limited application, these endpoints of risk estimation have routinely included unacceptable decreases in the abundance of one or more ecological populations of interest. The ecological consequences of undesired events that occur also lie within the domain of ecological risk assessment. However, assessments performed thus far have rarely addressed the ecological consequences of the disturbance or the probability (and rate) of recovery following disturbance.

This paper will review the current technical status of ecological risk assessment, offer suggestions for advancing this discipline, discuss the prospects for standardization of procedures and methods for ecological risk analysis, and finally, argue for the adoption of environmental planning to minimize the future need to assess ecological risks. Throughout this discussion, issues critical for the advancement of ERA will be identified and considered in relation to the continued technical evolution of ERA.

CURRENT STATUS

Several definitions of risk have been offered by risk practitioners (Table 1).

An efficient conceptual model of risk defines it as an ordered triplet (Helton 1993, Kaplan and Garrick 1981). Applying this model to ecological risk, the first element identifies the ecological phenomenon of interest, i.e., the assessment endpoint (USEPA 1992). The second element is an estimate of the conditional probability that the endpoint will occur in response to an ecological disturbance. The third element assesses the consequences of the occurrence of the endpoint. In nearly all applications, more than one ecological response is of interest. Thus, the model logically extends to a vector of ordered triplets; similarly, considerations of time or space can add additional dimensions to produce a matrix of triplets.

Previous assessments have focused on estimating ecological risks for different endpoints and disturbances

(Barnthouse et al. 1982, O'Neill et al. 1982, Bartell et al. 1988 , Cardwell et al 1993). Evaluating the ecological consequences of the occurrence of endpoints has received less attention. Increasing emphasis on risk to ecological resources in relation to RCRA/CERCLA enforcement, along with additional mandates such as the Natural Resources Damage Assessments (NRDA), is forcing valuation of ecological resources by risk estimators and risk managers. Nonetheless, calculating economic and cultural values of ecological resources at risk reamins difficult using traditional economic models (Kopp and Smith 1993).

TABLE 1--Definitions of risk relevant to ecologcial risk analysis.

Possibility of loss or injury...
The probability of loss or injury...
The conditional probability of an adverse event...
The product of the probability of an event and its consequences...
Consequence/time = events/time x consequence/event...
(Personal communication) Y.Y. Haimes, University of Virginia

OBSERVATIONS AND CONCERNS IN ECOLOGICAL RISK ASSESSMENT

One challenge in assessing ecological risks is that current quantitative capabilities in ecology and toxicology are quickly pushed to their limits (e.g., Suter 1981, 1992). Such limitations become evident in the process of risk estimation. Unacceptable risks can result from the expected severity of the disturbance in question, from high uncertainty, or their combination (O'Neill et al. 1982). A respectable goal in advancing ecological risk assessment will be to reduce the number of high-risk situations resulting from uncertainty or lack of information. Working towards this goal, the following sections discuss the need to consider ecological risk assessment in the context of ecological disturbance theory. The discussion continues with an examination of potential contributions to the development of ecological risk assessment that may derive from quantitative population, community, and ecosystem ecology.

Adding Ecology to Ecorisk Assessment

The potential development of ecological risk analysis will be determined in part by the continued transfer of advances in theoretical and applied ecology to the technical arsenal used in assessing risk. Ecological risk analysis used in a regulatory capacity must be based upon the most sound principles that ecology has to offer. The development of frameworks and guidelines for ERA (e.g., Cardwell 1993; Rowe 1989; USEPA 1989, 1992) can only benefit from the incorporation of state-of-the-art understanding of ecological systems.

A Subset of Ecological Disturbance Theory

The study of natural ecological disturbances (e.g., Pickett and White 1985, Allen and Starr 1982) is one area of basic ecological research that appears extremely relevant to ecological risk analysis. Ecological risk assessment is arguably a subset of basic ecological disturbance theory. An ecological risk can be thought of as ecological disturbance cast in a probabilistic framework and described as a conditional probability. Concepts and methods used to study ecological responses to natural disturbances should be explored for applications to ERA. Disturbance theory incorporated aggressively into the risk estimation process might prove valuable in formulating a framework or guideline for ecological risk assessment. In any case, ecological assessment for regulatory purposes should not develop independently from efforts in advancing basic understanding of ecological responses to natural disturbances.

Ecological Levels of Organization and Risk

One specific area for improving ERA requires an increase in sophistication concerning the concept of "levels" of ecological organization. If the concept is to be useful in practice, the salient points associated with different "levels" should be incorporated into the development of ERA. That is, the notion that the natural world is made up of landscapes that consist of ecosystems that contain communities of populations made up by individual organisms is overly simplistic, even misleading (Allen and Starr 1982, O'Neill et al. 1986).

The implicit nested model of nature ignores much of what modern quantitative ecology has to contribute to the development of ERA. The essential points that distinguish each level of organization change as the science evolves (McIntosh 1984). The following discussion points out potential contributions (and pitfalls) to the advancement of ERA that result from careful consideration of observing and measuring Nature from these different levels. Such contributions can be expected to change in relation to the continued development of the science of ecology.

Individuals

Individual organisms are conveniently bounded in space:time scales relevant to human observers, although individuals of several classes of organisms remain difficult to isolate and identify (e.g., grasses, fungi, corals). Furthermore, individuals of threatened or endangered species can be justifiably recognized as ecological resources worthy of protection. The ecological importance of individuals can only be assessed in terms of their contribution to the persistence and adaptability of the species, that is, some individuals (e.g., reproductive females) are ecologically and evolutionarily more important than others.[3]

Models of individual organisms may contribute substantially to understanding ecological response to toxic chemicals and other disturbances (Huston et al. 1989, Hallam et al. 1990, DeAngelis and Gross 1992). Model algorithms for individuals can combine bioenergetics, behavior, and life-history characteristics in ways that are cumbersome, if possible at all, using traditional modeling approaches. Simulations of many individuals might be used to describe a population-level response to disturbance.

Models of individuals are also attractive from a toxicological point of view. Physiologically-based pharmacokinetics (PB-PK) models can simulate the distribution of contaminants throughout an organism and estimate the rate of accumulation at target organs (Gerlowski and Jain, 1983). If modeled toxic effects can be related to physiological models that estimate growth or survival of contaminated individuals, more realistic integration of individual variability in exposure and response might result. Such integration may provide more realistic estimates of risk.

Clear delineation of what constitutes "individuality" in these models is often lacking and the mathematical formalism (e.g., the compound interest equations) applied to individual growth is equally, if not historically, valid for populations. This shortcoming is amplified by the absence of

[3] The concept of the individual has become misconstrued in the interpretation of standard toxicity tests (e.g., Suter 1992). These assays are not tests at the level of the individual organism. The assays evaluate the effects of a toxic chemical on a collection of individuals: the 48h-LC50 is not the concentration that kills one-half of an individual in two days of exposure, even though death is conveniently counted at the level of the individual. Rather, the toxicity benchmark implies a mortality rate, i.e., 50 percent of the collection of individuals per two days; individuals do not have a mortality (or reproductive) rate. Unfortunately, to say that the tests address populations is an ecological, if not a statistical, exaggeration.

model parameter values that truly characterize an individual. The values are typically random assignments of population-level measures. Correlations imposed on parameter values might help define an individual. However, in models developed thus far, such an approach has yet to be undertaken. An important consequence of these limitations is that population-level phenomena that "emerge" from the analysis of many individual simulations cannot be honestly assessed. Despite their limitations, individual-based models promise to substantially advance capabilities in assessing ecological risk, particularly for estimating risks posed to small numbers of individuals of endangered species.

Populations

Populations have received perhaps the most attention as ecological responses of interest in the development of ecological risk assessment (e.g., Cardwell et al. 1993, Suter 1992, Bartell 1990, Emlen 1989). However, population has come to mean a localized collection of individuals of the same species. Indeed, toxicity assays routinely imply this characterization of a population, that is, a population in a statistical sense. This view of a population has led to the selection of various fractional decreases in standing crop as responses in risk assessment (Bartell 1990, Bartell et al. 1992, Barnthouse et al. 1990, O'Neill et al. 1982). These decreases in population size have not been convincingly justified in relation to their impact on future production, maintenance, or survival of the assessed populations.

Populations can also be described in terms of the life history of the species in question. This perspective introduces, of course, considerations of age (size) classes, demographics, life tables, net reproduction, reproductive value - all of potential utility in defining ecologically meaningful responses for risk assessment. For example, Barnthouse et al (1990) focused on a 20 percent decrease in the recruitment of largemouth bass in relation to disturbance, yet this choice of response was not developed in a quantitative context of the production dynamics or sustainability of the bass population. Diminished net reproductive rates or reproductive values that carry an unacceptable risk of local extinction (e.g., Wissel 1988) appear to be the only ecologically justifiable responses for ecological risk assessment using this definition of population. Of course, societal concerns may certainly justify selection of other population-level effects for assessments.

In addition, populations can also be described genetically (Roughgarden 1979). Changes in the genetics of populations have been demonstrated in relation to toxic chemical exposures. It has been suggested that sensitive individuals in a population might be genetically similar -

the survivors might, as a result, compose a population with decreased capacity for adaptation to future stress. Diminished genetic diversity might portend an even greater response to the next disturbance. Changes in the population genetics of species that suggest an unacceptable risk in decreased adaptability might become the most important endpoints in ecological risk assessment. To date, genetic responses to disturbance have not been seriously addressed as endpoints in ecological risk assessment.

Community

Community and ecosystem have become used almost interchangeably in modern ecology (e.g., Suter and Bartell 1992). However, biotic communities have been distinguished as "...any assemblage of populations living in a prescribed area or physical habitat...they also have a compositional unity in that certain species will live together" (Odum 1971). Significant research efforts have been directed towards describing, measuring, and understanding the relationships (e.g., competition, food web interactions, mutualism, interference) that determine observed correlations among species composition in space and time. A fair summary might be that community ecology focuses on the response of species distributions to complex environmental gradients, and on the ecological interactions among species that forge community structure. Such emphasis has produced complex methods describing community structure and organization (Whittaker 1978a,b).

The interest in comparing the structure and organization of different communities stimulated, in part, the concept of species diversity and the many indices derived subsequently to quantify diversity. Indices that characterize community structure have been developed subsequently to describe and quantify community structural responses to disturbances (i.e., Karr et al. 1986). The potential utility of these indices for estimating ecological risk lies in summarizing complex community structure in a single number, which is also their major shortcoming. Issues similar to those confronting community ecologists in determining the most appropriate measure of diversity must be considered in the development and application of community indices used to advance current capabilities in ecological risk estimation (e.g. Hurlbert 1971).

Ecosystem

Methods in ecological risk analysis can profitably address ecosystem-level responses to disturbance. Ecosystems are fundamental units not only of basic ecology (Odum 1969, Smith 1975), but also ecological risk analysis (Levin and Kimball 1984; Bartell 1990; Bartell et al. 1992; O'Neill et al. 1982).

Ecosystem understanding continues to evolve (Forbes 1887, Tansley 1935, Lindeman 1942, Hutchinson 1948, Odum 1969, Allen and Starr 1982, O'Neill et al. 1986, DeAngelis 1992). Significantly, the ecosystem as merely habitat has been historically underemphasized in comparison to the emphasis on interactions and feedbacks among the physical, chemical, and biological components as the essential ingredient that distinguishes ecosystems (e.g., circular causal mechanisms, Hutchinson 1948, Patlen et al. 1976). One logical consequence of this emphasis is that ecosystem-level responses to disturbance should, by definition, address alterations to these interactions and feedback mechanisms. Unfortunately, the ecosystem concept has become primarily interpreted as habitat in current considerations of ecological risk (e.g., USEPA 1992).

Nature challenges risk analysts with middle number systems (Allen and Starr 1982, Weinberg 1975) that are inherently complex. The strength of each ecological perspective (i.e., level) lies in the nature of its set of simplifying assumptions that stimulate certain kinds of measurements and interpretation. But using these ecological concepts to their full advantage in ERA, particularly in identifying what is important to measure (i.e., endpoints), requires greater ecological sophistication than that offered by the simple nested model. It must also be remembered that simplifying our assumptions or simplifying our models does not simplify nature.

Extreme Events

The preceding discussion addressed the potential risks that might be assessed at different levels of ecological organization. Historically, ecological risk assessments have focused on non-catastrophic impacts.

Additionally, concepts and methods concerning ecological risk assessment should also consider extreme events. The analysis of extreme events estimates the probability of the occurrence of low frequency-high consequence events (Asbeck and Haimes 1984, Karlson and Haimes 1988, Mitsiopoulos and Haimes 1989). Extreme ecological endpoints might include for example, the probability of local extinction of a species or the complete functional breakdown of an ecosystem. Therefore, it is imperative that methods for estimating risks of extreme events be developed for ecological risk analysis (e.g. Fergon et al. 1989). Methods that relate conditional expectations to the statistics of extremes (e.g., Gumbel 1958) may provide more meaningful characterizations of risk by forcing attention on unlikely, but catastrophic events.

Parametric statistics might not provide the most effective means for estimating low probability events. These statistic focus on the mean of the statistical population. Thus, estimating extreme events is not best accomplished by using parametric methods. That is, 95 percent confidence estimates (or 99 percent) are not necessarily good estimates of extreme events, because these estimates are really quantitative statements about the mean. One simple example lies in the nature of the standard normal distribution, where the tails of the distribution extend theoretically to +/- infinity. Because the distribution must be truncated (at least to non-negative values) to make sense in most ecological applications, detailed analysis of the tails of distributions may provide inaccurate estimates of low probability events. That is, for less probable events, less data will be available to quantitatively characterize the tails of distributions.

Extreme events can be more accurately assessed by reformulating the underlying model to focus on the specific disturbances and ecological circumstances that increase the probability of such events. Probability density functions that describe risk can be partitioned into several conditional risk functions (Karlson and Haimes 1988): one for high frequency, low-consequence events; one for intermediate range events; and one for extreme and catastrophic events. The statistics of extremes demonstrate that the largest (or smallest) values of a distribution of random samples are also random variables whose probability distributions can be derived from the initial distribution (Gumbel 1958). The partitioned multiobjective risk method (PMRM) can be used to estimate the parameters that define the distributions of the extreme events (Karlson and Haimes 1988, Mitsiopoulos and Haimes 1989).

The PMRM provides a tool for a more comprehensive characterization of risk. However, the method is sensitive to the choice of the initial distribution. In many applications, it is not evident which distribution best represents the fundamental nature of the problem. This limitation can be addressed by examining the implications of different underlying distributions on the conditional risks of extreme events (Karlson and Haimes 1988).

ADVANCING CAPABILITIES IN ECOLOGICAL RISK ASSESSMENT

Examination of ecological risk assessments performed since 1980 reveals a focus on population-level responses to chemical disturbance (Bartell 1993). Risks have been estimated mostly using the quotient method; exposures measured in a contaminated system have been divided by a laboratory benchmark concentration. Probabilistic estimates of risk constituted less than 2 percent of the assessments reviewed. This review, while not claiming to be exhaustive, suggests several avenues for improving and advancing current capabilities in ecological risk assessment, including increased access and content of electronic data, the development of sequences of upwardly-scaled ecological models, operational connections of models to geographic information systems, and application of formal decision tools.

TABLE 2-- Critical issues in ecological risk analysis.

Topic	Status	Advancement
Ecology	Simplistic,population emphasis, nested model	Scaling,hierarchy,theory, landscape ecology, human ecology
Data	poorly known, scattered, inefficient use	increased electronic databases, efficient access to ecological and toxicological data
Models	poorly inventoried, quality largely unknown	systematic review of potential models, model validation studies
Assays	emphasis on comparative toxicology, mortality	process oriented assays, emphasis on extrapolation
Decisions	implicit, poorly stated, vague legislation	explicit criteria, link to planning, sustainability

<u>Electronic Data Bases</u>

Ecological risk analysis is data intensive. Quantitative estimates of site-specific risks quickly exhaust available ecological and toxicological data. In applying models for risk estimation, derivation of critical model parameters from values reported in the primary and secondary literature is time consuming, costly, and fraught with uncertainty. Repeated derivations of the same parameter in independent assessments compounds costs and frustration. With the exception of notable examples (e.g., Jorgensen 1984, 1979), compendia of ecological and toxicological data are largely absent. Clearly, one avenue for advancing capabilities in risk estimation lies in increased effort directed at constructing and maintaining electronic data bases. An important beginning has taken the form of a compendium of environmental data routinely collected by different government agencies and available for electronic access (USEPA 1992).

Another tactic to explore consists of assembling an electronic data base to accumulate and preserve data and results from case studies in ecological risk assessment. Following necessary "de-sensitizing," this collective experience in ecological risk estimation could become an invaluable resource for site characterization, exposure assessments, toxicity profiles, and ecological structure and process data. Such an electronic knowledge base could be used not only to assist in future risk assessments, but also to provide data of known accuracy and precision for use in model testing.[4]

Long term environmental monitoring can generate data sets for use in risk assessment. The USEPA Environmental Monitoring and Assessment Program (EMAP) was established to monitor the status and document trends of ecological resources (McKenzie et al. 1992). The results of monitoring will be summarized annually. While the EMAP was not designed for purposes of ecological risk assessment, the USEPA recognizes the potential contribution of EMAP data to the risk assessment process. Organizers of the EMAP also embrace the framework for ecological risk analysis as one approach for evaluating the results of long term monitoring. A critical issue in the continued development and implementation of the EMAP will be the ease of access to monitoring data. On-line access to EMAP data may be extremely useful in developing regional site characterizations, deriving model parameter values, or estimating initial conditions for ecological models used in risk estimation.

<u>Upwardly-Scaled Ecological Models</u>

Ecological models will play an ever increasing role in ecological risk analysis. Advances in ecological risk estimation will proceed commensurately with improved

---

[4] International research programs (e.g., BIOMOVS, VAMP) have been established with the express purpose of using results from previous studies of human exposure to radionuclides to compare and evaluate human dosimetry models (Hoffman et al. 1990). These projects have been active for several years and continue to the present. In blind tests (to avoid simple calibration), data from previous assessments or monitoring are used to construct target scenarios for international teams of modelers. Similar programs aimed at exposure and effects modeling for ecological risk are urgently needed to determine how good are present modeling capabilities and where to best direct future model development.

capabilities in modeling ecological systems at different levels of organization. Lessons learned in previous comprehensive modeling efforts (e.g., the US IBP, McIntosh 1984), combined with theoretical offerings from ecological scaling and hierarchy theory (Allen et al. 1984, O'Neill et al. 1986), support a hierarchical approach to model construction. These same considerations argue against comprehensive models that include disparately scaled state variables. For example, complex ecosystem models that force bacteria and fish (Park et al. 1974) or forest floor arthropods and overstory trees (Shugart al. 1974) into a common time step have historically produced results of mixed accuracy. With a time step of one day, the aquatic models tend to produce reasonable results for algae and zooplankton, while bacteria and fish dynamics remain difficult to reconcile with data. One day represents several generations of bacteria, but is insignificant in the lifespan of most fishes.

Hierarchy theory states that a phenomenon of interest at one level of organization will have a causal explanation at one level lower and ecological significance one level higher (Allen et al. 1984). A sequence of upwardly-scaled models might provide a solution to the scaling problem. The sequence might begin with a model of an individual organism. The algorithm for the individual could consider growth, behavior, and life history - essentially an autecological model. Ecological interactions (e.g., competition, predation) could be modeled as exogenous forcing functions or encounter probabilities. For chemical disturbances, detailed pharmacokinetics models might distribute the toxic chemical to site of action at the organ or tissue level of detail. Repeated simulations of many individuals could provide results that can be integrated to estimate aggregate parameters required by bioenergetics or demographic population models. More importantly, comparing population-level predictions of an individual-based model with results from a Leslie model or bioenergetics model might identify population-level model behaviors that were consistent with either modeling approach. Just as important might be the inconsistencies, or population dynamics that were largely a function of the selected modeling approach.

The upward sequence can be extended to the population-community-ecosystem interface. Models of individual populations could be developed to derive aggregate parameters for functionally defined ecological groups at the system level, e.g., primary producers, grazers, shredders, and so forth.

A sequence of ecological models constructed according to this approach might eventually permit a quantitative, process-level examination of the implications of individual-based pharmacokinetics model results or measured values of biomarkers in estimating ecological risks.

Identifying and Evaluating Models for Ecological Risk

Concerted efforts are required to determine the set of models currently available for ecological risk estimation. Clearly, the size of this set depends on the criteria used to identify potential members. Comprehensive models that simulate the combined fate and effects of contaminants in a probabilistic framework remain few (Bartell et al. 1988, Mancini 1983). Chemical or ecological models that might be adapted for estimating either exposure, effects, or risk are many. The number of models depends on the capabilities (and willingness) of assessors to modify existing models. The diversity of ecological topics addressed using models has lead to their proliferation (e.g., Patten 1968). The plethora of models also underscores the importance of the modeling process, rather than the model, in ecological research; models are developed, applied, published, and forgotten. To reduce needless duplication and inefficiency, model developers should devote greater energies to placing their creations in an historical modeling context. Systematic examination and analysis of the ecological modeling literature (e.g., Emlen 1989) are urgently needed to identify the set of models that can be usefully applied to ecological risk estimation.

Defining the set of useful models is simply a beginning. Model evaluation remains the critical next step in advancing ecological risk assessment. Models can always be pushed to the point of failure or offhandedly dismissed as too simple or too complicated. A fairer statement is that the accuracy of ecological models remains largely unknown. In contrast, significant efforts have continued for several years, on an international scale, in evaluating models used in assessing risks posed by radionuclides to human health (i.e., BIOMOVS, VAMP). To date, no corresponding effort exists for examining ecological models. Clearly, ecological analogs to the programs in human health are sorely needed. Credible models are required for credible risk assessments (Barnthouse 1992).

Innovations in Assays

Advances in capabilities for estimating ecological risks will depend predominantly on the design and implementation of innovative assays that measure ecological effects that can be extrapolated from unavoidably simplistic test conditions to complex natural environments. For example, acute or chronic toxicity tests measure mortality under controlled laboratory conditions. The success of direct extrapolations of such test results to expected mortalities in the field has been mixed. Field tests of extrapolations using disturbance regimes that would suggest either minimal toxic effects or massive mortalities have been more successful than tests of intermediate levels of disturbance. Yet, such intermediate disturbance regimes are likely to be encountered often in real world ecological risk assessments.

Toxicity tests designed to measure biological (ecological) processes may provide data that are more reliably extrapolated to non-laboratory situations. For example, tests that measure changes in physiological process rates (e.g., photosynthesis, respiration, feeding, etc.) in relation to exposure may produce more accurate estimates of the effects of sublethal exposures than attempts to extrapolate the results of current acute or chronic tests. Increased understanding of relations between physiological processes, modes of chemical toxicity, and effects on growth and survival is a critical issue in advancing current capabilities in ecological risk analysis.

Advances in Structure-Activity Relations

Structure-activity relations have become increasingly important for supplying estimates of chemical exposure (Bartell 1984) and effects (Suter 1992) parameters used to estimate ecological risk. However, the majority of applications have thus far used a fairly small subset of easily measured structural characteristics of chemical compounds. Continuing advances in increasingly detailed examination of the structural and functional chemistry, coupled to the increased availability of highspeed computers, promises advanced capability in using information derived from the fundamental chemistry of the compounds to predict their environmental behavior and their toxicity (e.g., likely mode of action, target organs, etc). Ecological risk analysis may serve as the interface between calculations in quantum mechanics and environmental toxicology.

Integrating Risk Models with GIS

Ecological risk assessment may be advanced by explicitly addressing the spatial characteristics of individual site-specific assessments. Ecological resources at risk have relevant spatial, as well as temporal, scales. Geographic information systems (GIS) are seeing increasing application in addressing environmental issues (Johnston et al. 1988). GIS tools greatly facilitate comparisons of patterns of population or resource distribution or animal movement with spatial-temporal distributions of disturbance (e.g., toxic chemical concentration).

An innovative approach in assessing risk involves the operational connection of dynamic dose-response models with GIS tools to characterize risks in a spatial context. In this approach, the GIS can store values of initial conditions and parameters required by an exposure or effects model. Subsequent model results can be stored and analyzed using the capabilities of the GIS. This hybrid approach permits mapping the results of the analysis back to the specific area of concern. This approach also permits incorporation of spatial attributes of ecological resources (e.g., immigration, emigration, home range, foraging territories, etc.) that have been essentially absent from ecological risk models. Difference in behavior among various life history stages or age (size) classes can be represented using this spatial approach and differential exposure of various life stages can be explored in relation to risk.

Additionally, the operational connection of GIS to dynamic models of chemical transport, degradation, and accumulation will permit more detailed descriptions of exposure, and thereby extend current methods that ignore spatial variability in exposure.

Formal Decision Making

Decision making is a science in itself (Baird 1989, Rubenstein 1975, Morgan and Henrion 1991). Methods have been developed to translate information of varying degrees of accuracy and precision into coherent decisions. To date, these methods have been largely unexplored in the development of ERA. Conscious efforts to apply and adapt formal decision making tools to problems specific to ERA stand the chance of making significant strides toward increased sophistication and credibility in ecological assessments.

Ecological risk assessments would appear to lie within the domain of decision making under uncertainty (Baird 1989). The complexity inherent to ecological systems prohibits their complete specification and characterization. Typical assessments are characterized by incomplete, even sparse, data. Natural variability combined with inadequate sampling frequently lend additional uncertainty to ERA. Decision making under uncertainty attempts to explicitly incorporate such inaccuracy and imprecision through its analyses and quantify the relative worth of new information in refining the decision.

One limitation in applying formal decision theory to ERA lies in the difficulty of constructing defensible cost or damage functions that can be used to objectively evaluate alternative risk management decisions. Considerable discussion has been directed towards establishing the worth of ecological resources (e.g., Cairncross 1992, Costanza 1991). However, a generally agreed upon system for such valuation remains nearly impossible to formulate in suitable detail to be of value in a formal decision framework. This lack of decision criteria is symptomatic of an even more important absence of an underlying conceptual model of the relation between humans and their environmental context.

PLANNING, SUSTAINABILITY, AND RISK ASSESSMENT

The inability to precisely define ecological cost or damage functions in risk assessments highlights a critical missing component in ERA, namely an underlying conceptual model of the desired (or necessary) relationship between humans and the environment (e.g., "the natural past," Bratton 1991). Just what is at risk? And why? The legislation that currently drives most of the assessments (e.g., RCRA/CERCLA) provides for after the fact estimates of ecological damage or reconstructions of historical environmental insults. Without some underlying model of a human-environmental status quo, meaningful criteria for risk assessment and remediation will remain elusive - cost or damage functions will remain difficult to derive and justify. These considerations emphasize the importance of placing individual assessments in proper spatial and land use context. For example, remediation of waste sites or landfills to levels of detection for specific chemical contaminants seem unjustified if adjacent property is contaminated to a similar degree, particularly if said property lies outside the purview of enforceable legislation.

The absence of realistic environmental goals guarantees that even perfectly accurate risk assessments will at worse merely chronicle further degradation of ecological resources, and at best serve as a kind of ecological damage control. In the absence of a plan, the environment will lose by default i.e., the current implicit status quo. Working actively towards environmental protection might justify risk-based decision making as a framework for NEPA.

Addressing ecological risks in a meaningful way leads quickly to considerations of landscape ecology and regional planning. Assessing risk is really assessing the symptoms of human dominated systems. These symptoms compel us to address the technically challenging questions concerning multiple pollutants, point and nonpoint sources, and politically and culturally charged questions concerning human population carrying capacity, environmental resources, and sustaining a quality life. A comprehensive and detailed discussion of sustainability is beyond the scope of this presentation. Nonetheless, it's plainly apparent that critical issues in ecological risk analysis must be evaluated and acted upon in the context of current and desired interactions between humans and their necessary, sustaining ecological resources.

STANDARDIZATION OF ECOLOGICAL RISK ASSESSMENT

The regulatory environment that continues to foster the development of ERA also argues for standardization of concepts, data, and methods for assessing risk. The likely inclusion and examination of ERAs in eventual RCRA/CERCLA litigations adds additional pressures for standardization. Two critical issues lie in determining where in the assessment process and to what degree standardization should occur.

The paradigm for human health risk assessment (e.g., the National Research Council "red book") may serve as a model for ERA standardization (NRC 1983). Human health risk assessment, as currently practiced, suggests operational consensus on what to estimate, the general structure of models to be used, the nature and values of input data, and finally, the form and presentation of the estimated health risks. By comparison, ERA is forced to address a greater diversity of endpoints from different ecological perspectives and with data that are sparse by human health standards. Experience in human health risk assessment suggests that some standardization of ERA will result simply from the accumulation of completed ecological risk assessments.

Guidelines that emanate from the Framework for Ecological Risk Assessment (USEPA 1992) will undoubtedly contribute to the standardization of ecological risk assessment. Thus, the contents of the Framework may help to preview the nature of future standardization. The Framework decomposes risk assessment into its component processes: problem formulation, exposure analysis, effects analysis, and risk characterization. Each process contributes a product for the overall assessment: conceptual model, exposure profile, effects profile, and risk estimates. In the very least, the Framework can contribute to standardization by identifying the necessary components of an ecological risk assessment. Upon review and refinement, the Framework will in all likelihood provide more detailed guidance concerning each of the assessment components.

SUMMARY AND CONCLUSIONS

Ecological risk assessment remains a dynamic and evolving discipline. Current capabilities in assessing ecological risks represent a preliminary integration of concepts and methods borrowed from several ecological and environmental sciences. The form and function of this integration have been shaped largely by the demands of specific environmental legislation, e.g., RCRA/CERCLA. Ecological risk assessment advances traditional environmental impact assessments by explicitly incorporating uncertainties throughout the assessment process and presenting ecological risks as conditional occurrence probabilities. The uncertainties associated with the risk estimation process can be exploited through iterative calculations to refine risk estimates as useful inputs to risk management.

The continued development of ecological risk assessment can benefit from careful consideration of several important issues outlined in this chapter. The nested model of levels of ecological organization is a simplistic representation of what modern quantitative ecology can offer to furthering technical capabilities for identifying and estimating ecological risks. That is, population, community, and ecosystem ecology, for example, emphasize different aspects of the same natural world. Each subdiscipline has developed different concepts and theory and correspondingly, different methods and measures. These salient contributions, not organizational nestedness, should be the focus in adding to risk assessment the best of what quantitative ecology has to offer. A sequence of upwardly scaled and hierarchically structured ecological models might result from adding ecology to risk assessment from this perspective. Assessing ecological risks can also be improved through advances in electronic storing and retrieving the diverse kinds of ecological and environmental data that enter into specific assessments. Innovations in bioassays that emphasize ecological responses that can be extrapolated to scales of concern in actual risk assessments will contribute significantly to the development of ecological risk assessment. For chemical stresses, further explorations of the information contained in the fundamental structure and chemistry of toxicants may lead to important advances in structure-activity relations for assessing risks. Geographic information systems and expert systems technologies should provide the operational foundations for integrating advanced ecological modeling and data analysis in a formal decision context for next generation risk assessment.

Finally, if ecological risk assessments are to have significant meaning beyond legislative compliance, a strategic framework must be instituted to provide an environmental context within which to assess and manage ecological risks. Sustainable environmental management appears as one strong candidate for providing a meaningful strategic context for future refinements of ecological risk assessment.

REFERENCES

Allen, T.F.H. and T.B. Starr. 1982. Hierarchy - perspectives for ecological complexity. University of Chicago Press, 310 pp.

Allen, T.F.H., R.V. O'Neill, and T.W. Hoekstra. 1984. Interlevel relations in ecological research and management: some working principles from hierarchy theory. USDA Forest Service General Technical Report RM-110. Rocky Mountain Forest and Range Experimental Station, Fort Collins, CO.

Asbeck, E.L.; Haimes, Y.Y. 1984. The partitioned multiobjective risk method (PMRM). Large Scale Systems 6:13-84.

Baird, B.F. 1989. Managerial Decisions Under Uncertainty. Wiley-Interscience, New York, 530 pp.

Balk, L., L. Forlin, M. Soderstrom, and A. Larson. 1993. Indications of regional and large-scale biological effects caused by bleached pulp mill effluents. Chemosphere 27:631-650.

Barnthouse, L.W. 1992. The role of models in ecological risk assessment: a 1990's perspective. Environmental Toxicology and Chemistry 11:1751-1760.

Barnthouse, L.W., D.L. DeAngelis, R.H. Gardner, R.V. O'Neill, G.W. Suter II, and D.S. Vaughan. 1982. Methodology for environmental risk analysis. ORNL/TM-8167. Oak Ridge National Laboratory, Oak Ridge, Tennessee.

Barnthouse, L.W., G.W. Suter II, and A.E. Rosen. 1990. Risks of toxic contaminants to exploited fish populations: influence of life history, data uncertainty, and extrapolation intensity. Environmental Toxicology and Chemistry 9:297-311.

Bartell, S.M. 1990. Ecosystem context for estimating stress-induced reductions in fish populations. American Fisheries Society Symposium 8:167-182.

Bartell, S.M. 1993. Thirteen (+1) years of ecological risk assessment in SETAC. Abstract in the Fourteenth Annual Meeting of the Society for Environmental Toxicology and Chemistry, November, 1993. Houston, Texas.

Bartell, S.M., R.H. Gardner, and R.V. O'Neill. 1988. An integrated fates and effects model for estimation of risk in aquatic systems. Aquatic Toxicology and Hazard Assessment: 10th Volume, ASTM STP 971, American Society for Testing and Materials, Philadelphia, pp. 261-274.

Bartell, S.M.; Gardner, R.H; O'Neill, R.V. 1992 . Ecological Risk Estimation. Lewis Publishers, Inc., Chelsea, Michigan, 233 pp.

Bratton, S.P. 1992. Alternative models of ecosystem restoration, pp. 170-189. In, Costanza, R., B.G. Norton, and B.D. Haskell (Eds.), Ecosystem Health, New Goals for Environmental Management. Island Press, Washington, DC.

Bulkley, J.W.; Barkholz, R.H. 1989. Application of extreme value theory to Great Lakes rise. In, Haimes, Y.Y. and E.Z. Stakhiv (eds.), Risk analysis and management of natural and man-made hazards. ASCE, New York, pp. 240-252.

Cairncross, F. 1992. Costing the Earth. Harvard Business School Press, Boston, Massachusetts, 341 pp.

Cardwell, R.D., B. Parkhurst, W. Warren-Hicks, and J. Volosin, Aquatic ecological risk assessment and clean-up goals for metals arising from mining operations1993...In, Bender, E.S. and F.A. Jones (eds.), Applications of ecological risk assessment to hazardous waste site remediation. Water Environment Federation, Alexandria, VA, pp. 61-72 .

Costanza, R. 1991. Ecological Economics. Columbia University Press, New York, 525 pp.

DeAngelis, D.L. 1992. Dynamics of Nutrient Cycling and Food Webs. Chapman & Hall, New York, 270 PP.

DeAngelis, D.L. and L.J. Gross. 1992. Individual-based Models and Approaches in Ecology. Chapman & Hall, New York. 525 pp.

Duckstein, L., A. Bardossy, T. Barry, and I. Bogardi. 1990. Health risk assessment under uncertainty: a fuzzy-risk methodology, . In, Haimes, Y. Y. and E. Z. Stakhiv (Eds.), Risk-Based Decision Making in Water Resources. American Society of Civil Engineers, New York pp.205-223.

Emlen, J.M. 1989. Terrestrial population models for ecological risk assessment: a state-of-the-art review. Environmental Toxicology and Chemistry 8:831-842.

Ferson, S. L. Ginzburg, and A. Silvers. 1989. Extreme event risk analysis for age-structured populations. Ecological Modelling 47:175-187.

Forbes, S.A. 1887. The lake as a microcosm. Bulletin Science Association of Peoria, Illinois, pp. 77-87.

Gerlowski, L.E. and R.K. Jain. 1983. Physiologically based pharmacokinetic modeling: principles and practice. Journal Pharmarascutical Science. 72:1103-1127.

Hallam, T.G., R.R. Lassiter, J. Li, and W. McKinney. 1990. Toxicant-induced mortality in models of Daphnia populations. Envrironmental Toxicology and Chemistry 9:597-621.

Helton, J.C. 1993. Risk, uncertainty in risk, and the EPA release limits for radioactive waste disposal. Nuclear Technology 101:18-39.

Hoffman, F.O. 1990. Conculsions of BIOMOVS Phase I, . In, BIOMOVS - on the validity of environmental transfer models. National Institute of Radiation Protection, Stockholm, Sweden,pp. 405-411.

Hurlbert, S.H. 1971. The nonconcept of species diversity: a critique and alternative parameters. Ecology 52:577-586.

Huston, M., W.M. Post, and D.L. DeAngelis. 1989. New models unify ecology. BioScience 38:682-691.

Hutchinson, G.E. 1948. Circular causal systems in ecology. Annals of the New York Academy of Sciences 50:221-246.

Johnston, C.A., N.E. Detenbeck, J.P. Bonde, and G.J. Niemi. 1988. Geographic information systems for cumulative impact assessment. Photogrammetric Engineering and Remote Sensing 54:1609-1615.

Jorgensen, S.E. (Ed.). 1979. Handbook of environmental data and ecological parameters. International Society for Ecological Modelling, Copenhagen, Denmark.

Jorgensen, S.E. 1984. Parameter estimation in toxic substance models. Ecological Modelling 22:1-11.

Park, R.A. (and 24 co-authors). 1974. A generalized model for simulating lake ecosystems. Simulation 23:33-50.

Patten, B.C., R.W. Bosserman, J.T. Finn, and W.G. Cale. 1976. Propagation of cause in ecosystems, pp. 457-579. In, Patten, B.C. (Ed.), Systems analysis and simulation in ecology. Volume IV. Academic Press, New York. 593 pp.

Peet, J. 1992. Energy and the Ecological Economics of Sustainability. Island Press, Washington, DC. 309 pp.

Pickett, S.T.A. and P.S. White. 1985. The Ecology of Natural Disturbance and Patch Dynamics. Acadenic Press. 472 pp.

Roughgarden, J. 1979. The Theory of Population Genetics and Evolutionary Ecology: an Introduction. MacMillan, New York, 634 pp.

Rowe, W.D. 1989. Alternative risk evaluation paradigms. In, Haimes, Y. Y. and E. Z. Stakhiv (Eds.), Risk Analysis and Management of Natural and Man-Made Hazards. American Society of Civil Engineers, New York, pp. 1-21.

Sargent, F.O., P. Lusk, J.A. Rivera, and M. Varela. 1991. Rural Environmental Planning for Sustainable Communities. Island Press, Washington, DC, 254 PP.

Shugart, H.H., R.A. Goldstein, R.V. O'Neill, and J.B. Mankin. 1974. TEEM: a terrestrial ecosystem energy model for forests. Ecologia Plantarum 9:231-264.

Smith, F.E. 1975. Ecosystems and evolution. Bulletin of the Ecological Society of America. 56:2-6.

Starfield, A.M. and A.L. Bleloch. 1991. Building Models for Conservation and Wildlife Management. Burgess International Group, Inc., Edina, MN. Suter, G.W.,II. 1992. Ecological risk assessment. Lewis Publishers, Inc. Chelsea, MI.

Tansley, A.G. 1935. The use and abuse of vegetational concepts and terms. Ecology 16:284-307.

USEPA. 1989. Risk assessment guidance for Superfund. Volume II. Environmental Evaluation Manual. EPA/540/1-89/001. U.S. Environmental Protection Agency, Washington, DC.

Kaplan, S. and B.J. Garrick. 1981. On the quantitative definition of risk . Risk Analysis 1:11.

Karlson, P.-O.; Haimes, Y.Y. 1988. Risk-based decision making of extreme events. Water Resources Research 24:9-20.

Karlson, P.-O.; Haimes, Y.Y. 1989. Risk assessment of extreme events: application. Journal of Water Resources Planning and Management 115:299-320.

Karr, J.R., K.D. Fausch, P.L. Angermeier, P.R. Yant, and I.J. Schlosser. 1986. Assessing biological integrity in running waters: a method and its rationale. Illinois Natural History Survey Special Publication No. 5., Champaign, Illinois.

Kopp, R.J. and V.K. Smith (eds.). 1993. Valuing natural assets - the economics of natural resource damage assessments. Resources for the Future, Washington, DC. 358 pp.

Levin, S.A. and K.D. Kimball. (Eds.). 1984. New perspectives in ecotoxicology. Environment Management. 8:375-442.

Lindemann, R.L. 1942. The trophic-dynamic aspect of ecology. Ecology 23:399-418.

Mancini, J.L. 1983. A method for calculating effects on aquatic organisms of time varying concentrations. Water Research 17:1355-1362.

Mitsiopoulos, J.; Haimes, Y.Y. 1989. Generalized quantification of risk associated with extreme events. Risk Analysis 9:243-254.

National Research Council (NRC), 1983. Risk Assessment in the Federal Government: Managing the Process. National Academy Press, Washington, DC., 189 pp.

Odum, E.P. 1969. The strategy of ecosystem development. Science 164:262-270.

O'Neill, R.V., R.H. Gardner, L.W. Barnthouse, G.W. Suter II., S.G. Hildebrand, and C.W. Gehrs. 1982. Ecosystem risk analysis: a new methodology. Environmental Toxicology and Chemistry 1:167-177.

O'Neill, R.V., D.L. DeAngelis, J.B. Waide, and T.F.H. Allen. 1986. A Hierarchical Concept of Ecosystems. Princeton University Press, Princeton, NJ. 186 pp.

USEPA. 1992. Framework for Ecological Risk Assessment. EPA/630/R-92/001. Risk Assessment Forum. U.S. Environmental Protection Agency, Washington DC.

USEPA. 1992. United States Environmental Protection Agency. Inventory of Exposure-related Data Systems Sponsored by Federal Agencies. EPA/600/R-92/078. Washington, DC.

Whittaker, R.H. 1978a. Classification of Plant Communities. Dr W. Junk bv Publishers, The Hague, Netherlands, 408 pp.

Whittaker, R.H. 1978b. Ordination of Plant Communities. Dr W. Junk bv Publishers, The Hague, Netherlands, 388 pp.

Wissel, C. 1988. Avoidance of ecological risk in optimal exploitation of biological resources, pp. 181-201. In, Wolff, W., C.-J. Soeder, and F.R. Drepper (Eds.), Ecodynamics: Contributions to Theoretical Ecology. Springer-Verlag, Berlin.

Ecotoxicology: Prediction and Assessment

John R. Vigna,[1] J. Kent Johnson,[2] and Burton C. Kross[2]

CASE STUDY: BIOASSESSMENT OF GLOVERS CREEK, WEST UNION, IOWA, USING THE USEPA'S RAPID BIOASSESSMENT PROTOCOL II

REFERENCE: Vigna, J. R., Johnson, J. K., Kross, B. C., "CASE STUDY: BIOASSESSMENT OF GLOVERS CREEK, WEST UNION, IOWA, USING THE USEPA'S RAPID BIOASSESSMENT PROTOCOL II," Environmental Toxicology and Risk Assessment - Third Volume, ASTM STP 1218, Jane S. Hughes, Gregory R. Biddinger, and Eugene Mones, Eds., American Society for Testing Materials, Philadelphia, 1995.

ABSTRACT: The Glovers Creek Watershed Protection Project aims to establish extensive agricultural conservation and management practices to protect the soil and water resources by limiting the amount of sediment, nutrients, and pesticides that enter the stream. In order to assess the effectiveness of these best management practices, biological, physical, and chemical components of water quality were examined using the Rapid Bioassessment Protocols For Use in Streams and Rivers as a template (Plafkin et al., 1989). The goal of this investigation is to examine the family-level macroinvertebrate RBP II and assess the biological condition of Glovers Creek in the early stages of the watershed protection project.

Bioassessment results indicate that Glovers Creek is moderately impaired relative to the chosen reference site. A paired-watershed approach is also examined. The shortcomings of RBP II are evaluated and suggestions are made to increase protocol applicability to this region.

KEYWORDS: biological monitoring, insects, macroinvertebrates, nonpoint source pollution, rapid assessment, stream

INTRODUCTION

Glovers Creek is a headwater stream located near West Union, Iowa (Figure 1). It is part of Iowa's put-and-take fishery program. As a trout stream, it is designated a Class "B" cold-water stream of high

[1] Environmental Specialist, Iowa Department of Natural Resources, Environmental Protection Division, 1004 W. Madison, Washington, IA 52353.

[2] Research Scientist and Associate Professor, respectively, University of Iowa, Department of Preventive Medicine AMRF-Oakdale, Iowa City, IA 52242-5000.

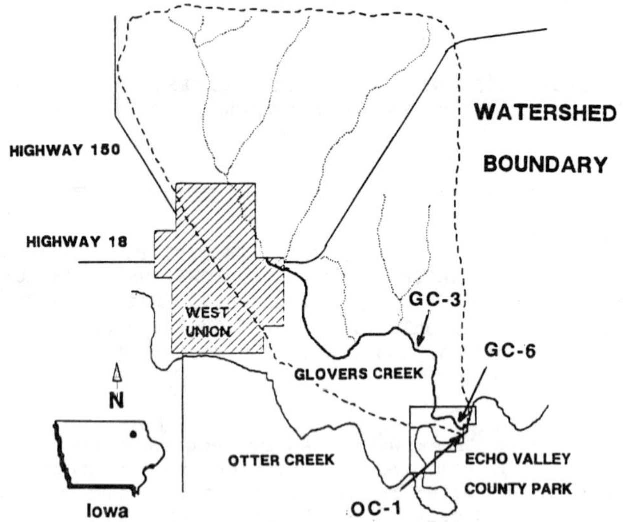

Figure 1.--Glovers Creek and Otter Creek.

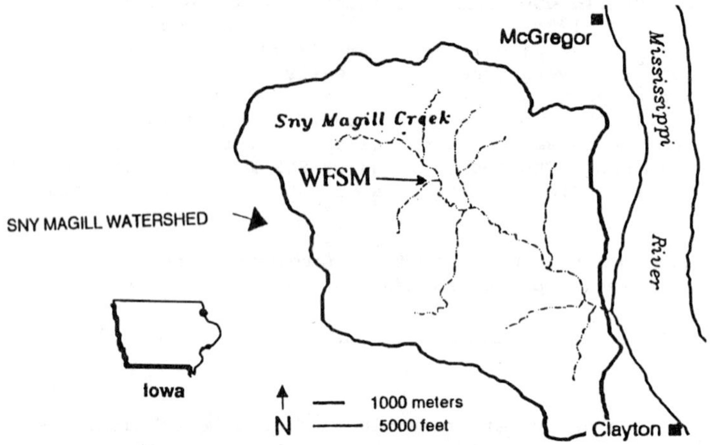

Figure 2.--Sny Magill Creek (Modified from Hallberg, 1992).

water quality. Under Iowa State law this stream is governed by an antidegradation policy which states that the existing water quality mu be maintained and protected (Iowa, 1990). But, a majority of the Glovers Creek watershed is agricultural. Therefore, the stream has th potential to receive a large quantity of nonpoint source pollution.

Nonpoint source pollution has recently received increased attention as a major contributor to the degradation of our Nation's waters. This attention follows the relatively successful reduction of point source discharges. The USEPA estimates that nonpoint sources of water pollution account for more than half of the pollutants entering our waters (USEPA, 1991). In a 1988 study of Iowa, 99% of the 8,320 river and stream miles (13,390 km) assessed were determined to be impacted by nonpoint sources (IDNR, 1988). Siltation and suspended solids top the list of pollution causes. Nutrients, organic enrichment, pathogens, and pesticides are also among the more commonly recognized agricultural pollutants (USEPA, 1990a).

Section 319 of the 1987 Clean Water Act and a recent call for the development of biological criteria for surface waters have prompted a serious look at nonpoint source pollution management and assessment (USEPA, 1990b). A biological means to assess agricultural control measures and agricultural impact on water quality is the next step in preserving two of Iowa's most treasured resources for future generations.

The Glovers Creek Watershed Protection Project was initiated in order to protect against water-quality degradation and to provide improved conditions to support the stream's recreational fishery while concurrently protecting agricultural resources. Best management practices such as terracing, conservation tillage, conservation reserve program, sinkhole easements, and animal waste management are being implemented. These best management practices limit the amount of sediment, nutrients, and pesticides that enter the stream, protecting the soil and water resources within the watershed. In order to assess the effectiveness of these best management practices, a bioassessment program was initiated.

Two sites on Glovers Creek, GC-3 and GC-6, were studied. One site on Otter Creek, OC-1, near the confluence of Otter Creek and Glovers Creek was studied for use as a control in a paired-watershed comparison between these two streams. The West Fork of Sny Magill Creek (Figure 2) was chosen as an ecoregional reference site to enable comparison of Glovers Creek to minimally impacted conditions. Macroinvertebrate and habitat data for the West Fork of Sny Magill Creek is part of the Sny Magill Watershed Nonpoint Source Pollution Monitoring Project. Data was utilized with permission from the University Hygienic Laboratory and the Iowa Department of Natural Resources.

Bioassessment methods and data interpretation followed the United States Environmental Protection Agency's Rapid Bioassessment Protocols For Use in Streams and Rivers (RBP)(Plafkin et al., 1989). The goals of this investigation were the following: (1) examine the RBP II (family-level macroinvertebrate identification) for applicability to an agriculturally-impacted cold-water stream in Iowa (2) initiate a biomonitoring program integrating biological, physical, and chemical means to address the effectiveness of nonpoint source control measures implemented within the watershed, and (3) assess the biological condition of Glovers Creek.

RAPID BIOASSESSMENT PROTOCOL II

The Rapid Bioassessment Protocols for Use in Streams and Rivers is a comprehensive reference assisting agencies in development of rapid bioassessment procedures (Plafkin et al., 1989). The document consists of five RBPs (I, II, III, IV, and V). RBP I, II, and III pertain to analysis of the macroinvertebrate community while RBP IV and V pertain to analysis of the fish community. Identical water chemistry parameters, physical characterizations, and habitat assessments are recommended to accompany the five protocols.

RBP II involves standardized macroinvertebrate field sampling and identification of major taxa. This multi-metric approach is an intensive survey where taxonomic identification is taken to the family-level. This approach has been supported by the RBP pilot study (Plafkin et al., 1989), and by some states, including New Jersey (Kurtenbach, 1990) and Maryland (Primrose et al., 1990), and Hilsenhoff (1988a) as a relatively sensitive approach to screening, prioritization, or determining water quality impairment over a large number of streams in a relatively short period of time.

Data analysis integrates community structure and function and into a single number that results in a bioassessment. This multi-metric approach provides a valid and meaningful assessment of an aquatic community. Eight metrics are used:

1. Taxa Richness
2. Hilsenhoff Biotic Index
3. Ratio Scrapers/(Scrapers + Filterers)
4. Ratio EPT /Chironomidae Abundance
5. Percent Contribution of Dominant Family
6. EPT index
7. Coefficient of Community Loss
8. Ratio Scrapers/Total Sample Size (CPOM sample)

Metric 3. was modified to a percentage rather than the ratio Scrapers/Filterers by recommendation of Barbour (et al., 1992). The other metrics remain as presented in the RBP document (Plafkin et al., 1989).

A numerical value is calculated for each metric. In general, these values are then compared in a ratio to values derived from an ecoregional reference site or control site. Scores of 6, 3, or 0 are assigned to specific comparison ranges to determine biological condition. Refer to Plafkin (et al., 1989) for a more detailed description of biological condition scoring.

Biocondition scores are plotted against habitat scores (Figure 3 and Figure 4). The sigmoid curve, in Figure 3 and Figure 4, represents the theoretical relationship between biological condition and habitat quality. Deviations from this curve can aid in discerning the causes of stream impairment other than habitat limitations (Plafkin et al., 1989). Three levels of impairment can then be determined: non-impaired, moderately impaired, and severely impaired.

DESCRIPTION OF STUDY AREA

Glovers Creek

Glovers Creek has a total drainage area of approximately 4,300 acres (17 km^2). Figure 1 illustrates the watershed area, stream location and sampling locations. The watershed consists of approximately 3,356 acres (13.6 km^2) of cropland, 300 acres (1.2 km^2) of pasture, 100 acres (0.4 km^2) of woodland, 150 acres (0.6 km^2) in the conservation reserve program, and 400 acres (1.6 km^2) of urban land (Fayette, 1989).

The Glovers Creek watershed consists of very hilly terrain having gradually sloping ridgetops and steep sideslopes (USSCS, 1978). Seventy-six percent of the watershed's cropland contains highly erodible slopes. Sinkholes are present: four within the watershed and about twenty within a half mile (0.8 km) of the watershed (Fayette, 1989).

Corn is the predominant crop. Conservation tillage is the most common best management practice used. Other conservation practices applied within the watershed include 650 acres (2.6 km^2) of conservation cropping, 200 acres (0.8 km^2) of contour strip-cropping, 300 acres (1.2 km^2) of contour farming, and 100 acres (0.4 km^2) of terraces (Fayette, 1989).

Glovers Creek is approximately two miles (3.2 km) in length. The stream consists mostly of cobble and gravel substrates with alternating riffles, pools, and runs. The stream corridor is mainly forested with a 0.4 mile (0.6 km) stretch of cattle access located just before it enters Echo Valley County Park. Glovers Creek is a tributary of Otter Creek and the confluence of the two streams is located within the park.

Site GC-3--This site is located just above a cattle stream-access approximately 0.4 miles (0.6 km) upstream from Echo Valley County Park on Glovers Creek.

Site GC-6--This site is located 0.75 miles (1.2 km) downstream from GC-3 and 500 feet (150 m) upstream of the confluence of Glovers Creek and Otter Creek. GC-6 is approximately 0.25 miles (0.4 km) downstream of the cattle access.

Otter Creek

The Otter Creek watershed is adjacent to the Glovers Creek watershed. Otter Creek is also a Class "B" cold-water stream. It is also stocked with trout. At its confluence with Glovers Creek, Otter Creek is approximately 6 miles (9.7 km) long and its watershed covers more than 16 square miles (41 km^2)(Larimer, 1957).

The watershed is mainly agricultural and corn is the major crop. Therefore, Otter Creek receives most of the above mentioned agricultural perturbations. In addition, before its confluence with Glovers Creek, Otter Creek runs through the West Union Country Club golf course, two poorly managed cattle feedlots, and receives effluent from the West Union wastewater treatment plant. The stream consists mostly of cobble and gravel substrates with alternating riffles, pools, and runs.

Otter Creek's effectiveness as a control is examined in the Discussion.

Site OC-1--This site is located on Otter Creek approximately 160 feet (49 m) upstream from the confluence of Glovers Creek and Otter Creek. OC-1 acts as the control site in a paired-watershed comparison of Glovers Creek and Otter Creek.

Sny Magill Creek

The Sny Magill watershed (Figure 2) covers a total of 22,780 acres (92.2 km^2) in Clayton County, Iowa. It is entirely agricultural and woodland without contribution by industry or urban areas (Hallberg, 1992).

Sny Magill Creek is also a Class "B" cold-water stream of high water quality (Link, 1986). It is also part of the Iowa DNR's put-and-take trout fishery program. The stream consists mostly of cobble and gravel substrates with alternating riffles, pools, and runs.

West Fork of Sny Magill Creek (WFSM)--WFSM was chosen as the ecoregional least-impacted reference condition for this study. This central tributary of Sny Magill Creek drains approximately 1,984 acres (8.0 km^2). The sampling site is located near the confluence of WFSM and Sny Magill Creek.

METHODS

On June 14, 1991, approximately 13 inches (33 cm) of rain resulted in a 100-year flood that affected the Glovers Creek and Otter Creek watersheds (Hillaker, 1991). The flood dramatically altered the stream corridor. Extremely high flows can decimate the benthic community (Hoopes, 1974). Therefore, it was decided that the flood would be a good starting point for observing water quality. The macroinvertebrate community was sampled in early November. This allowed the community five months to re-establish itself. Water sampling, physical characterization, and habitat assessment were performed between June and November 1991.

During the preliminary investigation of the biomonitoring program, macroinvertebrate sampling sites were selected. Specific criteria were followed to ensure that sampling locations had similar habitats to provide valid biological comparisons (Plafkin et al., 1989). Stream riffles were chosen as sampling sites because of their uniformity of physical parameters such as velocity, depth, and substrate size (Platts et al., 1983) and their highly diverse macroinvertebrate communities (Plafkin et al., 1989). Similar physical properties such as percent canopy and degree of substrate embeddedness were also considered during site selection (Bode, 1987).

A kick net (1250 µm, 8 mesh/cm) was used to collect insects from the riffles. Samples were taken from three 1-m^2 (3.3 ft^2) areas at each riffle. All insects recovered at each site were combined before preservation. The macroinvertebrate samples were preserved using a 70% ethanol solution (Hilsenhoff, 1987).

One hundred organism subsamples were removed in the laboratory. The subsampling procedure followed Appendix B of the RBP document (Plafkin et al., 1989) as a guide. Following family-level identification, approximately 10% of the organisms were sent to an experienced entomologist for verification.

The macroinvertebrate collection and identification for the West Fork of Sny Magill Creek (WFSM), the biological reference site, was performed by the University Hygienic Laboratory. They used a modified Hess bottom-sampler (505 µm, 0.5 mesh/cm)(UHL, 1992). Three 0.1-m^2 (1.1 ft^2) Hess samples were taken at WFSM. For data evaluation these three samples were combined and RBP metrics calculated.

Grab samples of water were taken at GC-3, GC-6, and OC-1 during this investigation. Special emphasis was given to rain-event water sampling in order to measure the nonpoint pollution episodes resulting from precipitation.

The stream area characterized was limited to one cross section at each macroinvertebrate sampling station. Stream widths were averaged from three, four, or five measurements, whichever was judged most representative. Depth measurements were taken at one transect across the stream where velocity was measured.

The RBP Habitat Assessment is composed of three categories: primary, secondary, and tertiary parameters. Primary parameters, which mainly involve bottom substrate characteristics, were evaluated at the sampling sites. Secondary parameters identify channel characteristics. Tertiary parameters identify riparian and stream bank structure effects on habitat quality. Secondary and tertiary parameters were evaluated upstream from the sample sites. More detailed explanations of the habitat assessment are presented in the RBP document (Plafkin et al., 1989) and the revised habitat assessment by Barbour and Stribling (1990).

Metric 8 was not included in this investigation. The coarse particulate organic matter sample (CPOM) pertains to the functional presence of Shredders. Two sampling trips resulted in very low numbers of Shredders. The litter available for sampling in the late Summer and Spring CPOM samples did not appear to be microbially degraded enough to allow for Shredder utilization. It has been concluded that even in the presence of riparian forests a majority of the CPOM input is seasonal, with most input occurring in the Fall. This seasonality along with the sample processing time required for only one metric resulted in the removal of metric 8 from the bioassessment.

RESULTS

Several analyses were performed on water samples. Analytes included temperature, pH, dissolved oxygen, biological oxygen demand, total suspended solids, total dissolved solids, alkalinity, hardness (total and calcium), total kjeldahl nitrogen, ammonia, major anions and cations, and herbicides (atrazine and alachlor). These results are not presented because the water quality is inherent in the aquatic community. The RBP II uses the macroinvertebrate community to assess the stream.

Table 1 shows physical parameters measured at each sample location. WFSM is a smaller stream than both Glovers Creek and Otter Creek as illustrated by its smaller stream width and lower flow. Otter Creek is the largest of the three streams. Riffle depth appears to be quite similar across all three streams. Flow measurements performed at two locations on Glovers Creek other than GC-3 and GC-6 resulted in an average flow of 5.1 ft^3/second (0.14 m^3/s).

TABLE 1--Physical Parameters.

Site	Average Width (feet)[1]	Average Depth (feet)	Velocity (feet/sec)	Flow (ft^3/sec)[2]
GC-3	14.7	0.33	0.65	5.1
GC-6	18.7	0.36	1.16	5.1
OC-1	28.5	0.53	0.81	8.2
WFSM[3]	7.6	0.46	...	1.8

1 1 ft = 0.3048 m
2 1 ft^3 = 0.0283 m^3
3 IDNR (1992)

WFSM macroinvertebrate data from the University Hygienic Laboratory's (UHL) pilot study (UHL, 1992) were utilized as well as water-quality data from the Iowa Department of Natural Resources/

Geologic Survey Bureau. Habitat-quality data were taken from a draft document (IDNR, 1992). All data were collected in the Fall of 1991 and were used with the permission of the IDNR.

No habitat reference site was identified during this investigation because habitat quality on Glovers Creek and Otter Creek is higher than WFSM (Table 2). The range indicating excellent habitat quality is 111 to 135. The range indicating good habitat quality is 75 to 102 (Plafkin et al., 1989). Since habitat quality is good to excellent for all sampling locations, the conservative assumption was made that the habitat score was 90% of a reference habitat when plotting the biological condition scores.

TABLE 2--RBP Habitat Assessment.

Site	Habitat Score
GC-3	116
GC-6	107
OC-1	99
WFSM[1]	90

1 Adapted from IDNR (1992)

Table 3 shows the RBP II metric results for GC-3, GC-6, OC-1, and WFSM. Table 4 and Table 5 show the results of the biological condition scoring. In general, a high score indicates a higher quality stream than a lower score.

TABLE 3--RBP II metric results.

RBP Metric	GC-3	GC-6	OC-1	WFSM[1]
Taxa Richness =	8	10	9	15
Family Biotic Index =	4.10	4.10	4.08	4.14
Scrapers/(Scrapers + Filterers) =	0.06	0.42	0.43	0.41
EPT/Chironomidae =	45.0	13.6	21.2	5.0
% Dominant Taxon =	77	37	48	43
EPT Index =	3	4	5	8
Coefficient of Community Loss =	...	...	...	...

1 Adapted from IDNR (1992)

The integration of habitat and biological condition data was performed by plotting their respective values in Figure 3. This provides the bioassessment results of this investigation. The % of Reference in Table 4 is plotted on the y-axis. The results in Figure 3 indicate that Glovers Creek and Otter Creek are moderately impaired relative to WFSM, the reference site. The percent comparisons under the

TABLE 4--RBP II biological condition scoring, WFSM as reference.

RBP Metric	GC-3	GC-6	OC-1	WFSM
Taxa Richness =	3	3	3	6
Family Biotic Index =	6	6	6	6
Scrapers/(Scrapers + Filterers) =	0	6	6	6
EPT/(EPT + Chironomidae) =	6	6	6	6
% Dominant Taxon =	0	3	3	3
EPT Index =	0	0	0	6
Coefficient of Comm Loss =	3	3	3	6
Biological Condition Score =	18	27	27	39
% of Reference =	46	69	69	100

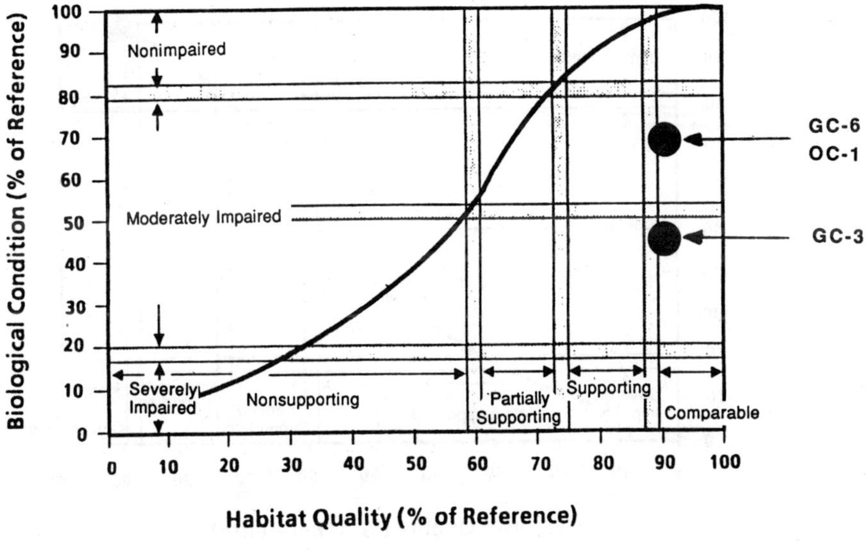

Figure 3--Biological condition, WFSM as reference.

curve on Figure 3 indicate differences from reference conditions resulting from water quality.

Table 5 shows the results of the biological condition scoring using the paired-watershed comparison of Glovers Creek and Otter Creek.Figure 4 illustrates the biological condition. The comparison indicates that no detectable differences exist in the level of impairment between the two streams.

TABLE 5--RBP II biological condition scoring, OC-1 as control.

RBP Metric	GC-6	OC-1
Taxa Richness =	6	6
Family Biotic Index =	6	6
Scrapers/(Scrapers + Filterers) =	6	6
EPT/(EPT + Chironomidae) =	6	6
% Dominant Taxon =	3	3
EPT Index =	6	3
Coefficient of Comm Loss =	6	6
Biological Condition Score =	39	36
% of Reference =	108	100

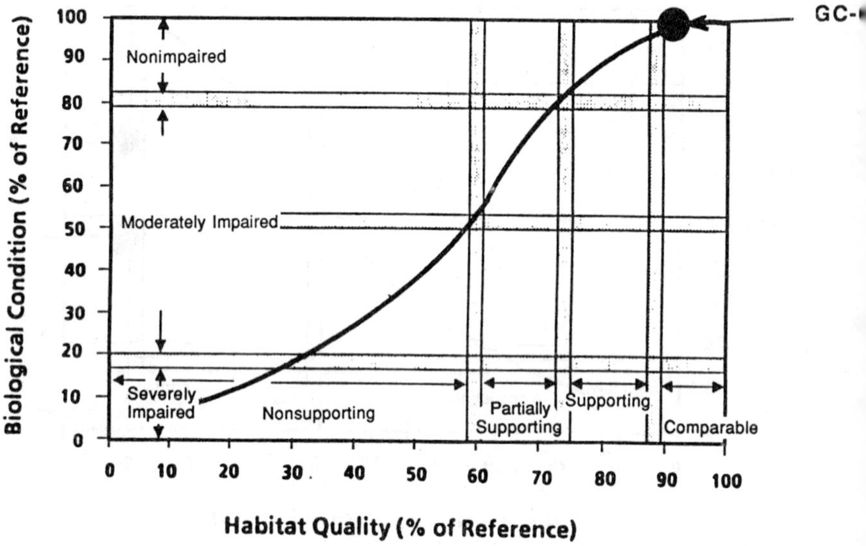

Figure 4--Biological condition, OC-1 as control.

DISCUSSION

One season of sampling was performed during this investigation. Since the Fall macroinvertebrate community is naturally diverse (Hilsenhoff, 1988b), the results should be a good representation of community characteristics. It should be noted that subsequent sampling is required to support the information presented here and assess invertebrate seasonality in the streams.

Post-flood macroinvertebrate recolonization occurred for five months before kick-net samples were collected. Hoopes (1974) states that, in a cold and infertile headwater stream in Pennsylvania, the stream macroinvertebrate community diversity was re-established four months after extreme flooding. The infertility of Hoopes' stream was identified by its very low total hardness concentrations (9-12 mg/L as $CaCO_3$). The streams in this study are quite fertile, with hardness values frequently exceeding 300 mg/L as $CaCO_3$. This greater productivity should have allowed for a shorter recolonization period. Therefore, five months should have been adequate time for full macroinvertebrate recolonization.

The mesh sizes are acceptable for both the kick net and the Hess sampler. Data comparisons are not likely to be biased in this investigation. Although, a long-term investigation may lead to erroneous comparisons if samplers of differing net sizes are used. The goal of further assessment is to use identical sampling equipment and field personnel to provide standardized sampling procedures.

An agriculturally-impacted surface water is likely to have a larger proportion of Filtering-Collectors. A large proportion of the samples contain the filter-feeding caddis-fly larvae (Trichoptera, Hydropsychidae). At each site, the dominant family was Hydropsychidae. Metric 5, percent dominant taxon, is a good indicator of Hydropsychidae over-abundance (Table 3). Nutrient and organic enrichment provide the food and attachment source necessary for the Filterers. In addition, algae was abundant during the time of sampling. Algae is a major source of attachment for Filterers.

Metric 4, EPT/Chironomidae may not be a metric to be considered further in this biomonitoring program. The over-abundance of Trichopteran larvae may give an inaccurately elevated biological condition of nonpoint source impacted streams.

Iowa is currently divided into four ecoregions. A majority of the state is identified as the Western Corn Belt Plains. Iowa is just touched in the northwest by the North Central Hardwood Forest Ecoregion, in the south by the Central Irregular Plains, and in the northeast by the Driftless Area Ecoregion (Omernik, 1987). Because of this highly generalized regional description of Iowa, the IDNR is working with the EPA to further delineate ecoregions in Iowa (Wilton, 1992). The Paleozoic Plateau in which the Glovers Creek and Sny Magill Creek watersheds are located could be a potential subregion of the Driftless Area Ecoregion. Potential reference streams were investigated within this region.

The reference site was selected as a relatively nonimpaired or minimally impacted ecological system within the same ecoregion as Glovers Creek and Otter Creek. This allows comparison of the study streams to attainable conditions. The reference watershed area and flow are within the recommended order of magnitude range (Hughes et al., 1986). The smaller size of WFSM ensures that the stream is less agriculturally impacted. Sites further down the Sny Magill watershed are considered to be susceptible to larger quantities of agricultural pollution due to larger drainage areas. The reputation of WFSM as a high-quality stream also prompted its use as a reference site.

Results indicate high-quality habitat at all the sites. It was determined that habitat is not a limiting factor to the biological community. Therefore, the differences between sites can be attributed to the water-quality differences inherent in the macroinvertebrate communities at the sites. It should be noted that the original version of the RBP Habitat Assessment is a general approach that may not be sensitive to all perturbations effecting the community being studied

(IDNR, 1992). Aware of these shortcomings, the Iowa Department of Natural Resources is developing a comprehensive and highly applicable habitat assessment for use in Iowa. In addition, Barbour and Stribling (1990) have published a refined version of the RBP Habitat Assessment.

In Figure 3, all sites are considered moderately impaired with respect to the reference condition. The low percent comparison of GC-3 to reference conditions is not necessarily a result of poorer water quality at the site. This site was sampled with only one kick net. The other sites were sampled by a composite of three kick nets. The single kick-net sample may have resulted in the sampling of a clumped distribution of organisms which is overcome by composite samples (Lenat, 1990). This, along with the greater presence of filamentous algae at this site may explain why there was such a dominance of Hydropsychidae larvae at GC-3 causing the lower percent comparison to the reference site. This location was included in this bioassessment because its use in future biomonitoring of Glovers Creek will be required.

Otter Creek was included in this investigation to determine the feasibility of a paired-watershed approach as a means to assess water-quality improvement on Glovers Creek. The size of the watersheds are within comparable size limits and the soil types and topography are similar. No intensive watershed protection has been implemented on Otter Creek's watershed. Therefore, changes that occur in Glovers Creek water quality due to the effectiveness of best management practices may be identified. Since Otter Creek will act as the control site, one would expect percent comparisons to increase upon improved conditions on Glovers Creek. Since the percent comparison shown in Table 5 is already one hundred eight percent, it is not certain that this bioassessment method will yield useful information. However, using a paired-watershed assessment would enable the project to be self sufficient, not relying on second-party data collection and reducing the amount of time spent on data collection and analysis.

Family-level identifications may not be as sensitive as species-level identifications to changes in water quality. This is true due to the fact that within a family there exist many genera/species of varying sensitivities. It should also be noted that functional feeding group classifications may actually breakdown at the family-level because at that point many generalizing assumptions have been made about feeding classes (Barbour, 1992). These generalizations are likely the cause of the similar biological conditions between GC-6 and OC-1 illustrated in Figure 3 and Figure 4.

CONCLUSIONS AND RECOMMENDATIONS

The highly variable and intermittent pollution episodes that occur in agricultural watersheds support the use of the biotic community to assess water quality. Although water sampling may not catch all the pollution episodes, the stream insect and fish communities will represent cumulative effects of the nonpoint source pollution over time.

The information gathered during this investigation has provided a preliminary framework for future investigation on Glovers Creek. RBP II was an initial indicator of macroinvertebrate community structure and function and water quality of an agricultural nonpoint source impacted stream in this region.

Several advantages and disadvantages of RBP II were identified during this investigation. The relative ease and quickness of generating a biological condition with RBP II makes it an attractive model for bioassessment activities. A technician with a relatively modest knowledge of identification keys and insect anatomy could easily become proficient in field methods and family-level macroinvertebrate identification. Regulatory offices or conservation departments with small budgets could use the RBP II to assess water quality on numerous streams in a short period of time.

Further investigation will require species-level identification. RBP III will have to be performed in order to fully accomplish the biomonitoring goals of this project. The species-level approach will provide the increased sensitivity needed to detect changes in water quality over time.

Comprehensive chemical analyses and additional studies, such as periodic 24 hour dissolved oxygen profiles and fish surveys are recommended to be performed. This information will increase the understanding of the limnology and improve interpretation of biological assessment results.

The ecoregional reference site and the paired-watershed approach are both important aspects of biomonitoring. Both methods will be studied further as additional data is collected.

ACKNOWLEDGEMENTS

Funding for this project was provided by the State of Iowa through the Iowa Department of Agriculture and Land Stewardship. Invaluable insight into habitat assessment, macroinvertebrate sampling, and identification along with the macroinvertebrate data pertaining to Sny Magill Creek were provided by the University Hygienic Laboratory Limnologists, J. Kennedy, M. Schueller, and M. Hausler. Additional bioassessment insight was provided by T. Wilton of the Iowa Department of Natural Resources. Appreciation is expressed to G. Hallberg and L. Seigley of the Iowa Department of Natural Resources/Geologic Survey Bureau for providing information pertaining to the Sny Magill Watershed Nonpoint Source Pollution Monitoring Project. Lastly, thanks go to K. Schmude, of the University of Wisconsin-Madison Department of Entomology, for providing insect verifications.

REFERENCES

Barbour, M. T. and Stribling, J. B., 1990, "Use of Habitat Assessment in Evaluating the Biological Integrity of Stream Communities," Proceedings, Biological Criteria: Research and Regulation, Arlington, VA, United States Environmental Protection Agency, Office of Water, EPA-440/5-91-005.

Barbour, M. T., 1992, April, Personal communication.

Barbour, M. T., Plafkin, J. L., Bradley, B. P., Graves, C. G., and Wisseman, R. W., 1992, "Evaluation of EPA's Rapid Bioassessment Benthic Metrics: Metric Redundancy and Variability Among Reference Stream Sites," Environmental Toxicology and Chemistry, Vol. 11, pp. 437-449.

Bode, R. W., 1990, "Development of Biological Impairment Criteria for Streams in New York State," Proceedings, Biological Criteria: Research and Regulation, Arlington, VA, United States Environmental Protection Agency, Office of Water, EPA-440/5-91-005.

Fayette Soil and Water Conservation District, 1989, Water Quality Protection Project Application, Water Protection Fund, Glovers Creek.

Hallberg, G. R., 1992, Sny Magill Watershed Nonpoint Source Pollution Monitoring Project Workplan, Draft Document, Iowa Geological Survey Bureau.

Hillaker, H. J., 1991, "Special Weather Summary," Climatological Data-Iowa, National Oceanic and Atmospheric Administration, Vol. 102, No. 6.

Hilsenhoff, W. L., 1987, "An Improved Biotic Index of Organic Stream Pollution," The Great Lakes Entomologist, Vol. 20, pp. 31-39.

Hilsenhoff, W. L., 1988a, "Rapid Field Assessment of Organic Pollution With a Family-Level Biotic Index," Journal of the North American Benthological Society, Vol. 7, No. 1, pp. 65-68.

Hilsenhoff, W. L., 1988b, "Seasonal Correction Factors for the Biotic Index," The Great Lakes Entomologist, Vol. 21, No. 1, pp. 9-13.

Hoopes, R. L., 1974, "Flooding, As the Result of Hurricane Agnes, and Its effect On a Macrobenthic Community In An Infertile Headwater Stream in Central Pennsylvania," Limnology and Oceanography, Vol. 19.

Hughes, R. M., Larsen, D. P., and Omernik, J. M., 1986, "Regional Reference Sites: a Method for Assessing Stream Potentials," Environmental Management, Vol. 10, No. 5, pp. 629-635.

Iowa Department of Natural Resources, 1988, State Nonpoint Source Assessment Report - Iowa 1988, Environmental Protection Division, Water Quality Planning Section.

Iowa Department of Natural Resources, 1992, Sny Magill Creek 319 Monitoring Project: 1991 Habitat Evaluation Results, Draft Report, Water Quality Section.

Iowa, State of, 1990, "Water Quality Standards," Iowa Administrative Code, Environmental Protection, Section 567, Chapter 61.

Kurtenbach, J., 1990, "A Method for Rapid Bioassessment of Streams in New Jersey Using Benthic Macroinvertebrates," Proceedings, Biological Criteria: Research and Regulation, Arlington, VA, United States Environmental Protection Agency, Office of Water, EPA-440/5-91-005.

Larimer, O. J., 1957, Drainage Areas of Iowa Streams, Bulletin No. 7, Iowa Highway Research Board, United States Geological Survey, Water Resources Division.

Lenat, D. L., 1990, "Reducing Variability in Freshwater Macroinvertebrate Data.," Proceedings, 1990 Midwest Pollution Control Biologists Meeting, Chicago, IL., April 10-13, 1990, United States Environmental Protection Agency, EPA 905/9-90-005.

Link, R. V., 1986, Northeast Iowa Rivers Basin Study- Pollution of Coldwater Streams Report, United States Department of Agriculture, Soil Conservation Service.

Omernik, J. M., 1987, "Ecoregions of the Conterminous United States," Annals of the Association of American Geographers, Vol. 7, No. 1, pp. 118-125.

Plafkin, J. L., Barbour, M. T., Porter, K. D., Gross, S. K., and Hughes, R. M., 1989, Rapid Bioassessment Protocols for Use in Streams and Rivers: Benthic Macroinvertebrates and Fish, Office of Water, Washington, D.C., EPA/444/4-89-001.

Platts, W. S., Megahan, W. F., and Minshall, G. W., 1983, Methods for Evaluating Stream, Riparian, and Biotic Conditions, General Technical Report INT-138, United States Department of Agriculture, U.S. Forest Service, Ogden, Utah.

Primrose, N. L., Butler, W. L., and Friedman, E. S., 1990, "Assessing Biological Integrity Using EPA Rapid Bioassessment Protocol II- The Maryland Experience," Proceedings, Biological Criteria: Research and Regulation, Arlington, VA, United States Environmental Protection Agency, Office of Water, EPA-440/5-91-005.

United States Environmental Protection Agency, 1990a, National Water Quality Inventory: 1988 Report to Congress, Office of Water, EPA-440-4-90-003.

United States Environmental Protection Agency, 1990b, Biological Criteria: National Program Guidance for Surface Waters, Office of Water Regulations and Standards, EPA-440/5-90-004.

United States Environmental Protection Agency, June 1991, "Commentary...", Nonpoint Source News-Notes, No. 13.

United States Soil Conservation Service, 1978, Soil Survey of Fayette County, Iowa, Soil Survey Report No. 96, United States Department of Agriculture.

University Hygienic Laboratory, 1992, Sny Magill Creek 319 Monitoring Project: 1991 Benthic Biomonitoring Pilot Study Results, Limnology Section.

Wilton, T., 1992, March, Personal communication, Iowa Department of Natural Resources, Water Quality Section.

John M. DeSesso[1]

GUIDANCE FOR PERFORMING ECOLOGICAL RISK ASSESSMENTS AT HAZARDOUS WASTE SITES

REFERENCE: DeSesso, J. M., **"Guidance for Performing Ecological Risk Assessment at Hazardous Waste Sites,"** Environmental Toxicology and Risk Assessment - Third Volume, ASTM STP 1218, Jane S. Hughes, Gregory R. Biddinger, and Eugene Mones, Eds., American Society for Testing and Materials, Philadelphia, 1995.

ABSTRACT: Potential risks to the environment have become considerably more prominent in the investigation of hazardous waste sites. The paradigm for conducting risk assessment, as articulated by the National Research Council, is geared primarily towards the assessment of potentially adverse health in humans. Subsequent detailed guidance published by the Environmental Protection Agency has also focused on the protection of the human health. In spite of the scientific complexity, potentially high costs of conducting ecological risk assessments, and lack of regulatory guidance, a relatively straightforward method for assessing ecological risks at hazardous waste sites has been developed. The method comprises a series of phases including a preliminary phase to gather information and formulate problems and three active phases. The active phases include (1) risk screening to estimate risk to keystone ecological receptors through an ecological toxicity quotient method; (2) initial investigations that may include field or laboratory work to assess the health of the community of exposed receptors through activities that may entail collection and analysis of tissue samples, bioassays, bioavailability studies or, if needed, a biodiversity study; and (3) detailed investigations that determine the potential adverse effects of contamination over several life cycles of the species of concern through population studies or studies of the life history-habitat requirements of given species. The method is designed to encourage evaluation of the results at the end of each phase so that remedial decisions can be made as expeditiously as possible. The entire three phases need not be completed in many cases.

KEYWORDS: Ecological risk assessment, ecotoxicology, hazard evaluation, terrestrial wildlife, regulatory toxicology, environmental contamination

---

[1] Principal Scientist, Energy, Resources, and Environmental Systems Division, Center for Environment, Resources and Space, The MITRE Corporation, 7525 Colshire Drive, McLean, VA 22102

The Superfund Amendments and Reauthorization Act of 1986 makes repeated reference to protection of human health and the environment. As a result, the Environmental Protection Agency (EPA) has written guidance for the protection of human health (EPA, 1989a) and the environment (EPA, 1989b). The methods outlined for human health assessment follow the paradigm for risk assessment as described by the National Research Council (NRC, 1983). This paradigm is rather complete for the human situation and has been shown to be adaptable for ecological risk assessment (NRC, 1993). Most of the guidance relating to environmental evaluation, however, has been devoted to describing specific types of ecological toxicity tests and how to interpret them rather than how to plan and execute the environmental assessment of a potentially contaminated area (EPA, 1988). While the Environmental Protection Agency is currently developing a framework for ecological risk assessment (EPA, 1992; Norton et al., 1992), detailed guidance is not yet available. The complexity of ecological systems has led to a variety of qualitative and quantitative methods that could be used depending on the conditions prevailing at a given site. EPA (1993a) has assembled and published different successful approaches to ecological risk assessments as case studies demonstrating the complex nature of ecological risk assessment. Because of this complexity, the available guidance for conducting ecological risk assessments at hazardous waste sites is much less explicit than that for human health.

Individuals charged with the assessment of risks to the environment at potentially contaminated sites require an approach for assessing ecological risks that guides them through the entire assessment process. The approach should (1) be predictive of ecological risks; (2) directly evaluate ecological effects while being as nondestructive of the environment as possible; (3) provide for the validation of these data such that the approach produces data that are capable of allowing decisions regarding the need for possible remediation to be made as expeditiously as practicable, and (4) protect the ecological community in the site environs.

The human health risk assessment paradigm can be modified to meet many of the needs of a successful ecological risk assessment methodology (NRC, 1993). The modification is necessary because human health risk assessment deals with a single species, and its goal is the protection of *individuals*, while the goal of ecological risk assessment is the protection of the *ecological community*, which is made up of individuals of multiple species that interact with each other and their habitats in very complicated ways. Consequently, the ecological risk assessment is a separate effort with unique data needs that are different from those of the human health risk assessment.

This document briefly summarizes the fundamentals of the risk assessment paradigm and describes a method for conducting ecological risk assessments at hazardous waste sites that was developed for the Air Force Center for Environmental Excellence to be used in the Installation Restoration Program. The stressors of concern in this method are usually chemical toxicants because chemical contamination is the major problem encountered at such sites. The method is based on the fundamentals of risk assessment and fulfills the needs for an ecological risk assessment methodology outlined above.

FUNDAMENTALS OF RISK ASSESSMENT

Risk assessment characterizes the probability that exposure to hazardous substances in the environment will produce adverse effects. Most of the effort in the development of risk assessment methods has been directed at human health risk assessment; however, the processes of the risk assessments performed for other biological organisms may parallel those of human health risk assessment and can be described in the similar terms.

Risk assessment consists of four components. The first component, hazard identification, involves determining whether the presence of a contaminant causes an adverse effect of sufficient importance that further investigation is warranted. The second component, dose-response assessment, characterizes the relationship between increasing doses of the hazardous substance and the incidence of the identified adverse effect and defines the smallest concentration of contaminant that will produce the adverse effect. Generally, information relevant to these first two components is available in the scientific literature. The third component, exposure assessment, measures or estimates the amount of the contaminant substance that comes into contact with receptors. This evaluation considers field measurements of the concentration of contaminant in various environmental media, the transport of contaminated media to receptors, and the duration, magnitude, and frequency of receptor contact. The, final component of risk assessment, risk characterization, combines the information from the preceding three tasks to (1) estimate the likelihood that the measured concentrations of the hazardous substance in the environment will cause the identified adverse effect in the receptors and (2) discuss the uncertainties associated with the risk estimates.

The quantitative assessment of risk is fraught with uncertainty due to the inability of the risk assessor to quantify all the information that must be used. While the concentration of each contaminant in sampled media can be measured with relative accuracy, the exposure concentration at the point of contact with a receptor is generally not measured and may be estimated by environmental transport modeling techniques. These models estimate exposure concentrations through the use of assumptions concerning physical characteristics of the media and the environmental behavior of the contaminants in the media. The unpredictable nature of receptor behavior that leads to (or avoids) exposure contributes to uncertainty in defining the magnitude, frequency, and duration of exposure. In addition, many toxicity data (especially for terrestrial organisms) are gathered from experiments that were conducted in laboratory animals using doses that greatly exceed anticipated environmental exposures. Thus, the expected incidence of a harmful effect at low doses are often based on observations at high doses. In addition, the expected harmful effects in one species (the receptor) often are based on observations in another species (often a laboratory species). These extrapolations and assumptions are sources of uncertainty in the risk assessment process.

From this description it should be clear that the goals of risk assessment are to determine the probability that adverse ecological effects have (or will) occur; to estimate the magnitude of the problem; and to express the uncertainties surrounding these estimates. Activities associated with deciding whether the mitigation of the problem through remedial action is warranted or selecting the appropriate remedial alternative are considered to be risk management activities and are distinct from risk assessment.

ECOLOGICAL RISK ASSESSMENT

Ecology is the study of the interactions of organisms with each other and with their environment. Estimates of risk to organisms other than humans and domesticated species fall within the purview of ecological risk assessment. Ideally, ecological risk assessment should estimate the potential for adverse effects that are manifested as changes in the diversity, health, and behavior of the constellation of organisms that share a given environment over time. The large number of ecological receptors at most sites and their complex interactions among themselves and their habitats make ecological risk assessments (ERAs) very complicated undertakings. While the following procedure is one way of approaching an ERA, different approaches or modifications of the described method may be suitable depending upon the particular investigation site.

The method described below accomplishes ecological risk assessment in phases that involve (1) estimating the effects (i.e., impact) to individual species, (2) evaluating the impact on the community of exposed species, and (3) determining the potential adverse effects of contamination over several life cycles of the species under study. These phases of ecological risk assessment are described in the following paragraphs. While these paragraphs describe a complete ecological risk assessment, other approaches, or modifications of the approach described herein, may be suitable, depending upon the particular site under investigation. It should be stressed that a decision concerning the need to continue with the assessment should be made at the end of each phase upon interpretation and review of the results by qualified professionals, including regulatory scientists.

Ecological risk assessments (ERA) should be performed on an ongoing basis starting in the earliest stages of remedial investigation. The individual steps performed during the ERA may need to be repeated several times. For example, risk characterization should be updated and refined throughout the ERA process as new information becomes available. Ecological areas included in the ERA should not be limited by the property boundaries of the study area if affected environments or habitats are located beyond the property boundaries. The following steps provide general guidance for the performance of an ERA. Although the steps are listed in sequential order, several steps may be performed simultaneously.

PRELIMINARY PHASE: INFORMATION GATHERING/PROBLEM FORMULATION (SITE SCOPING)

Background Information--Assemble all data that are relevant to the ERA of the study area, including historical information. From this information, identify all probable ecological contaminants, locate all likely sources and potentially contaminated media for each site (include maps), and estimate source size and volume. Quantify the contamination to the extent possible through concentration data for each relevant medium.

Habitat and Ecological Receptor Characterization--Identify and locate habitats and environments (both terrestrial and aquatic) on or surrounding the study area (include maps). This allows the assessors to compare locations of ecologically important areas with those areas in Background Information that were suspected of being contaminated.

The risk assessors should confer with local, state, and Federal Natural Resource Trustees to assist in establishing whether any of the areas identified above qualify as critical habitats or sensitive environments and to determine the identity of any important, threatened or endangered species that may inhabit or migrate through the study area. In the event that current detailed information concerning the species that are likely to inhabit or migrate through the study area, a field reconnaissance survey may be required.

The important species for which the risk assessment will be performed should be considered to be keystone species. Keystone species should be identified, in association with regulatory scientists, by applying criteria such as whether the species is important to the structure and function of the ecological community at the site (e. g., important prey); is an indicator of changes in the ecological community (States et al., 1978); or is valuable for commercial or recreational purposes. Those species that are threatened, declining, endangered, or of special concern are not suitable selection for keystone species because they must be protected as individuals.

Contaminant Identification--Identify site contaminants by determining the presence, ecological toxicity, environmental persistence, and bioaccumulation potential of all contaminants and, where appropriate, additivity, synergism, or antagonism between toxicants. Published research and ecological toxicity databases should be consulted first. Contaminants whose concentration in media result in exposures to ecological receptors that approach or exceed concentrations that cause toxicity are contaminants of concern (see Assessment Endpoints and Exposure Characterization). Where published ecological toxicity data are inadequate, bioassays may be necessary (see Phase II). Qualified professionals, including regulatory scientists and scientists with expertise relating to the media of concern, should be consulted before making the decision to conduct laboratory or field toxicity tests. See Data Gap Analysis for additional information.

Conceptual Site Model--Develop a conceptual model of the sites that identifies the source(s) of contamination, the likely migration pathways, and the extent of contaminant migration based on information such as topography, hydrology, geology, and geochemistry of the area and the physical properties of the contaminants (e.g., volatility, water solubility). The purpose of the conceptual site model is to determine whether ecological receptors are exposed to contaminants.

For ecological risk assessments, the environmental transport media of greatest interest are surface water, sediments and soil because these are the media that are most frequently in contact with the organisms of concern. While surface water and sediment are of primary interest to aquatic ecosystems, terrestrial ecosystems involve all three media. The reason that surface water and sediments are of concern in terrestrial assessment is because many terrestrial receptors contact them for such reasons as drinking, development through some of their life stages (e.g., tadpole stage of frogs and toads, larval stage of dragonflies), and living in or near the water (e.g., beaver, muskrat, some snakes). Consequently, areas of contaminated soil and territories near contaminated surface water bodies as well as near contaminated soils are likely to require terrestrial risk assessment. In addition, certain types of terrestrial environments are likely to be affected by contaminated air. While, in general, the concentrations of contaminants found in the air pathway do not pose a great risk to animal species, forests and lichen can be exquisitely sensitive to airborne contamination (Grodzinski and Yorks, 1981; Bordeau et al., 1990). Thus, when terrestrial ecological assessments are conducted at or near forested areas, the air may be an important environmental transport medium for certain classes of receptors.

Background Concentrations--Establish background concentrations of all potential ecological contaminants found at the study area. Background concentrations of contaminants should be determined from samples collected at the same time and from the same media as the contaminated samples, but from nearby uncontaminated locations with similar physiography. Aromatic and halogenated organic substances are assumed not to exist in the natural environment (i. e., they have a background of zero). Despite this, ambient background concentrations greater than zero may be used if the contamination is caused by general human activities (e. g., vehicular traffic near roadways) rather than by site-related activities.

Potential contamination by inorganic substances may be difficult to interpret because inorganics occur widely in nature and exhibit great ranges of normal concentration. Consequently, background concentrations of inorganic substances are sometimes difficult to establish. The concentrations of inorganic substances are generally compared to the concentrations found in reference area samples using an appropriate statistical procedure (e. g., "t" test) and an appropriate metric (e. g., 95% upper confidence limit or maximum value). Because of the great normal variations of chemical concentrations in soils, there are times when comparing site concentrations of inorganics to national average or regional average background concentrations is appropriate (LaGoy and Schulz, 1993).

Field Survey--A field survey should be conducted by a qualified ecologist (with expertise in the types of habitats and/or environmental media present at the site) to check the validity of all ecological information obtained above (e. g., locations and types of habitats), to select keystone species or habitats where applicable, and to verify the appropriateness of the conceptual site model. The locations of all wetlands and surface water bodies (including intermittent water bodies and drainages) should be verified to ensure the accuracy of the maps used in the preceding steps.

Data Gap Analysis--Based on the results of the ERA to this point, identify any additional environmental data that will be needed to assess ecological risk to the study area. Plan and conduct sampling and analyses (including background samples), where appropriate, to provide missing information. Care should be taken to ensure that the most appropriate data are collected and that sufficient data will be collected to support any remedial decision. EPA (1993b) has recently published useful guidance for the setting of "Data Quality Objectives".

PHASE I: ECOLOGICAL SCREENING/ECOLOGICAL TOXICITY QUOTIENTS

Measurement Endpoints--Establish appropriate, measurable endpoints (e.g., observable toxic effects in target species) for all ecological contaminants of concern. Depending upon the dose of a given substance, a spectrum of undesirable effects may be observed that ranges from relatively benign effects at lower doses (e.g., dryness of the mouth) to serious or life threatening effects at higher doses (e.g., cardiac arrhythmia). Consequently, the dose of a contaminant to a given receptor that causes a relatively minor, reversible toxic effect (e.g., shaking and listlessness) is likely to be much lower than the dose of the same substance that is lethal in the same species. Since effective concentrations may be reported and listed in databases for several adverse effects of a substance, care must be taken to ensure that the endpoint selected for use in ecological risk assessment is one that is biologically relevant for potential ecological damage. Examples of biologically relevant endpoints include death, retarded growth, reduced fecundity, and overt signs of toxicity (Suter, 1990). The concentrations of contaminants that cause biologically relevant endpoints have been termed critical toxicity values (CTVs).

Determine the effective dose of each contaminant of concern (i.e., the concentration that produces significant impact in the target species). Where data for a specific species or endpoint are unavailable, other toxicity data (e.g., LC_{50}or LOEC/LOEL)[2] may be used to derive a surrogate for effective concentration. For example, EPA ambient water quality criteria or other NOEL-type data may be used. However, the distinction between the concepts of effective concentration (one that produces a significant effect, e. g., LC_{50}) and a "safe" concentration (one that does not produce an effect, e.g., NOEL/NOEC)[3] should be considered in the interpretation of the assessment results. (See discussion in UNCERTAINTIES).

---

[2] LC_{50} is the concentration of contaminant that causes 50 percent of exposed test organisms to die. LOEC (often determined for aquatic organisms) is the "lowest observed effect concentration"; LOEL (often determined for terrestrial organisms) is the "lowest observed effect level."

[3]NOEL is the "no observed effect level"; NOEC is the "no observed effect concentration"

Effective concentrations are determined under controlled conditions in either laboratory or field toxicity tests that examine specific endpoints. Many of these are available in the scientific literature or in databases. Thus, there is a source of effective concentrations for many substances in a variety of species. However, the species of test organism in which the effective concentrations were measured must be noted. Differences in sensitivity to hazardous substances among species of organisms are well known as confounding factors in risk assessment. In addition to species differences, pronounced variation in response to hazardous substances has been reported for laboratory and feral test organisms of the same species and for laboratory organisms that are exposed in the field and feral organisms that are used in the laboratory (Schaeffer and Beasley, 1989). These facts must be considered as a possible explanation for cases when the ecological toxicity quotient predictions calculated in Phase I do not agree with the field observations made in Phases II or III.

Exposure Characterization--Characterize exposure (present and future potential) based on (1) contaminant concentrations in media samples collected from the site (2) the environmental fate and transport of contaminants as predicted by the physical model developed above, (3) the magnitude and frequency of exposure for each keystone species/habitat, (4) any ecological food chain considerations, including bioaccumulation potential, and (5) the effects of seasonal variations on the exposure scenario.

The exposure concentration of the site contaminants in environmental transport media should be measured at or near the presumed point of contact with receptors or estimated from modeling of contaminant migration. Literature values may be available for both plant uptake factors and bioaccumulation factors. When there is insufficient information about contaminant uptake and absorption efficiencies of receptors, exposure concentration values are used to estimate the amount of uptake (dose).

Other factors that must be considered in the estimation of dose to receptors include the duration of the exposure and the frequency with which the receptor comes into contact with the contaminant. Duration of exposure can be affected by the environmental removal of contaminants (e.g., through decomposition by photo-oxidation or bacterial degradation, or through leaching and eventual transport to another location). Computer models of the environmental fate and transport of contaminants may be useful for predicting future exposures.

In the event that the contaminant is stable in the environment, as is often the case, the dose estimate will only be affected by the frequency of contact that the receptor has with the contaminated media. Frequency of contact can be related to receptor mobility because both direct contact with the contaminated media and ingestion thereof can be directly related to the amount of time the receptor remains in the contaminated area. (Receptor mobility is considered below in Ecological Toxicity Quotients.)

Ecological Toxicity Quotients--Develop preliminary ecological risk characterizations (pERC) for each keystone species for each ecological contaminant of concern. Include a discussion of the level of confidence, assumptions, and uncertainties for each pERC. Where threatened or endangered species are being characterized, the acceptable risk will be lower than for the general ecological community because these species must be protected on an individual basis. The pERC should be quantitative, whenever possible. This can be most readily accomplished by using the ecological toxicity quotient method. The general formula for an ecological toxicity quotient for receptors that are continuously exposed (e.g., aquatic organisms, sediment and soil invertebrates) follows:

$$\text{Ecological Toxicity Quotient} = \frac{\{\text{observed contaminant concentration}\}}{\{\text{effective concentration or surrogate}\}}$$

An important characteristic of ecological receptors that should be considered in exposure assessment is their mobility relative to the area of contamination. The mobility of a receptor can be indexed to the average foraging range of a typical member of the species under consideration. For example, adult plants (by definition), soil organisms, and most flightless invertebrates can be considered to be stationary due to the small area within which they live their lives. Small vertebrates (including some species of fish, amphibians, reptiles, many terrestrial and some volant avian species, and small arboreal and burrowing mammals) constitute a category of mobile receptors whose foraging area is likely to be up to several acres. A final group of transient receptors is made up of larger vertebrates including grazing species (e.g., deer, moose), predators (e.g., coyote, wolf, fox, bear), most volant birds, and raptors (e.g., hawk, eagle, falcon). The foraging areas of transient species are likely to be several square miles.

The sizes of the foraging ranges vary considerably among terrestrial and some aquatic receptors as discussed above. The calculation of ecological toxicity quotients for terrestrial receptors should be modified to account for the effect of receptor mobility on the frequency and duration of contact with contaminated media. When the foraging area exceeds the area of contamination, a correction factor that accounts for less than full-time exposure is required. A suggested method calculates a fractional exposure (calculated as the ratio of the contaminated area to foraging area) that is designated the mobility factor, θ. The value of θ will range such that $1 \geq \theta > 0$. When applicable, the mobility factor would appear in the formula for an ecological toxicity quotient(ETQ) as follows:

$$\text{ETQ} = \theta \frac{(\text{exposure concentration})}{(\text{effective concentration or surrogate})}$$

When NOEL-type values are used as a surrogate for effective concentration, the ecological toxicity quotient will have a significantly more conservative meaning as an indicator of risk. Both current and future risks (based on environmental fate and transport modeling data or anticipated future activities) should be calculated.

When appropriate dose-response data are available, they should be included in the assessment. When the ecological toxicity quotients of contaminants with steep dose-response curves approach unity, they are of more concern than the ecological toxicity quotients of other contaminants.

In the event that ecological receptors are exposed to multiple chemicals, it is appropriate to assume (in the absence of information that shows synergism or antagonism of contaminants) that the effects caused by the contaminants are additive. Thus, the ecological toxicity quotients for each contaminant should be summed to provide an ecological toxicity index. If the magnitude of the ecological toxicity index is less than unity, the probability of an adverse ecological impact is negligible; if the ecological toxicity index is between unity and ten, ecological damage is possible; if the ecological index exceeds ten, ecological damage is likely (Barnthouse et al., 1986). These values may be useful in prioritizing sites for further investigation or immediate remedial action.

Human Activities Impact--Address the impacts of human activities on the environment at the study area. This should include any ongoing or proposed remediation (whether undertaken for human health, ecological, or aesthetic reasons) that may affect the ecological resources at or near the study area.

The preceding approach quantitates the potential for risk to individual species independent of the interactions among species. It is limited by the number of species considered and the availability of information on the toxicity of the contaminants. The potential for adverse effects to the entire ecological community must be inferred from information derived from the keystone species (a subset of the extant species in the community) or from surrogate species. The results of the Phase I investigation should be evaluated by qualified professionals, including regulatory scientists, to determine whether additional field work is required. Field and laboratory investigations are discussed in Phases II and III. The Data Quality Objectives process, mentioned in Data Gap Analysis, should be followed.

Phases II and III are carried out to resolve the problems formulated at the end of Phase I and to fill data gaps. The type of investigation or field work to be performed depends upon problems that must be solved at the site under investigation. Examples of the types of investigation that might be carried out in each phase at a given site are provided below. It should be stressed that the descriptions are examples of the kinds of investigation that could be carried out. Some sites will require only one or two of these investigations; others may require different kinds of investigation than those listed below. The type of investigation should be guided by the problem to be solved, not by strict adherence to written guidance.

PHASE II: INITIAL INVESTIGATIONS

Confirmatory Samples--The procedures described up to this point have been largely nondestructive. No ecological receptors have been killed, nor have sensitive environments been disturbed to any great extent. Upon the completion of Phase I, it may be deemed important to either confirm or quantify exposure to contaminants that had been based on modeling, to determine bioaccumulation, or to reduce the uncertainties of assumptions. Accomplishment of these tasks will require sampling and analysis of biota (tissue analysis) and/or media for contaminant concentrations. Decisions with regard to pursuing this avenue of investigation should be made cautiously. Field and laboratory efforts should be carefully planned and executed in order to reduce the uncertainties associated with the Phase I analyses. Because tissue analyses are frequently expensive and may be subject to large variations in measured contaminant concentrations, the proposed sampling and analysis plan should be scrutinized carefully before being implemented.

It should be noted that for ecological receptors that may be eaten by humans (i. e., game fish, fowl, and mammals), tissue samples taken for human health risk assessment may not be appropriate for ecological risk assessment. The tissue samples collected for use in human health risk assessments are usually edible flesh (primarily muscle), whereas the samples needed to confirm the presence or absence of contaminants in ecological receptors be whole body samples, or should at least include adipose tissue (body fat).

Toxicity Testing--A toxicity test (bioassay) to evaluate effects in a keystone receptor or surrogate species may be necessary under certain conditions. Possible examples include when the site contaminants have no published ecological toxicity data, or when the only available toxicity data are in species from distantly related taxa, or if a combination of contaminants suggests synergism (more than additive toxic effect). Bioassays are conducted on test organisms by exposing them to varying concentrations of contaminants in order to assess whether they are adversely affected by the contaminants, in what way, and at what concentrations. Bioassays are usually conducted in a laboratory setting, although they can be performed on the site using resident species. Decisions about the necessity of a bioassay, and the appropriateness of its design, should be made in concert with regulatory scientists.

Bioavailability--Bioavailability tests expose test organisms to contaminated media from the site to determine whether or not toxic effects are observed. This may be important because toxicants must be absorbed by an organism in order to exert systemic adverse effects. While chemical analyses of environmental media can demonstrate the presence or absence of a contaminant in the media, and laboratory bioassays can determine if the pure contaminant is toxic to test organisms, neither of these procedures demonstrates that the contaminant *as it exists in environmental media* is absorbed into the ecological receptors. In other words, these tests do not measure the "bioavailability" of contaminants. Some contaminants, like metals under certain conditions, may bind so firmly to other environmental constituents that they cannot be absorbed by receptors, thereby precluding the induction of toxic effects. This means that at sites with a single, or only a few contaminants, it is important to know whether the contaminants are bioavailable. As in the case of bioassays, the decision to perform a bioavailability test and discussions about its design should be made in concert with regulatory scientists.

Biological Diversity--The status of the ecological community at a site can be measured by determining the biological diversity of the area affected by contamination compared to the biological diversity of a nearby similar but unaffected area. The results of a biological diversity analysis can be used to support the findings of the ecological quotient-based risk assessment. The biological diversity type of assessment is similar in design and approach to human epidemiology studies. It is retrospective rather than predictive. When quantitative risk estimates are available, conclusions from a biological diversity analysis can be confirmatory and can be carried out as a second phase of the ecological risk assessment as discussed below.

Analysis of the biological diversity of a given region must be preceded by careful definition of (1) the boundaries of the territory to be studied and (2) the period of time during which the community will be measured. For the purpose of an ecological assessment, an equally important consideration is the identification of a nearby control area that is not contaminated but that exhibits nearly identical physiographic, topological, and climatic characteristics. The biological diversity analysis can take the form of a complete census in which all extant species are identified and the total numbers of individuals of each species are counted. The number of different species identified (species "richness") and the total number of individuals in each species (species "evenness") taken together provide an indication of biological diversity for the community in question. Comparison of the measurements made at the control and contaminated sites can provide a qualitative measure of the ecological similarity between the two sites.

Interpretation of the significance of differences in measurements between the sites is not always straightforward. When a large number of species is present, the analysis becomes excessively complex. The populations within ecological communities are dynamic; under normal conditions, changes in their distribution are expected to occur from time to time. For this reason, the detection of change by itself does not necessarily mean that contaminants are exerting biological effects. If a difference from background is detected, and if the ecological toxicity quotient is equal to or greater than unity, a change in diversity strengthens the confidence that can be placed in the quantitative risk assessment. Similarly, no change in biological diversity coupled with an ecological toxicity quotient that is less than unity bolsters the conclusion that the contamination is not exerting an adverse effect.

The suggested, practical alternative to a complete census is to monitor the distribution of selected species. While this approach ignores some species within a territory, it is more incisive because a smaller number of carefully selected species will be monitored and any changes from background should be relatively easy to interpret. Selected species should include any species whose abundance or other characteristics contribute to the perceived value of an area (e.g., sequoias in California redwood forests; species of commercial or recreational importance), and a suite of species whose status reflects the general health of the community. In general, the selected species will include those species for which ecological quotients were calculated in Phase I. The predictions of the species-specific ecological toxicity quotients can be confirmed by direct observation of the number and health of that species. In addition, the health status of those species for which ecological toxicity quotients are not available will confirm or contradict the accuracy of ecological damage predicted by the calculated ecological toxicity quotients. Effects not anticipated by the ecological toxicity quotients calculated in Phase I may become apparent in Phase II. If the results from Phases I and II disagree or are unable to lead to a decision regarding the need for (or extent of) remediation, further investigation may be required as described in Phase III.

In the event that an appropriate reference site is not available, gradient analyses of site contaminants versus observed adverse effects in keystone or other target ecological receptors could be conducted.

PHASE III: DETAILED INVESTIGATIONS

Population Studies--In the event that there is either an apparent decline in population size of a species that is deemed important in the presence of a low ecological toxicity quotient and no contaminant found in tissue samples; or no apparent effect on population size in the presence of a high ecological toxicity quotient (predicted effect), a more detailed study may be required. This may take the form of a population study (for organisms with a relatively short life span).

Population studies involve taking a census of the number of individuals in each life stage for selected species at several time points over the course of one to several life cycles or seasons. These studies can be expanded by including observations of the health or intoxication of individuals at different life stages for each time interval. The temporal aspect of the study design is likely to provide insight into any age-related or life-stage-specific sensitivities of the organism in question. This type of study is analogous to prospective epidemiology studies. While it is true that, in general, population studies are both time-consuming and expensive, they are one of the few types of study that can be performed when the ecological receptor of concern is endangered, threatened or declining because they do not require destruction of individuals. (See also Life History and Habitat Relationships below.)

Confounding factors that may affect the interpretation of the analysis include unusual extremes of climate such as drought, heat waves, excessive rain or flooding, or untimely frost, that could cause deviations from the expected numbers of individuals. The confounding factors can affect the species under study directly (e.g., temperature affecting hatching rate, floods that drown larvae) or indirectly (e.g., die-offs of prey, increased or decreased presence of predators).

Alternatively, computer driven population models have been developed that predict the effects of contaminants by means of mathematical formulae (Suter, 1993). The advantage of these models is the relative low cost and quick implementation. However, the models are relatively simplistic in the ways that they portray the interactions of species and environment (especially with respect to the types of confounding factors listed above), leading to some question about their accuracy.

Life History and Habitat Relationships--Population studies are not always feasible, especially if the subject species is long-lived, as is the case with many vertebrate keystone or threatened/endangered species. The health of these species can still be assessed if one knows (1) the behavior and habits of the species in question during its life phases, and (2) the species' habitat requirements for each of these life phases. For instance, species often have different habitat requirements for foraging, mating, nesting, rearing of young, and protection from predators. Destruction of a habitat that is critical for a given phase of a species' life can interrupt its life cycle. Interruption of the life cycle will adversely affect not only individuals but also the population. In an appropriately designed field investigation, a qualified, professional ecologist can infer the well-being of the population by studying the presence, areal extent, and condition of the required habitats. If site contamination has caused the decline or demise of a required habitat, then, depending upon the species and the availability of similar habitat nearby, inferences can be drawn about whether the population is likely to suffer adverse consequences. For species with extremely restrictive habitat requirements, like the spotted owl or the snail darter, any destruction of habitat will be of great concern.

UNCERTAINTIES

At times, safety factors have been applied to toxicity values for the purpose of comparing the results of different types of study design or comparisons between species. For instance, it has been recommended that LOEL data be divided by a safety factor of 5 for comparison to NOEL data (Lewis et al., 1990). Similarly, if the toxicity data are derived from a subchronic study, a safety factor of 5 is applied to chronic data (Lewis et al., 1990). Oftentimes, toxicity data will not be available for receptor species because the available data were derived in laboratory settings. In such cases, data from laboratory species of a different taxon have been divided by a safety factor. For example, the results of Suter and Rosen (1988) suggest that, for marine fish and crustaceans, the literature toxicity value should be divided by a safety factor of 5 when extrapolating between species within the same genus; when extrapolating between species of the same family the toxicity values should be divided by 10; when extrapolating between species of the same order, a safety factor of 20 should be applied. It should be noted that while approach of applying a universal safety factor is easy to use, it is simplistic and its use should be discouraged except for screening purposes. Techniques are available for quantifying the uncertainties associated with such extrapolations (Suter, 1993) and these will be applied to quantify the uncertainties for each ecological toxicity quotient.

When multiple toxicity values for the same endpoint in a given species are listed in databases or in the literature, the lowest value found is likely to be overly conservative. In such cases, it is appropriate to use the geometric mean of the values (EPA, 1986).

Assessment of ecological risks possesses other dimensions, compared to human health risk assessment, that add further uncertainty to the assessment. Not only are multiple species involved, each of which may be subject to overt, as well as insidious, toxicological effects caused by contaminants, but also interactions among the species at the assessment site could potentially be perturbed, thereby adversely affecting the health of the ecosystem as a whole. Among the subtle adverse effects that may not be discovered by traditional toxicity testing are seemingly minor physiological and/or behavioral changes that may result in reduced fecundity, altered rates of maturation of individuals leading to a decrease in the number of adults available for mating, any changes that may affect the ability of the species in question to compete for food or to avoid predation, or avoidance of certain contaminants resulting in emigration.

The high degree of complexity and numerous potential direct and indirect interactions that may affect ERAs require that the protocol for an ERA of a given site remain flexible. The exact procedures are not possible to predict *a priori*. However, as early results in the ERA are gathered and interpreted, new and testable hypotheses may emerge that will guide the completion of the assessment. Generally, as targeted or detailed investigation increases, uncertainty decreases.

CONCLUSION

The preceding method is a relatively straightforward procedure for assessing ecological risks that has been used at contaminated sites on Air Force Bases. The method is predictive of potential ecological effects and minimally destructive of sensitive environments. The method is executed in a series of phases. At the end of each phase, a decision should be made about whether the need exists for additional information (i. e., continued investigation). In some cases, decisions about the need for remediation can be made without completing all three phases of the assessment.

It should be stressed that at all times, the impact of investigations performed for an ecological risk assessment should be fully understood before beginning any type of invasive analysis. For instance, if the target receptors are among the endangered or other important species, are tissue samples really necessary? Will the investigators disrupt or permanently damage a particularly sensitive environment or a critical habitat during the course of the investigation? If the answer to either of the preceding questions is affirmative, will the adverse impact be a lasting one? How long will it take the damaged territory to recover? The obtaining of some kinds of ecological information may cause more harm to the receptors than the presence of contaminants.

Similarly, the impact of any proposed human activity, such as remediation of the site, should be assessed for any harm that may befall the site. In cases such as contaminated sediments in a sensitive wetlands, more damage may result from the dredging of the sediments to cleanse the area of contamination than from leaving the contaminants *in situ* and merely monitoring the neighboring areas for signs of possible contaminant migration. Clearly, in cases such as those just mentioned, no amount of guidance or detailed methodology will serve as a replacement for common sense.

REFERENCES

Barnthouse, L. W., G. W. Suter II, S. M. Bartell, J. J. Beauchamp, R. H. Gardner, E. Lindner, R. V. O'Neill, and A. E. Rosen, 1986, User's Manual for Ecological Risk Assessment, Publication No. 2679, ORNL-6251, Environmental Sciences Division, Oak Ridge National Laboratory, Oak Ridge, TN.

Bordeau, P., G. C. Butler, D. Calamari, J. W. Gillett, V. Landa, P. Sheehan, G. Persoone, R. Truhaut, and P. Wells, 1990, "Short-Term Tests in Ecotoxicology," Short-Term Toxicity Tests for Non-Genotoxic Effects, SCOPE 41 IPCS Joint Symposia 8, P. Bourdeau, E. Somers, G. M. Richardson and J. R. Hickman eds., New York: John Wiley & Sons pp. 49-55.

Environmental Protection Agency (EPA), 1986, Standard Evaluation Procedure, Ecological Risk Assessment, PB86-247657, Hazard Evaluation Division, Washington, DC.

Environmental Protection Agency (EPA), 1988, Review of Ecological Risk Assessment Methods, 1988, PB89-134357, Prepared for EPA by ICF, Inc., Fairfax, VA.

Environmental Protection Agency (EPA), 1989a, Risk Assessment Guidance for Superfund, Volume 1, Human Health Evaluation Manual (Part A) Interim Final, EPA/540/1-89/002, Office of Emergency Remedial Response, Washington, DC.

Environmental Protection Agency (EPA), 1989b, Risk Assessment Guidance for Superfund, Volume II, Environmental Evaluation Manual Interim Final, EPA/540/1-89/001, Office of Emergency Remedial Response, Washington, DC.

Environmental Protection Agency (EPA), 1992, Framework for Ecological Risk Assessment, EPA/630/R-92/001, Prepared by the Risk Assessment Forum, Washington, DC.

Environmental Protection Agency (EPA), 1993a, A Review of Ecological Assessment Case Studies from a Risk Assessment Perspective, EPA/630/R-92/005, Prepared by the Risk Assessment Forum, Washington, DC.

Environmental Protection Agency (EPA), 1993b, Data Quality Objectives Process for Superfund: Interim Final Guidance Review Draft, EPA/540/R-93/071, Office of Emergency Remedial Response, Washington, DC.

Grodzinski, W. and T. P. Yorks, 1981, "Species and Ecosystem Level Bioindicators of Airborne Pollution: An Analysis of Two Major Studies," Water, Air, and Soil Pollution, Vol. 16, pp. 33-53.

LaGoy, P. K. and C. O. Schulz, 1993, "Background Sampling: An Example of the Need for Reasonableness in Risk Assessment," Risk Analysis, Vol. 13, pp. 483-484.

Lewis, S. C., J. R. Lynch, and A. I. Nikiforov, 1990, "A New Approach to Deriving Community Exposure Guidelines from 'No-Observed-Effect-Levels,'" Regulatory Toxicology and Pharmacology, Vol. 11, pp. 314-330.

National Research Council (NRC), 1983, Risk Assessment in the Federal Government: Managing the Process, National Academy Press, Washington, DC 20460.

National Research Council (NRC), 1993, "A Paradigm for Ecological Risk Assessment," in Issues in Risk Assessment, National Academy Press, Washington, DC 20460, pp. 243-271.

Norton, S. B., D. J. Rodier, J. H. Gentile, W. H. Van der Schalie, W. P. Wood, and M. W. Slimak, 1992, "A Framework for Ecological Risk Assessment at the EPA," Environmental Toxicology and Chemistry, Vol. 11, pp. 1663-1672.

Schaeffer, D. J. and V. R. Beasley, 1989, "Ecosystem Health: II. Quantifying and Predicting Ecosystem Effects of Toxic Chemicals: Can Mammalian Testing Be Used for Lab-to-Field and Field-to-Lab Extrapolations?" Regulatory Toxicology and Pharmacology, Vol. 9, pp. 296-311.

States, J. B., P. T. Hang, T. B. Shoemaker, L. W. Reed, and E B. Reed, 1978, A System Approach to Ecological Baseline Studies, FQS/DBS-78/21, U. S. Fish and Wildlife Service, Washington, D. C.

Suter II, G. W., A. E. Rosen, 1988, "Comparative Toxicology for Risk Assessment of Marine Fishes and Crustaceans," Environmental Science and Technology, Vol. 22, pp. 548-556.

Suter II, G. W., 1990, "Endpoints for Regional Ecological Risk Assessments," Environmental Management, Vol. 14, pp. 9-23.

Suter, G. W. II, 1993, Ecological Risk Assessment, Lewis Publishers, Chelsea, MI.

Greg Linder,[1] Mike Bollman,[1] Chris Gillett,[1] Ricky King,[1] Julius Nwosu,[1] Suean Ott,[1] David Wilborn,[1] Gray Henderson,[2] Thomas Pfleeger,[3] Thomas Darrow[4], and David Lightfoot[5]

A FRAMEWORK FOR FIELD AND LABORATORY STUDIES FOR ECOLOGICAL RISK ASSESSMENTS IN WETLAND AND TERRESTRIAL HABITATS: TWO CASE STUDIES

REFERENCE: Linder, G., Bollman, M., Gillett, C., King, R., Nwosu, J., Ott, S., Wilborn, D., Henderson, G., Pfleeger, T., Darrow, T., and Lightfoot, D., **"A Framework for Field and Laboratory Studies for Ecological Risk Assessments in Wetland and Terrestrial Habitats: Two Case Studies,"** Environmental Toxicology and Risk Assessment - Third Volume, ASTM STP 1218, Jane S. Hughes, Gregory R. Biddinger, and Eugene Mones, Eds., American Society for Testing and Materials, Philadelphia, 1995.

ABSTRACT: Field surveys are frequently required during an ecological risk assessment for a hazardous waste site. Depending upon habitat type, field and laboratory methods that were developed for hazard evaluation lend themselves directly to the ecological risk assessment process. For example, wetlands are frequently impacted by various anthropogenic chemicals, and field and laboratory methods have been developed to help focus laboratory testing routinely planned in site evaluation. Here we compare and contrast the field and laboratory methods used in evaluating wetlands that occurred in markedly different geographic settings and were impacted by two different, but relatively simple contaminant sources. Both field studies were completed as part of the baseline ecological risk assessment process, one being located at Milltown Reservoir wetlands in western Montana and the other in the high desert of south central Oregon. In conjunction with chemical analyses of soil, sediment, and water samples, biological and ecological evaluations yielded an integrated evaluation of ecological effects and exposure at each site, which is critical information for any baseline ecological assessment. Overall, the field activities at each site illustrate the role that laboratory and field screening methods play in ecological management of waste sites.

---

[1]ManTech Environmental Technology, Environmental Research Laboratory, 200 S.W. 35th Street, Corvallis OR.

[2]University of Missouri, Columbia, MO.

[3]US Environmental Protection Agency, Environmental Research Laboratory, 200 S.W. 35th Street, Corvallis OR.

[4]Lewis and Clark College, Portland, OR.

[5]University of New Mexico, Albuquerque, NM.

KEYWORDS: soil contamination, wetlands, ecological risk assessment

---

Ecological risk assessment has recently gained a more prominent role in hazardous waste site evaluations (US EPA 1991; Suter 1993), and this increased role has been reflected in technical guidance to assure that reliable, yet cost-effective methods are used in the process (Warren-Hicks, *et al*. 1989; US EPA 1991; Linder, *et al*. 1992). Field methods for chemical analysis, particularly for screening purposes, have been developed and are relatively routine in their application in waste site assessment (Fribush and Fisk 1991). But, biological methods are not nearly as widely used, despite biological tests and survey methods being readily available, well developed and standardized (Warren-Hicks, *et al*. 1989; ASTM 1992). As previously summarized (Parkhurst, *et al*. 1989), both chemically-based and toxicity-based approaches may make significant contributions to ecological assessments for hazardous waste sites. When used together, chemical and biological test and survey methods can directly evaluate ecological endpoints pertinent to risk assessment. From an ecotoxicological perspective, ecological effects and exposure assessments are complex interrelated functions which yield estimates of hazards, and potentially risks, associated with environmental contaminants in various matrices sampled at a waste site. Here, we briefly summarize field and laboratory methods used to support an integrated approach to ecological risk assessment, using two wetland habitats as examples. In particular we provide a synopsis of field and laboratory activities that were common to each site, and illustrate site-specific differences in survey and testing methods that were inherent to each.

Background and History: Montana Field Site

Milltown Reservoir is on the Clark Fork River in western Montana, six miles east of Missoula, Montana. The reservoir was formed in 1907 following the construction of a hydroelectric facility located on the Clark Fork River immediately downstream from its confluence with the Blackfoot River. Since construction of the dam, a wetland habitat has been created. Because of the upstream copper mining activities in the Clark Fork River watershed, Milltown Reservoir has accumulated a large volume of sediment enriched with heavy metals and metalloids, including arsenic, cadmium, copper, lead and zinc. The Milltown Reservoir wetland was initially identified under CERCLA (Comprehensive Environmental Response, Compensation, and Liability Act) in 1981 after community well-water samples were found to have arsenic levels that ranged from 0.22 to 0.51 mg/L; the EPA recommendation for potable water supplies suggested that arsenic not exceed 0.05 mg/L. Within an ecological context, however, the impact of the contaminated wetland soils and sediments on the indigenous wildlife and vegetation characteristic of the site was unclear.

Background and History: Oregon Field Site

Alkali Lake, Oregon is located in south central Oregon (elevation ca 1300m). When seasonally recharged or during wet years, Alkali Lake is characteristic of many Great Basin lakes, being relatively shallow and highly alkaline. During dry years, the lake recedes and the exposed lake bed presents extensive evaporative deposits of sodium carbonate. Between 1969 and 1971 over 25,000 drums containing herbicide formulations (primarily, 2,4-dichlorophenoxyacetic acid [2,4-D], MCPA [2-methyl-4-chlorophenoxyacetic acid], and related chlorophenoxy herbicides) were hauled from a Portland, Oregon production facility to a storage facility located immediately west of Alkali Lake. In November, 1976 the storage facility was converted to a disposal site, and the drums were placed into shallow (1 m), unlined trenches, crushed, and buried on the playa near Alkali Lake. Unfortunately, in addition to releasing the materials to the soil, groundwater contamination resulted from these disposal activities, since a relatively shallow aquifer (1 to 3 m below ground level) existed in the closed-basin around the Alkali Lake playa. Prior to these preliminary studies, the ecological effects associated with this contaminated soil and aquifer were poorly understood.

METHODS

As part of the ecological assessment at each site, a variety of terrestrial and aquatic laboratory tests or field survey methods were critical to each wetland evaluation (Table 1). While this overview must limit detailed descriptions of laboratory and field methods, those methods applied at each site reflected site-specific contingencies whenever possible. For example, amphibian work at the Montana site used standard methods (ASTM 1992), but also tested surrogate species (bull frog, Rana catesbeiana) that were more relevant to ecological interpretation (Linder, *et al.* 1991). In contrast, if amphibian work had been identified as critical to the high desert site, an alternative surrogate (spadefoot toad, Scaphiopus intermontanus) would have been appropriate. Despite differences in contaminant sources, each assessment considered ecological effects potentially associated with:

- phytotoxicity and contaminant uptake by plants;
- adverse biological effects expressed by soil macroinvertebrates;
- adverse biological effects expressed by sediment macroinvertebrates;
- adverse biological effects expressed by terrestrial and wetland vertebrates; and
- preliminary evaluations of food-chain contamination.

Overall, the field activities for the ecological assessment at each site illustrate the role that field surveys and biological testing play in the ecological assessment process.

Table 1. Summary of field survey and test methods used at study sites.[1]

Ecological assessment component	**Candidate field survey or test methods**	**Methods potentially applicable to Oregon field site, Alkali Lake disposal area**	**Methods potentially applicable to Montana field site, Milltown Reservoir wetlands**
Phytotoxicity and contaminant uptake by terrestrial and wetland plants, and field surveys for *in situ* effects and vegetation communities	Standard laboratory phytotoxicity tests for seed germination, root elongation, and plant vigor	Seed germination, root elongation, and plant vigor tests with lettuce	Lettuce seed germination and root elongation; plant vigor tests with lettuce and *Hydrilla verticillata*
		Alternative site-specific tests species, including alkaline tolerant plants and native species such as *Sacrobatus vermiculatus* (greasewood)	Plant vigor tests using alternative species, including native species (*Potamogeton pectinatus*, or sago pondweed)
	Field tests for seed germination and plant vigor	Field testing limited in preliminary studies, and seed collections gathered for laboratory testing	In-field seed germination tests with standard laboratory test species and plant vigor tests using sago pondweed
	Field surveys for vegetation communities	Field surveys for evaluating *in situ* effects (e.g., plant health) and vegetation mapping for baseline evaluations	Wetlands delineation and survey of facultative and obligate wetland plants
	Field and laboratory measurements of soil physicochemical properties	Soil texture, organic matter, pH, cation exchange capacity, base saturation, extractable acidity, extractable nutrients, N-P, electrical conductivity, water retention, bulk density, infiltration capacity, hydraulic conductivity	Soil texture, organic matter, pH, cation exchange capacity, base saturation, extractable acidity, extractable nutrients, N-P, electrical conductivity, water retention, bulk density, infiltration capacity, hydraulic conductivity
Biological effects in soil macroinvertebrates, and field surveys of *in situ* effects and soil communities	Standard laboratory tests using earthworms, nematodes, ants, or isopods	Laboratory tests with nematodes, harvester ants or isopods; soil community tests (microbial or nematodes) using soil cores	Laboratory tests using nematodes or earthworms; soil community tests (microbial or nematode) using soil cores
	Field tests using earthworms, ants, or isopods	Field tests using harvester ants or isopods	In-field testing with earthworms
	Field surveys for soil communities	Field collections of frequently captured surface- and subsurface-dwelling invertebrates and vegetation-inhabiting invertebrates	Field collections of frequently captured surface-dwelling and vegetation-inhabiting invertebrates

Ecological assessment component	Candidate field survey or test methods	Methods potentially applicable to Oregon field site, Alkali Lake disposal area	Methods potentially applicable to Montana field site, Milltown Reservoir wetlands
Biological effects in sediment macroinvertebrates, and field surveys of *in situ* effects and benthic communities	Standard laboratory tests using benthic macroinvertebrates	Laboratory tests using alkaline tolerant sediment- or water column-dwelling invertebrate (e.g., brine shrimp)	Laboratory tests using *Hyallela azteca* and *Chironomus riparius*
	Field tests using benthic macroinvertebrates	No field tests currently available for alkaline sediments or surface water	*In situ* testing with aquatic macroinvertebrates such as *Daphnia magna*
	Field surveys for benthic communities	Field survey collections of sediment-dwelling larval invertebrates and brine shrimp community and contaminant residues evaluation	Field collections of benthic communities for sediment quality triad analysis
Biological effects in terrestrial and wetland vertebrates, and field surveys of *in situ* effects and wetland communities	Standard laboratory tests using small mammals, birds, or amphibians	Candidate methods include laboratory tests using small mammals, birds, or amphibians	Laboratory testing with amphibians (or terrestrial vertebrates)
	Field tests using terrestrial vertebrates	Candidate field methods using small mammals, birds, and amphibians	*In situ* testing with amphibians
	Field surveys for terrestrial vertebrate communities	Field surveys for small mammals and other terrestrial vertebrates; collection for analysis of gut contents	Terrestrial vertebrate surveys and collections for contaminant residues analysis
Preliminary food-chain contamination evaluation	Designed feeding trials using pertinent test species (e.g., terrestrial or wetland vertebrates)	Candidate studies address sediment-dwelling benthic invertebrate and shorebird food-chain contamination evaluation	Candidate studies address vegetation consumption by small mammalian herbivores

[1] Methods referenced in ASTM 1992; U.S. EPA 1989a; Linder, *et al.* 1992.

Synopsis of Biological Methods at Montana Field Site

In the preliminary ecological survey for Milltown Reservoir wetlands, terrestrial vegetation assessments were accomplished through a wetlands delineation (Federal Interagency Committee 1989) and standard plant tests for soil contamination evaluations (seed germination, root elongation, and plant vigor; see Warren-Hicks, *et al.* 1989; Linder, *et al.* 1992). In emergent zone habitats, plant and animal tests were conducted in laboratory and field (Warren-Hicks, *et al.* 1989; Linder, *et al.* 1992; ASTM 1992). *In situ* tests were conducted using amphibians, and submerged aquatic vegetation was also evaluated in emergent zone habitats (Linder, *et al.* 1992). In upland areas earthworm and seed germination tests were completed on-site and in the laboratory. Root elongation tests using groundwater were also completed. Additionally, surface soils were sampled for metals analysis (US EPA 1986) and characterizations of soil quality (Page, *et al.* 1982). In order to determine food source contamination for site-specific receptors like small mammals, samples of native vegetation and terrestrial invertebrates were collected and analyzed for target analytes (cadmium, copper, zinc, lead, and arsenic). For aquatic food-chains, samples of aquatic biota, including fish, aquatic insects, and plants, were collected and analyzed for target analytes. Sediment samples were also collected from emergent zone habitats and analyzed to characterize the extent of metal contamination in depositional areas in the wetland.

Subsequent to these preliminary studies, the methods directly applicable to a biological assessment at Milltown Reservoir wetlands were fully described, and included additional tests to evaluate sediments (Pascoe and Blanchet 1993). A detailed discussion of the activities related to the assessment of sediments and surface waters exceeds the scope of the present discussion, which will briefly consider only the vegetation evaluations with wetland and upland plants (see "Synoptic Summary: Montana Field Site") that were completed subsequent to preliminary work at Milltown.

Synopsis of Biological Methods at Oregon Field Site

As part of the preliminary ecological survey for Alkali Lake, terrestrial plants and invertebrates were sampled in various seasons. Aquatic invertebrates were also sampled at various times of the year, and representative species were identified and analyzed for tissue residues of target analytes (2,4-D and chlorophenols). Vegetation measurements taken during the survey determined cover and qualitative evaluations of plant health. In conjunction with survey samples for vegetation, terrestrial invertebrates were sampled using a combination of pit-fall traps and net surveys; for terrestrial vertebrates, small mammals were trapped and gut contents were analyzed to evaluate food sources. In addition to small mammal surveys, habitat use by birds was also noted; shore birds were surveyed and seasonal patterns in habitat use were recorded. With these preliminary field results target species were identified, and conceptual food-chain models were developed for risk assessments for terrestrial vertebrates. Vegetation patterns were also evaluated for their future role in long-term site monitoring.

RESULTS AND DISCUSSION

Synoptic Summary: Montana Field Site (Pascoe and Blanchet 1993)

Soil characterization and chemical analysis. Within an ecological assessment, biological effects measured in toxicity tests must consider interactions, or potential interactions, between the soil matrix and metals in the soil, particularly with respect to bioavailability. Soil pH, percent total nitrogen and percent organic material were measured on soil samples collected at Milltown during the study. Soil texture analysis was also completed, and DTPA (diethylenetriaminepentaacetic acid, 0.025M)-extractable metals were evaluated as a physicochemical analog of bioavailable metals. With these characteristics of the soil matrix available, potential confounding effects associated with soil physicochemical properties could be identified, and interpretations of metal toxicity could be developed with more confidence.

Soils at Milltown were heterogeneous across the site. Within-sampling unit variability was relatively limited, though subtle geochemical differences in soil were indicated when plant test results were analyzed. Organic material was variable across Milltown but was relatively invariant within defined sampling strata. Total nitrogen, soil pH, and cation exchange capacity (CEC) also varied across the site, but were similar within sampling strata. These soil data were valuable for interpreting biological effects associated with soil metal content.

Vegetation Evaluations. During preliminary field and laboratory studies, seed-germination testing was completed using site soils. Both on-site methods (Nwosu, *et al.* 1992) and laboratory methods (Warren-Hicks, *et al.* 1989; Linder, *et al.* 1992) were employed in these soil contamination evaluations. No unexpected phytotoxicity was observed. On the basis of the preliminary field and laboratory results, additional test matrices (i.e., sediments) were then considered, and alternative test methods were evaluated during subsequent field survey and testing activities. In these efforts, groundwater samples were collected at selected sites across the wetland and were tested using the root-elongation procedure. Emergent zones in the wetlands were also evaluated using laboratory and field methods that tested marsh plants as well as a standard, submerged aquatic vascular plant (*Potamogeton pectinatus* and a standard test species *Hydrilla verticillata*, respectively).

The root-elongation tests that were completed on groundwater samples collected at Milltown were consistently not acutely toxic, suggesting that groundwater coincident with the rhizosphere would generally not be acutely phytotoxic. While not acutely toxic, at some locations groundwater was clearly inhibitory to root elongation, as measured using the standard laboratory test species. Field surveys completed in conjunction with the sampling and laboratory testing, however, did not suggest that this biological effect was currently being exhibited at these sampling locations.

In addition to root-elongation testing for groundwater evaluations, field and laboratory testing with aquatic vascular plants was completed with an indigenous, emergent vascular plant, sago pondweed (Potamogeton pectinatus), as well as the standard test species Hydrilla verticillata (Linder, *et al*. 1992). In general, emergent-vegetation testing in laboratory and field suggested that biological effects, when evident, were sublethal. The in situ testing with sago pondweed indicated no adverse effects for growth endpoints (root and shoot length); physiological markers (peroxidase activity [POD]) indicative of plant stress (Byl and Klaine 1991) were similarly unremarkable. Indigenous plant samples (Elodea spp.) were also collected concurrent with in situ testing and were analyzed for POD activity. Statistically significant differences among sites were noted across Milltown sampling locations and may be indicative of general plant stress. In parallel laboratory exposures, no consistent pattern was noted with respect to growth endpoints (root and shoot lengths and chlorophyll **a**) for either species when tested with bulk sediments. While morphologic endpoints related to growth suggested no acute toxicity in laboratory or field exposures with sediments, differences in POD activity across Milltown may reflect the spatial variability in metals that are differentially bioavailable (Byl and Klaine 1991).

For evaluating the potential for metal incorporation into garden plants grown in Milltown soils, two interrelated greenhouse exposures using field-collected soil or exposed sediment samples were completed. One was a qualitative study regarding normal plant growth, from germination through seedling, and from maturity through senescence, and suggested if germination and early seedling survival were not impaired, a typical life cycle could be completed under ideal garden conditions. However, a second quantitative early-seedling-growth and plant-vigor test (Linder, *et al*. 1992) suggested that soils collected from some depositional areas may yield biological effects that would not be detected in seed-germination and root-elongation tests. For example, companion work completed on Milltown samples with these routine plant-toxicity tests suggested that adverse effects may be associated with soils collected from old "oxbow" reaches along the river. In historic depositional areas, growth reduction was noted.

In contrast to these controlled greenhouse- and laboratory-exposures with commercial garden varieties, field surveys saw no widespread effects on vegetation in the sampled area. In part, the physicochemical characteristics of the soils across Milltown may explain the variation in growth reduction, particularly in those areas occasionally associated with reduced plant vigor in laboratory tests. The geochemical heterogeneity of soils across Milltown was apparent, even in sampling units that were similar with respect to texture. While all Milltown soils are xerofluvents, the soils ranged in texture from loams to silty loams to occasional silty-clay loams, and presented CECs that could, in part, contribute to the differential bioavailability of metals. Generally, soils with higher CECs ($\geq$ 30mEq/100gram soil) were more likely to be associated with subacute effects, and frequently gave rise to adverse effects in plant tests. Variability at relatively lower

CECs could be associated, in part, with subtle differences in soil texture, as well as organic content and geochemistry.

Earthworm evaluations. Earthworm tests performed on-site and in the laboratory (Linder, *et al*. 1992) showed no significant acute toxicity. Subtle biological-response data (e.g., morphologic and dermatopathologic effects) from laboratory and field tests were occasionally encountered in soils with elevated total metals, however. For example, these tests suggested that total lead and total copper in Milltown soils were associated with sublethal effects in exposed earthworms. Differential bioavailability of metals may be considered a possible source of spatial variation in these sublethal effects.

Preliminary studies using amphibians. Laboratory tests for acute and chronic toxicity to amphibians were completed on Milltown surface-water during the preliminary study. Results from these tests were spatially variable, but consistent within sampling units. No significant acute toxicity was found in tadpoles exposed to site samples in the laboratory for 96 hours. Also, compared with laboratory work using defined metal mixtures and single-metal exposures, chemical analysis of these site-samples suggested that metal concentrations were not sufficient to cause acute effects. Chronic effects measured on Milltown surface-water samples were generally noted by altered growth, though only a limited number of embryos demonstrated effects in a statistically significant manner. Although gross malformations were occasionally noted, these chronic endpoints were frequently subtle (e.g., mild abdominal edema, hyperpigmentation). No contaminant-specific malformations were noted in these exposures.

Preliminary survey of linear food-chain contamination. In preliminary linear food-chain analyses, metals were clearly being bioaccumulated in small mammals sampled at Milltown; relative to the comparative literature, metal residues in carcasses or selected organs of these herbivores were not elevated. There was no indication of metal biomagnification in these herbivores. Observations regarding health and status of resident small-mammal populations were also considered in the evaluation of risks associated with metal exposures. Upon gross examination, external features were generally unremarkable in all animals collected at Milltown.

Synoptic Summary: Oregon Field Site (U.S. EPA 1993)

Chemical analysis of soil, sediment, groundwater, and biological materials. In order to adequately characterize exposure, representative samples of soil, sediment, and groundwater were collected and analyzed for the target compounds, 2,4-D and the dichlorophenols. Groundwater was grossly contaminated with 2,4-D (contaminanted samples exceeded 1800 ppm) and the dichlorophenols (contaminanted samples exceeded 3,000 ppm 2,4-dichlorophenol and 400 ppm 2,4,6-trichlorophenol), as indicated by samples collected along sampling transects along the playa. Soils and sediments at various locations in the playa were also contaminated, but to a much lesser extent than groundwater, ranging from no-detectable amounts to concentrations of 2,4-D in excess of 90 ppm. Sediment-dwelling invertebrates (e.g., black fly larvae) and soil-dwelling invertebrates collected coincident with soil and sediment samples frequently presented residues of target compounds. For example, harvester ants collected on the playa had 1.0 to 6.0 ppm (dry weight) 2,4-D, and dipteran larvae collected from alkaline depressions on the playa presented 2,4-dichlorophenol residues ranging from no-detectable amounts to 0.4 ppm (dry weight). The majority of plant tissues were negative for 2,4-D, but presented 0.05 to 1.0 ppm 2,4- dichlorophenol in live plants collected on the playa.

Vegetation sampling and survey. The Alkali Lake area supported a relatively simple flora dominated by greasewood (*Sarcobatus vermiculatus*) on silty and clay soils. Suspected adverse impacts from previous chemical waste disposal activities were apparent at various locations near Alkali Lake, particularly near, and immediately west of the disposal site. Most of the greasewood shrubs in these areas were dead or in relatively poor health, but no additional extensive stands of dead shrubs were observed in the immediate vicinity, including highly alkaline depressions distant (within 0.5 miles) from the chemical disposal site. There were few, if any, biological indications of exposure in the areas surrounding the playa. Seasonal influences on potential ecological effects associated with the disposal site were tracked, primarily through a floristic survey and evaluations of vegetation cover. Vegetation surveys may be applicable to long-term studies at Alkali Lake, and vegetation should be evaluated periodically for potential contaminant-related effects. Changes in vegetation patterns near the disposal site may indicate an expansion, contraction or movement of soil-groundwater contaminants.

High desert wetlands, like those associated with Alkali Lake, range in area from a few square meters to approximately 0.25 Ha, and the persistence of surface water in these high desert regions is probably the most important environmental factor determining plant species composition. Wetlands having limited periods of inundation support vascular plants such as desert saltgrass (*Distichlis spicata*), while areas still flooded in late summer and autumn support stands of bulrushes (*Scripus acutus*). High desert wetlands are a valuable asset to the area and represent a species diverse "island" within the surrounding high desert landscape. The high plant-species richness and the presence of water make these areas very active biologically, and a variety of invertebrates and vertebrates use them as a critical component of their life cycles. At present, these habitats appear to have been little affected by the activities associated with the waste site, but future surveillance may be indicated, particularly if groundwater flow is not clearly understood.

Sampling for soil- and vegetation-inhabiting invertebrates. Terrestrial invertebrates were abundant and diverse at all sites sampled near the disposal site, but seasonal trends in species composition and numbers were apparent. In late spring and early summer, the observed species composition appeared typical of high desert habitats throughout the

Great Basin. *S. vermiculatus* shrubs supported large numbers of individuals and species of vegetation-dwelling insects. The composition and densities of foliage insects differed little among all sites sampled; the only notable difference among sampling units was spider mites occurred in great abundance on *S. vermiculatus* shrubs at the disposal site. High densities of spider mites may result from plant stress, reduced plant vigor, or decreased numbers of natural predators (D. Lightfoot, Univ. New Mexico, Albuquerque NM; pers. comm.).

Ground-dwelling arthropods were also abundant and diverse at all sites during late spring and early summer with ants being the most abundant ground-dwelling arthropods. The harvester ants, *Pogonomyrmex salinus* and *P. owyheei*, were especially abundant. *P. salinus* nest mounds were common at the disposal site, while *P. owyheei* appeared to be more abundant in the surrounding areas. This difference in species occurrence was probably due to habitat preferences and not contaminant related.

In late spring and early summer tenebrionid beetles were also common at all sampling locations. One species, *Eleodes pilosa*, was particularly abundant at the disposal area, while another species, *Eleodes n. nigra*, was most prevalent in the areas surrounding the disposal site. Again, these patterns probably result from natural edaphic features and should not be interpreted as contaminant-related. Ground-dwelling caterpillars of noctuid moths were abundant, and several species were trapped at all sampling locations.

Relative to late spring and early summer, terrestrial invertebrates were generally less abundant and diverse in the autumn survey. Overall insect densities were generally less than earlier in the year. Such seasonal differences in terrestrial insects in the Alkali Lake region should be considered normal, and not necessarily indicative of hazardous waste effects. Greasewood supported large numbers of individuals and species of insects, even at the disposal site. The composition and densities of foliage insects differed little among all sites sampled. Lepidoptera larvae and mirid plant bugs were less abundant than in late spring and early summer, and spider mites were absent on greasewood at the disposal site during the autumn sampling period.

In contrast, grasshoppers were more diverse and abundant in the autumn. Overall, grasshoppers were a numerically dominant group of insects at the Alkali Lake site. For example, *Aeloplides minor*, a grasshopper which lives and feeds on shrubs in the family Chenopodiaceae, and membracid treehoppers (*Lieosycta ferruginipennis*) were common on greasewood in the autumn, but absent or reduced in numbers relative to the late spring and early summer. Asilid robber flies (*Efferia basingeri*) were common at all terrestrial sampling sites in the autumn, and were representative predators of nearly all flying insects, except for the larger grasshoppers. Harvester ants were abundant in the autumn; however, their numbers were much lower than in late spring and early summer.

Overall, the Alkali Lake study site was found to support a rich, but seasonally variable, invertebrate fauna. Certain taxa were particularly abundant and might be considered as target species. Ants, tenebrionid beetles, and noctuid moth larvae were common ground-dwelling arthropods, and may be important for future consideration because they may transfer hazardous chemicals to higher trophic levels. In addition, ants may be important because they transport soil, especially deep soil particles to the surface. Ants and various families of moth larvae were also abundant foliage arthropods.

Aquatic invertebrate sampling. Although limited in biological diversity, the aquatic invertebrates most widely available as potential food sources at Alkali Lake included aquatic flies (Ephydridae and Dolichopodidae), water beetles (Dyticidae and Hydrophilidae), shore bugs (Saldidae), and brine shrimp (Artemiidae; Artemia salina). Their abundance closely tracked habitat availability, which in its simplest statement means that aquatic environments -- most frequently the ephemeral alkaline waters of the Alkali Lake basin -- must be present for their numbers to be sufficient to be likely prey items in the diet of a terrestrial vertebrate. Clearly, these ephemeral habitats are most frequently present in spring and early summer at West Alkali Lake. As the work at Alkali Lake illustrates, dry winters, as well as late season periods in any year, would be associated with relatively low numbers of aquatic invertebrates. In contrast, wet winters and extended periods of available ephemeral surface waters would correspond to relatively high population numbers. The data collection may be critical to evaluating the changing patterns in food availability throughout the year.

Small mammal trapping survey and gut analysis. While ecological indicators (Angus 1991) are currently being evaluated as critical components in ecological assessment, various potential receptors at Alkali Lake may be considered along these lines, especially within a food-chain contamination evaluation. A preliminary food-chain analysis for small mammals at Alkali Lake was considered, and small mammal trapping was completed. Deer mice (Peromyscus maniculatus) were captured most frequently across all sample units. Stomach analysis was completed on small mammal specimens trapped at various sites on, near, or far-field from the disposal area. Stomach contents were sorted as broad food categories: seeds, vegetation, and insects. Depending upon time of year, small mammals were apparently feeding on vegetation and insects in varying proportions, depending upon the trap location. For example, insect parts were commonly observed in stomach contents sampled from deer mice trapped near the perimeter of the disposal site in late spring and early summer, while vegetation was the predominant food source in autumn.

When given a food-chain contamination scenario for small mammals (Sullivan, *et al.* 1987; Tasca, *et al.* 1989), calculations using empirical data suggest acute exposures are unlikely to occur through dietary exposures (food plus coincidental ingestion of soil) in deer mice. Also, on the basis of past work completed at the site (T. Darrow, Lewis and Clark College, Portland, OR; unpublished data), no reproductive effects (e.g., embryotoxicity and teratogenicity) have been apparent in small mammals living on and around the disposal site at Alkali Lake.

CONCLUSIONS

Montana field site. The wetlands at Milltown Reservoir represent a single operable unit within the Superfund regulatory process. But, to be considered in ecological contexts, the wetland should be viewed as a part of the Clark Fork River watershed. Nonetheless, these preliminary studies have been incorporated into the baseline risk assessment being developed for the wetlands, and have suggested future work in the continuing ecological risk assessment process. For example, soils and sediments at Milltown wetlands may be characterized as having greater metal loads than the surrounding watersheds, although the historic and current release and movement of metals may be quite dissimilar. At Milltown wetlands, the measures of exposure-point concentrations suggest that metals, and specifically target analytes -- arsenic, cadmium, copper, lead, and zinc -- occur at greatest concentrations in deposition zones located throughout Milltown wetlands. On the basis of total metal concentrations, it may be said that soils and sediments are both metal-enriched, though biological assessments suggest that only a small, and variable, fraction of that metal is biologically available and associated with subtle biological effects. Clearly, these deposition areas may warrant additional study, or at a minimum should be monitored to ensure that adverse effects do not develop with time.

As potential sources of metal, the soils and sediments, as well as the associated water column, must be considered in light of the potential biological and ecological receptors inhabiting Milltown wetlands. While diverse in their selection, the biological tests applied during the field and laboratory efforts at Milltown wetlands fall short of anticipating all the receptors potentially at risk. For example, while terrestrial vertebrates such as small mammals have been considered, the comparative-toxicity data base is clearly incomplete. Evaluations of vegetation completed at Milltown wetlands may have missed soil microbial effects. In summary, an understanding of the potential effects of metals on communities and populations at Milltown wetlands must be developed by inference, based upon these quantitative estimates of effects made during the ecological assessment.

The biological assessments at Milltown wetlands suggest that little, or no acute toxicity or adverse biological effects are occurring now. Consistently, and regardless of the field- or laboratory-test methods used, biological assessments at Milltown wetlands could not characterize acute toxicity; however, evidence of subtle biological effects was noted in samples collected from depositional areas. Future remediation plans should weigh the potential biological and ecological impacts associated with remediation efforts against of the current impacts associated with elevated metals in soils and sediments. While the current subtle effects and potential effects should not be understated in the risk-assessment, currently any widespread physical alteration of wetland habitats may not be justified on a technical basis. Future site monitoring should address problems that may occur with remediation at Milltown wetlands and at upstream operable units, and in particular should consider the long-term effects of metal exposures on vegetation in depositional areas. Also, indirect effects associated with future management plans (e.g., habitat alterations associated with "no action" or sediment dredging alternatives) should be considered as a potential consequence of the metals that presently occur in the soils and sediments at Milltown wetlands.

The data gathered from laboratory and field work at Milltown wetlands has reduced the uncertainty associated with the baseline ecological risk assessment, and has suggested that biological and ecological effects, if present in the wetland, were subtle. The uncertainty associated with historic data or data collected in the current assessment at Milltown wetlands must be stressed, e.g, were surrogate test species (in either laboratory or field) sufficient for the biological assessment? Questions like these must be considered proximate sources of uncertainty in the ecological risk-assessment process at Milltown wetlands, and in any management decision derived in part from these studies. At Milltown wetlands:

- The preliminary survey of linear food-chain contamination showed evidence of metal bioaccumulation in small mammalian herbivores. Bioconcentration of metals was also occurring in emergent vegetation in some reaches of the deposition zones within Milltown wetlands, but biomagnification of metals in herbivores did not appear to be a problem for the endpoints considered. Field surveys at Milltown wetlands did not contradict these assessments, but the sparse comparative-toxicity data available, particularly for chronic endpoints, must be considered as a source of uncertainty.

- Vegetation tests, especially those used in evaluating water collected from the rhizosphere, suggested that no acute effects were associated with groundwater and surface water, but subtle growth-related effects were occasionally observed in samples collected from deposition zones at Milltown wetlands. These subtle indications were noted in both laboratory tests using emergent vegetation and in standard root-elongation tests. Again, field surveys found no sign of altered vegetation patterns and reduced cover was evident only in those areas that had previously been physically manipulated.

- Earthworm evaluations in both field and laboratory were consistently negative for acute toxicity, suggesting that soil macroinvertebrates may not be at great risk as long as the current soil conditions exist. (This is provided that earthworms are good sentinel species for assessing soil health.) Soil microbial communities, however, were not adequately described and should be evaluated when methods are available.

- Preliminary studies using amphibians suggested that subtle biological effects may be found at Milltown wetlands, but qualitative field surveys did not support any conclusions that those effects would be prominent nor adverse.

- Preliminary studies using bacterial tests yielded results consistent with the balance of biological-tests used at Milltown wetlands, but may not be representative of the soil community there.

- Preliminary plant studies suggested that garden crops bioconcentrate metals. Bioconcentration of metals in plants differs depending upon the plant species and anatomical feature considered (e.g., root versus leaf).

- Characterization and metal analysis of Milltown wetlands soils, sediments, and biota indicated that metals have accumulated in various environmental matrices, and that Milltown wetlands is spatially quite heterogeneous with respect to metal deposition. Within-sample unit variation was relatively less than across Milltown wetlands variation, and metal deposition was consistent within topographic settings. Soils within sample units were relatively homogeneous.

Oregon field site. While the present work was designed primarily for data collection and survey, its role within an ecological risk assessment for Alkali Lake has become essential. The critical early phases (problem formulation, and pilot investigations for exposure and ecological effects assessment; see U.S. EPA 1991) of the ecological risk assessment process have been addressed, and existing data needs have been identified, which should allow more adequate characterizations of uncertainty during the risk assessment process. Baseline exposure and ecological effects assessments can now be developed and based upon site-specific data, and any future data needs may be clearly identified. For example, within the ecological effects assessment, field surveys and literature reviews have been considered, but by design little toxicity assessment has been completed. Future work could be developed to address this data gap, and additional comparative literature regarding contaminant effects could then be gathered for evaluating site-specific toxicity data. Whether future work regards these specific data needs, the baseline ecological assessment at Alkali Lake provides empirical information upon which decisions can be based.

Numerous technical recommendations can be identified as a result of these baseline data collections. While the studies at Alkali Lake were preliminary and not developed as a risk assessment, the information should be considered in developing management plans for Alkali Lake, including any future ecological risk assessment. On the basis of historical information and the completed field reconnaissance, the following may be relevant to future management decisions regarding Alkali Lake:

- With the baseline information gathered during these preliminary studies, efforts should be continued to evaluate vegetation pattern changes at Alkali Lake. The biological information subsequently generated in such a monitoring program could potentially benefit future evaluations of the effects of groundwater quality on vegetation. These should be completed using, for example, plant vigor tests modified to use representative species, e.g., Sacrobatus vermiculatus.

- Periodic soil sampling should be included in a monitoring program to evaluate soil contamination and the changing spatial patterns of the groundwater plume.

- Additional aquatic invertebrate sampling should be considered in conjunction with an evaluation of shorebird diet and foraging activities at Alkali Lake, particularly during the nesting season (e.g., spring and early summer field activity). Modified standard tests (ASTM 1992) using nestling shorebird exposures may be beneficial to evaluations of risks to this terrestrial vertebrate.

Future work at Alkali Lake must reflect management and policy related issues relevant to site managers, and field and laboratory efforts can directly address issues regarding risk characterization and uncertainty. Ecological risk assessments then could be developed more soundly and site management more adequately implemented.

Preliminary studies and ecological risk assessment. In general, an ecological assessment may be considered an integrated evaluation of ecological effects and exposure, and linkages among chemical contaminants, adverse ecological effects, and ecological toxicity may be evaluated during the site-assessment process using quantitative methods. As illustrated by these two examples, both laboratory tests and field methods may be beneficial to an ecological risk assessment. Designed preliminary studies may help focus more costly efforts that involve replicated, or larger-scale field and laboratory studies, as well as monitoring programs. These larger-scale studies may be more rigorous in a statistical sense, but effective use of preliminary studies may help identify, eliminate, or prioritize targets or habitats that should be considered in more costly risk assessment studies.

REFERENCES

Angus, T.H. 1991. Criteria for choosing indicator species for ecological risk assessments at Superfund sites. 101/F-90/051. U.S. Environmental Protection Agency, Office of the Administrator, Washington, D.C.

ASTM. 1992. Annual book of ASTM standards, Volume 11.04, American Society for Testing and Materials (ASTM), Philadelphia, PA.

Byl, T.D. and S.J. Klaine. 1991. Peroxidase activity as an indicator of sublethal stress in the aquatic plant *Hydrilla verticillata* (Royle). In Plants for Toxicity Assessment: Second Volume, ASTM STP 1115, J.W. Gorsuch, W.R. Lower, W. Wang, and M.A. Lewis, Eds., American Society for Testing and Materials, Philadelphia, PA, 1991. pp. 101-106.

Federal Interagency Committee for Wetland Delineation. 1989. Federal manual for identifying and delineating jurisdictional wetlands. U.S. Army Corps of Engineers, U.S. Environmental Protection Agency, U.S. Fish and Wildlife Service, and U.S.D.A. Soil Conservation Service, Washington, D.C. Cooperative technical publication, 76pp.

Fribush, H. and J. Fisk. 1991. Field analytical methods for Superfund. In Proceedings of Second International Symposium on Field Screening Methods for Hazardous Waste and Toxic Chemicals, Las Vegas, Nevada, pp. 25-30.

Linder, G., J. Wyant, R. Meganck, and B. Williams. 1991. Evaluating amphibian responses in wetlands impacted by mining activities in the western United States. In Fifth Biennial Symposium on Issues and Technology in the Management of Impacted Wildlife, Thorne Ecological Institute, Boulder, CO. pp. 17-25.

Linder, G., E. Ingham, C.J. Brandt, and G. Henderson. 1992. Evaluation of terrestrial indicators for use in ecological assessments at hazardous waste sites, EPA/600/R-92/183, U.S. Environmental Protection Agency, Environmental Research Laboratory, Corvallis, OR.

Nwosu, J., H.C. Ratsch, and L.A. Kapustka. 1991. A method for on-site evaluation of phytotoxicity at hazardous waste sites. In Plants for Toxicity Assessment: Second Volume, ASTM STP 1115, J.W. Gorsuch, W.R. Lower, W. Wang, and M.A. Lewis, Eds., American Society for Testing and Materials, Philadelphia, PA, 1991. pp. 333-340.

Page, A.L., R.H. Miller, and D.R. Keeney, Eds. 1982. Methods of soil analysis. Part 2: Chemical and microbiological properties, Second Edition. American Society of Agronomy Monograph 9. Madison, WI.

Parkhurst, B., G. Linder, K. McBee, G. Bitton, B. Dutka, and C. Hendricks. 1989. Toxicity tests. In W. Warren-Hicks, B. Parkhurst, and S. Baker, Jr. (eds.). Ecological assessment of hazardous waste sites. EPA/600/3-89/013, U.S. Environmental Protection Agency, Environmental Research Laboratory, Corvallis, OR, pp. 6-1 - 6-66.

Pascoe, G.A. and R.J. Blanchet. 1993. Baseline ecological risk assessment: Milltown Reservoir operable unit, Milltown Reservoir Sediments Sites. Prepared by Environmental Toxicology International, Inc. for U.S. Environmental Protection Agency, Region 8, Helena, MT.

Sullivan, J.R., T.J. Kubiak, T.E. Amundson, R.E. Martini, L.J. Olson, and G.A. Hill. 1987. A wildlife exposure assessment for landspread sludges which contain dioxins and furans. pp. 406-414. In Proceedings of Tenth Annual Madison Waste Conference. Department of Engineering Professional Development, University of Wisconsin-Madison. Madison, WI.

Suter, II, G. 1993. Ecological risk assessment. Lewis Publishers, Inc. Chelsea, MI.

Tasca, J.J., M.F. Saunders, and R.S. Prann. 1989. Terrestrial food-chain model for risk assessment. pp. 111-116. In Superfund '89, Hazardous Material Control Research Institute, Tenth National Conference and Exhibition, Washington, D.C.

U.S. EPA. 1986. Testing methods for evaluating solid waste. U.S. Environmental Protection Agency, Office of Solid Waste and Emergency Response, Washington, D.C., SW-846.

U.S. EPA. 1991. Ecological assessment of Superfund sites: An overview; ECO Update, Vol. 1, Number 2. U.S. Environmental Protection Agency, Office of Solid Waste and Emergency Response, Office of Emergency and Remedial Response, Hazardous Site Evaluation Division (OS-230), Washington, D.C., Publication 9345.0-05I.

U.S. EPA. 1993. Technical report for the Alkali Lake ecological assessment, Phase I reconnaissance. Prepared by ManTech Environmental Technology, Incorporated for U.S. Environmental Protection Agency, Environmental Research Laboratory, Corvallis OR. 72pp.

Warren-Hicks, W., B. Parkhurst, and S. Baker, Jr., Eds. 1989. Ecological assessment of hazardous waste sites. EPA/600/3-89/013. U.S. Environmental Protection Agency, Environmental Research Laboratory, Corvallis, OR.

Geoffrey B. Matthews[1], Robin A. Matthews[2], and Wayne G. Landis[2]

Nonmetric Clustering and Association Analysis: Implications for the Evaluation of Multispecies Toxicity Tests and Field Monitoring[3]

REFERENCE: Matthews, G. B., Matthews, R. A., and Landis, W. G., "**Nonmetric Clustering and Association Analysis: Implications for the Evaluation of Multispecies Toxicity Tests and Field Monitoring,**" Environmental Toxicology and Risk Assessment-Third Volume, ASTM 1218, Jane S. Hughes, Gregory R. Biddinger, and Eugene Mones, Eds. American Society for Testing and Materials, Philadelphia, 1995.

ABSTRACT: Many techniques developed by computer scientists in the field of artificial intelligence (AI) are currently being used as standard, state-of-the-art technology. These techniques have proven their value and validity in medicine, geology, agronomy, and astronomy time and again, often beating human experts at their own game. We present here an analysis tool for multispecies data based on nonmetric clustering, an AI technique developed specifically to aid in the interpretation of complex ecological data sets. This technique uses AI search to find an appropriate and meaningful characterization of a multivariate system. After appropriately characterizing the system in this fashion, the relationship between this characterization of the system and the critical environmental variables (pollution, toxicity, *etc.*) can be quantitatively analyzed to aid in the assessment of the effects of the environment on the system. *A priori* endpoints or indices are not necessary; the data are allowed to determine the variables that best separate treatment from controls.

We have now tested this methodology over a series of multispecies toxicity tests using a variety of stressors. During the initial blind testing the methodologies could pick treatment groups with high accuracy. When knowledge of treatment group is available, oscillations in the similarity of the treatments to the controls are apparent.

---

[1]Professor, Computer Science Department, Western Washington University, Bellingham, WA 98225.

[2]Professor, Huxley College of Environmental Studies, Western Washington University, Bellingham, WA 98225.

[3]This research is supported by USAFOSR Grant No. AFOSR-91-0291 DEF.

Much recent debate in toxicological studies has focussed on appropriate endpoints for multispecies toxicity tests and biomonitoring schemes. We suggest that the search for endpoints appropriate to the entire field of toxicity testing is a fruitless search. We recommend instead an approach that standardizes the common sense approach: different situations, even within a single experiment, call for different endpoints. Typically, the toxicologist, if called upon for an expert opinion, will examine multivariate data, and extract from that data a few critical species. The behavior of these species will give an adequate (though perhaps not complete) picture of the toxic effects. Which species are selected, and whether it is their mortality, behavior, or biomass that is important, will always vary from case to case. We call, therefore, for more research into the automation of the process typically performed by the expert. The selection of species, as well as other parameters, as significant for a particular experiment or field study, can be done automatically by computer algorithms. To be blind to the utility of these tools in the field of toxicology is to work by hand, over and over again, problems which could be solved in a twinkling with their aid.

KEYWORDS: artificial intelligence, ecotoxicology, statistics, expert systems, multispecies tests, field monitoring

Introduction

Modern ecotoxicology often assumes that ecosystem level functional indices are desirable. Such an index would tell us what numbers to measure, which mathematical formulae to use on them, and the position of the cutoff point between healthy systems and troubled ones. This would introduce "objectivity" into what is now done with intuitive assessments. However, the state of an ecological community is an inherently complex object, and probably cannot be captured by a few linear indices. Remaining with the traditional human "best judgement," on the other hand, also has problems, such as subjectivity, prejudice, and the difficulty of comprehending the innate complexity of ecological systems. Fortunately, there is a middle ground for dealing with complex systems, between mathematical formulae and intuition. The middle ground is provided by computerized data exploration, using tools from artificial intelligence, pattern recognition, and scientific visualization. In other scientific domains, such as medicine, astrophysics, particle physics, meteorology and geology, such tools have been in widespread use for years. The key to their success is that the human expert and the software tools are partners in the exploration of the data. The computer by itself, of course, has no semantic understanding of the data. But, equally, the unaided human may be blind to the many patterns implicit in the data.

Much of the work in computer-aided data exploration, however, has the wrong focus for ecotoxicology. Data sets generated, for example, by meteorological models of a thunderstorm, typically have millions of data points densely scattered through a well-defined three-dimensional model. The complexity is in the sheer number of data points and their interactions. In ecologically interesting situations, on the other hand, only a few dozen or hundred data points are in hand, from widely separated places in space and time, and each point records data on dozens or hundreds of species. This results in a relatively small number of points scattered through the huge volume of n-dimensional space (where n is the number of different species counted). Even a modest number of dimensions raises severe problems for conventional analysis techniques, and human intuition. For example, if some large number of points is scattered uniformly over a 10-dimensional hypersphere with radius one, then a hypersphere inside, of radius 3/4, will contain only 5% of the points. Clearly, sampling 10 or higher dimensional space can miss important things. Further, a lot of the time data points are missing, or incomplete.

The nature of the problem is that usually we have too many dimensions. Ten or twenty sampling points with, perhaps, fifty species, is underdetermined. There is no way to draw meaningful conclusions about the nature of the community as a whole (all fifty dimensions), from the smattering of points. What is required is *data reduction*, the dimensionality of the data has to be brought down to the point where ten or twenty points can tell us something. One methodology for this is based on *projections* of the data, such as factor analysis, principal components analysis, correspondence analysis, or, more generally, projection pursuit (Huber, 1985). There are many algorithms for finding good projections, and even a suggestion that *all* projections be examined in a "grand tour" of the data (Asimov, 1985). However, rotating at about 10° per second, a reasonable speed for careful observation, a grand tour of only four dimensions would take about three hours (Huber, 1985), and so computer-aided projections are the only real alternative.

While such projections are valuable in reducing the dimensionality of the data, they all suffer from a problem of comprehensibility. Since arbitrary linear and nonlinear transformations of the data matrix are allowed, the meaning of the resulting two-dimensional projection can be obscure, and difficult to grasp intuitively.

Another possibility for data reduction is provided by careful experimental design. Measuring too many parameters can be just as misleading as measuring too few. The problem with this approach, however, is that in many circumstances the correct parameters are not known in advance. Indeed, our understanding of ecological systems and their response to toxic stress is still in its infancy. What is needed is a tool to help the analyst in finding important and significant parameters in new situations.

The tradition of machine learning (ML), within artificial intelligence, has been addressing these problems for some time. The goal of an ML system is, not only to identify patterns in the data, but to come up with an efficient and intuitive characterization of them. Efficient and intuitive, in this context, imply that the characterization is not overly complex, that it uses simple logical combinations of descriptions rather than mathematical formulae, and that it is expressed in terms of attributes that are not contrived. This has been formulated as the *comprehensibility postulate*:

> The results of computer induction should be symbolic descriptions of given entities, semantically and structurally similar to those a human expert might produce observing the same entities. Components of these descriptions should be comprehensible as single "chunks" of information, directly interpretable in natural language, and should relate quantitiative and qualitative concepts in an integrated fashion (Michalski, 1983).

It is the primary failing of traditional statistical approaches, as well the "neural net" approach, to solving ML problems that they ignore the comprehensibility postulate.

In this paper, we present nonmetric clustering, a specialization of ML, faithful to the comprehensibility postulate, which we have been employing fruitfully on a wide variety of ecosystems. After its details are explained, some consequences for environmental policy making are outlined.

Machine Learning

As a simple example, consider the data in Table 1 (Quinlan, 1983). In this set,

Height	Hair	Eyes	Class
short	blond	blue	+
tall	blond	brown	–
tall	red	blue	+
short	dark	blue	–
tall	dark	blue	–
tall	blond	blue	+
tall	dark	brown	–
short	blond	brown	–

Table 1: Data set problem for identification and characterization.

we are given three "positive" individuals and five "negative" individuals and their characteristics on three attributes. The problem is to come up with a means of distinguishing the "positives" from the "negatives" based on height, hair, and eye color. There are many possible ways of distinguishing them, but one nice one might be:

> Positives either have red hair, or blond hair and blue eyes.
> Negatives either have dark hair, or blond hair and brown eyes.

There are several things to notice about this characterization of the positives and negatives.

First, the data are both categorical and numeric. The beauty of ML approaches to these problems is that they apply equally well to either kind of data. To make a regression, or linear discriminant, categorical data would have to be numerically coded somehow. A loglinear model can be used on categorical data, but then the numeric data would have to be fit in. In an ML approach, numeric attributes, such as height, are simply recoded into a number of discrete bins, such as small, medium, and large. Such categories can be as fine or as coarse as desired, and in all events are more comprehensible than an uninterpreted number.

Second, not all the original attributes are used in the description. Height, it turns out, is superfluous, and is omitted from the description.

Third, compound descriptions are created using logical operations, "and" "or" and "not", rather than mathematical formulae. A linear discriminant, for example, describes by adding up numbers and then determining if the result is greater or smaller than some cutoff point. The logical descriptions are much more natural and intuitive for humans, and lead to understanding of the data in a way that mathematical combinations cannot.

Fourth, even with only three attributes and eight points, there are a lot of different logical descriptions that have to be considered to get the best one (or even a

C1	A	B	C	D	E	F	C2
+	1	2	1	2	2	1	+
+	1	2	2	1	1	2	−
+	1	2	1	2	2	1	+
−	2	1	2	1	1	2	−
−	2	1	1	2	2	1	+
−	2	1	2	1	1	2	−

Table 2: Synthetic data for nonmetric clustering, with two possible clusterings.

good one). With real data sets the combinatorial complexity of finding a description would rapidly swamp a human investigator. A computer aid is essential.

Fifth, no artificial attributes are used. The use of "indices" or "ordination" techniques attempts to introduce a new attribute, defined mathematically in terms of the original ones, and then use the values of these indices or components to describe the classes. The ML description uses the same attributes (height, hair, and eyes) that were used in the design of the sampling program, and thus, the description of the classes will have direct meaning to the investigator, without the need to learn a new vocabulary. Such descriptions, which use simple logical combinations of the original attributes, are called "conceptual" descriptions (Michalski and Stepp, 1983).

Nonmetric Clustering

Nonmetric clustering (NMC) is an ML tool designed to search for conceptual descriptions of ecological data sets. The NMC methodology has been implemented in a computer program called Riffle (Matthews and Hearne, 1991). Unlike the simple example above, Riffle does not work from a preexisting set of class labels (such as + and −). Given a data set, Riffle attempts to two things simultaneously: Group the points into clusters (classes), and find the simplest possible conceptual description of those clusters. Since the points are not previously assigned to classes, Riffle is free to give the points any class label at all. However, the class labels must be such that they can be simply captured in a conceptual description, based on the original attributes (measured parameters), and, further, such that they, in turn, capture as much information as possible about the original attributes.

Consider the synthetic data in Table 2, where six points have been sampled for six attributes. One potential clustering, denoted C1, has two simple conceptual descriptions, each based on a single attribute, either A or B. C, D, E and F can be regarded as superfluous for this clustering. Another potential clustering, denoted C2, also has simple characterizations, but in terms of attributes C, D, E, and F, with A and B as superfluous. While both clusterings have simple conceptual descriptions, C2 should be preferred because it captures more information about the points than C1.

	A1	A2	A3
B1	5	3	1
B2	1	4	2
B3	7	0	5

Table 3: A contingency table to illustrate calculation of Guttman's λ.

One way to express this algorithmically is that there are *more* good conceptual descriptions of the classes in C2 than there are of the classes in C1. The computer program Riffle will prefer C2 to C1 for this reason.

To find the best clustering possible, for a given data set, the algorithm works by examining a great number of possible clusterings, like C1 and C2, above, and numerically ranks their conceptual adequacy. All data points are repeatedly reassigned to clusters, and then the conceptual association between clusters and attributes is reevaluated. When an assignment of points to clusters is found that outranks all others, it is reported as the most natural clustering.

We will now briefly discuss how conceptual adequacy is ranked, and also make some remarks on the particular strategy used in Riffle to convert numeric to categorical variables.

Numerically ranking conceptual descriptions

To begin with, assume all attributes are categorical. Nonmetric clustering measures the association between a clustering (which, itself, is a categorical variable) and another categorical variable by means of a contingency table test. A frequency table of cluster-number *vs.* categorical-value is set up, and the number of data points in each cell is counted in order to measure the association between cluster and variable. The most famous contingency table test is probably the χ^2 test, but the χ^2 test has some undesirable properties when it comes to interpretation and comprehensibility. Nonmetric clustering uses Guttman's λ to measure the association in the table (Goodman and Kruskal, 1954).

Guttman's λ is a measure defined on the basis of "optimal predictions". Consider, for instance, the contingency table represented in Table 3. Twenty-eight individuals have been sampled, and their values on attributes A and B have been tabulated. For concreteness, A can be regarded as "height" and B as cluster-number. A larger sample size would always be desirable, but we have no recourse other than to regard the proportion of points found in any cell as the best estimate of the probability of finding a new point also to be in that cell. Now suppose we need to predict which value on attribute B a new sample is likely to have. In the absence of any further information, there are nine B1's, seven B2's, and twelve B3's, so we would guess B3, and expect to be right about 12 out of 28 times, giving us an error expectation of 16 out of 28, or about 57%. We will call this the *absolute error rate of B*. Now, however, suppose we are given a new data point, and are told its value for attribute A. How will we predict B, and what will our expected error rate be when conditioned on this knowledge? Well, 13/28 of the time the new point will be A1, and we should then guess B3, and expect to be right 7/13 of the time. Similarly, 7/28 of the time it will be A2, and we will guess B2, and be right 4/7 of the time, and 8/28 of the time it will be A3, we guess B3, and are right 5/8 of the time. Predictions of B conditioned on A, then, should be correct $(13/28)(7/13)+(7/28)(4/7)+(8/28)(5/8)\approx 57\%$ of the time, and the *error rate of B conditioned on A* is 43%. The *reduction in error* is $57-43$, and the *proportional reduction in error* is $(57-43)/53\approx 26\%$. In comprehensible terms, we expect to be wrong about 26% fewer times if we know A. The proportional reduction in error when predicting A conditioned on B can be computed similarly. The absolute error rate of A is $(28-13)/28\approx 54\%$, the error rate of A conditioned on B is $1-[(9/28)(5/9)+(7/28)(4/7)+(12/28)(7/12)]\approx 43\%$, and the proportional reduction in error is $(54-43)/54\approx 20\%$. Each of these proportional reductions in error is a measure of how well knowledge of one attribute aids the prediction of the other. A symmetric measure of association can be obtained by simply averaging the two conditioned measures, giving the symmetric λ, of 23%.

Formally, λ can be defined as follows. For a contingency table with proportional entries ρ_{ab}, let $\rho_{\cdot b}=\sum_a \rho_{ab}$, $\rho_{a\cdot}=\sum_b \rho_{ab}$, $\rho_{am}=\max_b \rho_{ab}$, $\rho_{mb}=\max_a \rho_{ab}$, $\rho_{\cdot m}=\max_b \rho_{\cdot b}$, and $\rho_{m\cdot}=\max_a \rho_{a\cdot}$. Then the reduction in error of b with respect to a is

$$\lambda_b=\frac{\sum_a \rho_{am}-\rho_{\cdot m}}{1-\rho_{\cdot m}}$$

and the reduction in error of a with respect to b is, similarly,

$$\lambda_a=\frac{\sum_b \rho_{mb}-\rho_{m\cdot}}{1-\rho_{m\cdot}}$$

The symmetric form, which averages these two cases, becomes

$$\lambda=\frac{1}{2}\frac{\sum_a \rho_{am}+\sum_b \rho_{mb}-\rho_{\cdot m}-\rho_{m\cdot}}{1-\frac{1}{2}(\rho_{\cdot m}+\rho_{m\cdot})}$$

Obviously, the more strongly two attributes are associated, the higher the value of λ, and *vice versa*. Some other properties of λ (Goodman and Kruskal, 1954) are:

- λ lies between 0 and 1, inclusive, except when the entire population lies in a single cell of the table, in which case it is indeterminate.

- λ is 1 if and only if all the population is in cells no two of which are in the same row or column.
- Independence is sufficient, but not necessary, for λ to equal 0.
- λ is unchanged by permutations of rows or columns.

Elsewhere we have found λ to be an excellent measure of qualitative association, in that it accords well with human intuitions and is much more "stable" than χ^2 (Chen, 1992). Using λ to calculate the association between cluster-numbers and categorical attribute values is faithful to the comprehensibility postulate: an attribute is a good description of a clustering if knowledge of the attribute helps predict cluster, and *vice versa*.

Integrating qualitative and quantitative data

The frequency table approach works well for categorical variables, but what about numeric variables? Nonmetric clustering takes a pragmatic approach to these: if we assume that the data are going to be adequately described by a clustering into a finite number of clusters, then there are really only a finite number of values of a numeric parameter to consider, one for each cluster. All other variations in a numeric parameter can be assumed to be due to variance within the clusters. Accordingly, we can divide up the range of a numeric parameter into discrete parts. We can do this nonmetrically by simply choosing quantile points, but a more flexible arrangement allows the "splits" between categorically different values to be selected by the algorithm as it runs. How this is accomplished is illustrated in Figure 1. Here we have marked two clusters with open and filled circles, and the categorical division of two dimensions into "high" and "low" values are shown by the dividing gray lines. The point marked with an "X" is troublesome, as it does not fit well with either of the two clusters, and keeps us from obtaining a λ value of 1.0 for this data set. We could move the vertical line to the right, changing our division between "long" and "short", to try to include X in one cluster, but that would raise more problems by the inclusion of some points from the other cluster. Similar problems occur if we try to raise the horizontal line, changing our definition of "light" and "heavy". to try to include X in one cluster, but that would raise more problems by the inclusion of some points from the other cluster. Similar problems occur if we try to raise the horizontal line.

The computer program Riffle will keep adjusting these split lines up and down to achieve better associations between cluster and numeric attribute. In other words, what counts as "small" or "large" can be redefined by the algorithm as it investigates the data. At the same time, the algorithm is free to reassign the points themselves to different clusters. Both of these reinterpretations of the data are tried over and over, to

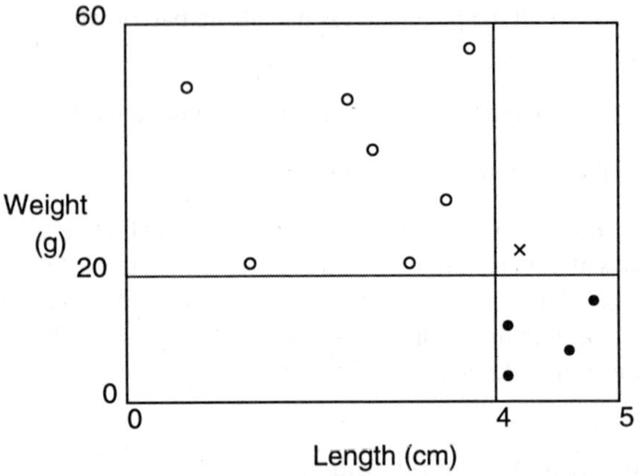

Figure 1: Twelve data points in two dimensions. Clusters are indicated by open and filled circles. Split values shown by gray lines. The point marked with an "X" cannot be included in either cluster by moving the split values without introducing further problems.

maximize λ. The algorithm stops when it cannot improve the association between clusters and attributes any more.

This clustering methodology has a number of advantages over traditional clustering methods:

- It does not combine counts from dissimilar taxa by means of sums of squares, or other *ad hoc* mathematical techniques.
- It does not require transformations of the data, such as normalizing the variance.
- It works without modification on incomplete data sets. Since each attribute has its λ-association with the clustering evaluated independently, the fact that some points have some values for some attributes, and other points for other attributes, is irrelevant. Attributes are *not* directly combined.
- It can work without further assumptions on different data types (*e.g.*, numeric, categorical, species counts, presence/absence data, *etc.*).
- Significance of an attribute to the analysis is not dependent on the absolute size of its count. For instance, a taxon having a small total variance, such as rare taxa, can compete in importance with common taxa, and taxa with a large, random variance will not automatically be selected, to the exclusion of others.

- It provides an integral measure of "how good" the clustering is, *i.e.* whether the data set differs from a random collection of points, by means of the size of the λ values for each attribute.

- It can, in some cases, identify a subset of the attributes that serve as reliable indicators of the physical environment. In our research the indicator species selected by Riffle often proved to be more reliable than indicators based on a linear discriminant (Matthews et al., 1991a; Matthews et al., 1991b).

The major disadvantage of the Riffle program is that, in order to find a clustering of the data points with the desirable qualities listed above, a massive search through thousands of potential clustering candidates is made before settling on the "right" one. Even after this search, there is no guarantee that Riffle finds the optimal clustering, in the sense outlined above. However, in our research, involving datasets with one or two hundred dimensions and points, Riffle does find an excellent clustering in a reasonable amount of time. For larger datasets, supercomputers and/or more heuristic searches may be required.

Riffle has been applied successfully in a number of ecological and toxicological situations. For example, in a study of urban runoff in a small stream (Matthews et al., 1990), Riffle was able to identify a community of macroinvertebrates that was associated with clean water regardless of season al variation. Many of the species in the community were quire rare, and would have been overlooked without the use of Riffle. In studies of jet fuel toxicity in microcosms (Landis et al., 1993a; Landis et al., 1993b), Riffle was able to identify communities of species associated with toxic dose. Over the sixty days of the experiment the communities changed, from communities distinguished predominantly by their predator/prey ratios (*Daphnia* and algae) to communities distinguished predominantly by the makeup of their detritivores (Ostracods, *etc*). These patterns in the data suggested new hypotheses and further experiments that would not have been conceived without Riffle's aid.

Association Analysis: a Significance Test from the Clustering

If the data analyzed have natural groups, such as treatment groups or sites, a significance test can be derived from the known groups and the generated clusters. Under the null hypothesis, clusters generated from the data will have no association with the known treatment groups. Thus, if the generated clusters closely match the treatment groups, with less than one or five percent probability under the null hypothesis, then a significant effect has been found. We have used nonmetric clustering and association analysis on a variety of multivariate experiments and find it to be comparable in sensitivity to many metric tests that make more assumptions about the underlying distributions of the data (Landis et al., 1993b).

Implications for Ecological and Ecotoxicological Tests

The fact that nonmetric clustering and association analysis (NCAA) adheres to the comprehensibility postulate has numerous consequences for the analysis of ecological data, and for policy. When establishing policy for mitigation or restraint, the ecologist is forced into the position of deciding what is "good" and what is "bad," or natural *vs.* unnatural, or pristine *vs.* polluted, or healthy *vs.* unhealthy. The development of various ecological indicators (diversity indices, indicator species, biomarkers, *etc.*) has proceeded by fits and starts, primarily because ecosystems are complex and rarely reproducible, and so a simple division into good and bad ecosystems is not feasible. Instead, each new system must be approached on its own terms, and ecological and toxicological experts must begin to understand it afresh and derive new concepts each time.

A computational induction from the data alone using ML techniques has a number of advantages.

1. Machine learning is free from prejudice. Too often natural ecologists are forced to rely on traditional indicator species, or traditional measures of diversity, rather than taking a fresh look at each new system. Machine learning software does not remember the past, although the possibility is always open to incorporate prior information by, for example, weighting the dimensions.

2. Machine learning is adaptable. There is no need to establish policy based on a few preselected species, or on one mathematical technique. A variety of techniques, and all possible species, can be incorporated into a single ML tool which will sort through them and return with an objective picture of the ecosystem based on the most interesting species and the most informative tools.

3. Machine learning is interactive. Because the concepts derived by computational induction are faithful to the comprehensibility postulate, they can be examined by human experts. The machine is not a "black box" which must either be trusted implicitly or thrown out completely. Refinements in the ML algorithm can be visualized, based on experiments, and reincorporated into future generations of the ML computational tools.

4. Machine learning is not constrained like expert systems. Unlike expert systems, which attempt to encapsulate a particular human's expertise in a computer system, ML tools attempt to derive new expertise, new categories and concepts, derived from the data themselves. The only constraint on an ML system is the comprehensibility postulate, requiring that all new ideas be expressible in human terms. Beyond that, anything goes.

5. Machine learning is inexpensive. One of the primary motivations behind the surge of interest in expert systems was that a computer program represents a large initial investment, but a very small marginal cost subsequently, compared to professional consultation with a human expert. ML systems, once developed, are marketed like any other software, and can be duplicated and reused, in identical form, on any site.

Because of these advantages, we can recommend a new direction in ecotoxicological policy. There is a middle ground between reliance on completely objective, simple, numerical cutoffs, on the one hand, and largely subjective, naked faith in consensus human judgement, on the other. Rather, policy must be made only after extensive interaction between human experts and their ML assistants. Without ML and the associated computational induction, the human expert cannot be sure that some important concepts not are being overlooked. The human's compromises and policies should only be made after the minimal step of consulting with an ML system. Such man-machine consultations must become part of policy, or else we are condemned to base judgements on only partial information, on oblique, narrow, and slanted views into the data. We therefore call for ecotoxicologists to review the large ML literature, and begin to establish standards for human-computer interactive analysis of ecological systems.

Future Work: Dynamic Ecosystem Change

While our system of nonmetric clustering and association analysis does well with a variety of environmental data, we are currently seeking a much-needed extension of our ideas. At present, each data set is treated statically, as an independent point in time. In reality, environmental systems are extremely sensitive to their history. What is needed is a conceptual description of ecological systems that pays particular attention to the dynamic nature of systems over time. On the one hand, time could simply be viewed as another measured attribute; however, it is obvious that this attribute holds a special place. Time series analysis, as it is currently practiced, is almost entirely a univariate technique, primarily concerned with trends and cycles. What is required is a multivariate technique that makes sense of multivariate trends in patterns. One straightforward approach is to consider the state of a multivariate system as a multivariate vector, and the change over time as simply another vector connecting the state at one time with the state at another. In this view, we could define velocity, curvature, torsion, and a host of other vectors which would, in some sense, characterize the changes of the system over time. However, we must look instead for a description of change that does not violate the comprehensibility postulate. For a conceptual clustering, we must look for a *conceptual shift*, and have a concise notion of what this means. When we have decided the terms under which conceptual shifts are described, we can then build an ML tool that will assist us in our search for understanding. We believe that a conceptual shift in the character of a community or ecological system will be far more significant than any simple change in the numbers of species.

Conclusion

Machine learning promises to revolutionize the practice of environmental policy, by making the marriage of human and computer expertise a reality. We anticipate computerized "policy assistants" that will create an atmosphere of understanding and familiarity with the most difficult data. We have presented here, as an illustration, our own technique of nonmetric clustering and association analysis, which we have used repeatedly in gaining deeper insights into ecological and toxicological data. The computer tools of machine learning present a new alternative to past practices, one which is at the same time more friendly and more objective, and one which will, sooner or later, be indispensible to our field.

References

Asimov, D. (1985). The grand tour. *SIAM Journal of Scientific and Statistical Computing*, 6:128–143.

Chen, C. (1992). The measurement of clustering tendency in machine learning. Master's thesis, Western Washington University, Bellingham Washington.

Goodman, L. A. and Kruskal, W. H. (1954). Measures of association for cross classifications. *Journal of the American Statistical Association*, 49:732–764.

Huber, P. J. (1985). Projection pursuit. *Annals of Statistics*, 13:435–475.

Landis, W. G., Matthews, R. A., Markiewicz, A. J., and Matthews, G. B. (1993a). Multivariate analysis of the impact of the turbine fuel jet-a using a standard aquatic microcosm toxicity test. *Environmental Sciences*, 2(3):113–130.

Landis, W. G., Matthews, R. A., Markiewicz, A. J., and Matthews, G. B. (1993b). Multivariate analysis of the impacts of the turbine fuel jp-4 in a microcosm test with implications for the evaluation of ecosystem dynamics and risk assessment. *Ecotoxicology*, 2:271–300.

Matthews, G. and Hearne, J. (1991). Clustering without a metric. *IEEE Transactions on Pattern Analysis and Machine Intelligence*, 13(2):175–184.

Matthews, G. B., Matthews, R. A., and Hachmöller, B. (1991a). Mathematical analysis of temporal and spatial trends in the benthic macroinvertebrate communities of a small stream. *Canadian Journal of Fisheries and Aquatic Sciences*, 48(11):2184–2190.

Matthews, R. A., Matthews, G. B., and Ehinger, W. J. (1991b). Classification and ordination of limnological data: a comparison of analytical tools. *Ecological Modelling*, 53:167–187.

Matthews, R. A., Matthews, G. B., and Hachmöller, B. (1990). Ordination of benthic macroinvertebrates along a longitudinal stream gradient. In *Annual Conference, North American Benthological Society*, Blacksburg, Virginia.

Michalski, R. S. (1983). A theory and methodology of inductive learning. *Machine Learning, An Artificial Intelligence Approach*, pages 83–134.

Michalski, R. S. and Stepp, R. E. (1983). Learning from observation: Conceptual clustering. *Machine Learning, An Artificial Intelligence Approach*, pages 331–363.

Quinlan, J. R. (1983). Learning efficient classification procedures and their application to chess end games. In Michalski, R. S., Carbonell, J. G., and Mitchell, T. M., editors, *Machine Learning, An Artificial Intelligence Approach*, pages 463–482. Morgan Kaufmann, Los Altos, California.

Models in Ecological Risk Assessment

Scott Ferson[1] and Thomas F. Long[2]

CONSERVATIVE UNCERTAINTY PROPAGATION IN ENVIRONMENTAL RISK ASSESSMENTS

REFERENCE: Ferson, S., and Long T. F., **"Conservative Uncertainty Propagation in Environmental Risk Assessments,"** Environmental Toxicology and Risk Assessment - Third Volume, ASTM STP 1218, Jane S. Hughes, Gregory R. Biddinger, and Eugene Mones, Eds., American Society for Testing and Materials, Philadelphia, 1995.

ABSTRACT: Toxicological risk analysis is at a crossroads. The traditional approach using worst case analysis is widely regarded as fundamentally flawed since it yields conclusions that are often strongly biased and presumed hyperconservative. Probabilistic analysis using Monte Carlo simulation can yield overly optimistic conclusions when used without information about the correlation structure among variables. What is needed is a conservative methodology that makes no assumptions unwarranted by empirical evidence. To be conservative means both that the estimated risk is not systematically lower than the actual impact, but also that the uncertainty around the estimate is not narrower than justified by the available data. An appropriate methodology is dependency bounds analysis which computes bounds on the distributions for arithmetic operations on random variables when only their marginal distributions are known. Used in a risk analysis, it yields conservative results because it does not depend on knowledge about the correlation structure among all of the variables used in the analysis.

KEYWORDS: dependency bounds, conservativism, correlation, Monte Carlo, risk analysis, worst case, probabilistic arithmetic

For the most part, the quantitative methods of toxicological risk assessment have been based on deterministic models (USEPA 1987). These models have been pressed into service in making assessments about the impacts by all manner of environmental contamination on the health of humans and the functioning of ecological systems. However, deterministic models fundamentally ignore the variability of nature and cannot reflect our uncertainty about its workings. The resulting assessments are insensitive to the variation that exists in the natural world and, consequently, they pretend that our knowledge of nature is perfect. It has been difficult with such assessments to produce meaningful estimates of environmental hazards and their risks. Perhaps not surprisingly, deterministic assessments have come under sharp criticism (Roberts 1990). This criticism has led to a reconsideration of the methodology that should be used in environmental risk assessments.

[1] Senior Scientist, Applied Biomathematics, 100 North Country Road, Setauket, NY 11733

[2] Senior Toxicologist and Section Chief, Toxicology Section, Division of Environmental Health, Illinois Department of Public Health, 525 West Jefferson, Springfield, IL 62761

WORST CASE ANALYSIS

The traditional approach to estimating human health risks associated with environmental contaminants has been to estimate exposure from all or at least the most important exposure pathways. In the case of carcinogens, for example, the estimate of total exposure is then multiplied by a potency factor that yields the risk that disease or death will result from that exposure. Since we know there will be variability in exposure among individuals, we try to estimate an upper bound on potential exposure so as to be conservative with respect to our calculation of the overall risk from the contaminant. Likewise, susceptibility or sensitivity to exposures varies among individuals as well. By choosing a value for the potency factor that is likely to be an upper bound, the hope is to estimate the risk to the most susceptible individual who receives the highest exposure. This approach, dubbed worst case analysis (or MEI for maximally exposed individual), has obvious advantages from the perspective of a prudent regulator charged with safeguarding the public health.

Worst case analysis has been widely criticized (Roberts 1990). One of the main criticisms is that there is no direct way to determine how uncertainty in one or more of the inputs would affect the reliability of the final answer. The result of a worst case analysis is a single number, with no associated information about its uncertainty. This means that doing a 'what if' study can be cumbersome since it requires repeating the entire analysis. As a result, such sensitivity studies are usually limited in scope because the analyst must design and implement them specially.

The worst case approach to risk assessment purposely uses extreme values for some of its variables so as to make the overall risk estimate conservative. Another common criticism (Roberts 1990; Finkel 1990; Paustenbach 1989; Nichols and Zeckhauser 1988; Karstadt 1988) attacks the very heart of this approach. An input to a worst case analysis is a single fixed number that bounds the most extreme values likely to occur, and so, by design, it is not representative of the variable it purports to measure. These values are subsequently used in calculations to estimate risks. Although it may be reasonable to find the best estimate of a sum of two numbers by adding the best estimates for each of them together (cf. McKone and Ryan 1989), this is definitely not a reasonable way to find extreme values.

For example, consider the sum of two quantities A and B. When the quantities have any variability or uncertainty, as they almost always do, they are statistical distributions even though we may try to characterize them with single scalar numbers. To emphasize that convolutions of random number distributions form a kind of arithmetic, we use the expression 'random number' to mean the distribution of a random number. The mean of the distribution of the sum $A+B$ can be estimated as the sum of the means of the respective distributions of A and B. Although this approach works for the mean, it does not work for percentiles. But risk analysts are using extreme estimates in their computations. Suppose, for instance, that to be conservative we represent the value of A by the 95th percentile of its distribution. This implies that only 5% of the population is more extreme than this value. Continuing this idea, we also represent the value of B by its 95th percentile. We then use these values to estimate the sum of the quantities. Note, however, that the probability that the actual sum is no more extreme than this estimate is *not* 0.95, but rather 0.9975, assuming the two distributions are independent. Consequently, the sum of the two quantities is now considerably more conservative than the original level of 95%.

Of course, practitioners of worst case analysis realize that this occurs. Indeed, they are doing it on purpose to make risk estimates that are certainly conservative. However, the results of this approach are risk estimates that are very difficult to interpret. Just how extreme a final outcome is depends on the number of extreme values that happen to be combined in the arithmetic of the risk analysis. Clearly this can lead to results that are artifactual in the sense that they depend, not on the properties of chemistry and biology, but on the details of how we study them. For instance, the level of conservativism (how extreme it is with respect to its actual distribution) of the final estimate of risk from an analysis with half a dozen inputs could be different by several orders of magnitude compared to a result from an analysis with a few dozen inputs. Added to this, not all of the parameters in a risk analysis are replaced by their extreme bounds; sometimes means or other 'best estimates' are used when the extreme value seems inappropriate or would yield wildly biased results. Unfortunately, which parameters get extreme values and which are given best estimates is more a product of tradition or the idiosyncratic choice of the individual analyst than the result of serious justification.

Practical experience seems to show that the results of worst case analyses can be hyperconservative. As an example, the National Wildlife Federation (1989) estimated the risk of cancer from the consumption of sport fish by simply combining high estimates of certain persistent contaminants in Lake Michigan with a high estimate of fish consumption by sport fishermen, together with the potency factors derived by USEPA. Their resulting estimate of risk was equivalent to that suffered by a pack-a-day smoker (Frome and Checkoway 1985). Despite the fact that humans have been exposed to these chemicals over the last four decades, no consistent increase in cancer rates in the exposed population is readily observable despite the high risks estimated. The danger of hyperconservativism includes time-consuming litigation, direct and indirect costs to the marketplace and misdirection of scarce societal resources.

The degree of conservativism is not regulated in the worst case approach. It seems to us that the real problem is not that the approach is hyperconservative, but that it has an uncontrolled level of conservativism. If worst case analysis gave consistent answers that were simply very pessimistic about, say, the number of potential deaths that would result from a given concentration of substance in the environment, we could still rank chemicals by their respective risks and make regulations that cost-effectively protected the public health. But the results of worst case analyses for different assessments are not guaranteed to be indicative of the likely actual outcomes, or even their rank order. The degree of conservativism can be radically different in different analyses. As a result, risk analysts and regulators cannot reliably compare a statement from one risk analysis with statements from other analyses. This strongly limits the usefulness of these results in any kind of planning or decision making. It makes it virtually impossible to construct sensible regulations from the results and leads to regulatory embarrassments associated with worst case analysis.

Many analysts routinely compute both the worst case prediction and 'best estimate' prediction (based entirely on medians or means) in the hope of finding reasonable bounds of the worst likely outcome. While this is prudent, these intervals still cannot be compared across studies because of the unquantified conservativism in worst case analyses.

PROBABILISTIC ANALYSIS VIA MONTE CARLO METHODS

If it is essential to environmental risk analysis to be able to project the uncertainty about model parameters through complex calculations, how should the uncertainty be factored into a risk analysis? It seems it would be better simply to recognize the variability and uncertainty in the parameter values from the outset and propagate their effect through the calculations to see the best estimate as well as the range of possible risks. This would allow conclusions about which eventualities can be discounted as unlikely and which to take more seriously. This approach answers the need for simultaneous calculation of best estimate and worst case predictions: it computes these as special cases while finding the chances of an outcome of any size. Adding to the attractiveness of the approach, there are convenient software tools available for probabilistic analysis based on Monte Carlo simulation including @RISK from Palisade Corporation (Newfield, NY), Crystal Ball from Decisioneering (Denver, CO) and Demos from Lumina Decision Systems (Palo Alto, CA).

Despite considerable discussion (Roberts 1990) and wide recognition of the fact that a full-blown probabilistic analysis is warranted in any serious risk assessment, and despite the wide availability of microcomputer tools for performing such analyses, there has been an unmistakable reluctance on the part of regulators to embrace the Monte Carlo approach (USEPA 1992; Norton et al. 1988). This may be due to simple regulatory inertia, but it may also have deeper causes. One significant drawback of the approach is that it requires a great deal of data to estimate the underlying probability distributions and cross correlations of the variables of interest.

Ignoring correlations among variates can yield non-conservative results.

Some researchers (e.g., Smith et al. 1992) have suggested that it may be acceptable for Monte Carlo methods to ignore correlations among the variates because the means of the resulting convolutions are insensitive to the presence of correlations of moderate strengths. However, it is not only the means that are of interest in risk analysis. Indeed, the *tails* of the distributions which represent extreme impacts (such as very high doses) are particularly of interest. Monte Carlo methods that ignore the interdependencies among variates can *strongly underestimate the probability of these extreme events*. In this sense, the results of a Monte Carlo analysis that routinely assumes zero correlations among the variables may yield non-conservative results which are too optimistic about the narrowness of uncertainty for a risk estimate.

How much of a difference can unknown correlations make? Let us consider an example. Suppose A is a uniformly distributed random variable, say, between zero and one. If B is another random number with the same distribution, then, so long as A and B are *independent*, their sum is a triangular distribution between zero and two with a modal value of one. In this case, the variance of both A and B is 1/12, and the variance of their sum is 1/6. If the two variates are not independent, however, then the sum will not necessarily have a triangular shape. In fact, if the correlation is one, the sum will be a uniform distribution between zero and two. The variance in this case will be 1/3. On the other hand, if the correlation between the two variates is negative, a Monte Carlo analysis that ignores correlation can exaggerate the dispersion of the result. For instance, if the correlation is −1, the sum of A and B is a degenerate distribution with zero variance centered at one. In fact, there are infinitely many possible distributions that could be the result of adding A and B together even though they seem to be well specified. The variances of possible results range from zero to one third. Thus we see that a naive application of Monte Carlo analysis chooses, rather arbitrarily, a single distribution with a particular variance and shape that, by construction of this example, are in no way justified by data.

The story is similar for multiplication, except that the distribution shape and range of the possible variances are different. Subtraction and division are just the opposite; strongly negative correlations yield the greatest dispersion in the result and positive correlations yield narrower distributions. Other mathematical operations have their own idiosyncratic response to correlations. If the operands are more complicated than identically distributed uniform random numbers, the chore of keeping track of the effect in some complex mathematical expression involving these random variates becomes very burdensome if one is constrained to using Monte Carlo methods. With each operation, the probability of extreme events may be underestimated. Since the number of mathematical operations in real-world risk assessments range in number from a few to a several dozen, the opportunity for overly optimistic calculations to corrupt the assessment is substantial.

Given that this loss of conservativism can occur, one would assume that correlations would be widely recognized as a necessary input into any serious risk assessment using Monte Carlo analysis. Most analyses, however, have been conducted without empirical information about correlation structure, presumably because of the considerable cost of the sampling effort needed to estimate correlations. Some have sought to rationalize this practice. Studying normal and lognormal distributions, Smith et al. (1992) studied the effect from correlations of different strengths on the mean, variance and fractiles of sums and products. They present expressions for computing the bias from neglecting correlations as rules of thumb which could provide guidance to risk analysts. Unfortunately, however, the formulas are rather cumbersome, and even in the circumstances under which they apply, the formulas offer little intuition for the analyst. In an odd use of the word, the authors suggest that in some cases correlations may be "safely" ignored, by which they mean that little overall precision in the final distribution of risk is gained by the additional effort necessary to estimate correlations. It is clear, however, that correlations cannot be safely ignored if safety is measured by freedom from grave errors such as underestimating the risks of adverse consequences.

<u>Deconvolutions cannot be determined with Monte Carlo methods.</u>

An important aspect of the Monte Carlo approach is that one can take a deterministic approximation formula and, by simply varying the inputs, use it to estimate the statistical distribution of the result. This use implicitly assumes that the arithmetic of random numbers (i.e., distributions) is equivalent to that of real numbers. Unfortunately, this assumption is not true.

We give a simple example that illustrates an important discrepancy. In the domain of real numbers, if $A+B=C$, one can conclude from this that $B=C-A$. However, this is *not* the case for random numbers. Fig. 1 gives an example in which A, B and C are now random numbers, depicted as cumulative distributions. A and B are uniformly distributed between one and two, and between three and four, respectively. Their sum C is a triangular random number between four and six. But if only C and A could be observed empirically, we might try to estimate B as the difference $C-A$. However that difference does not equal the B we started with. Although the central tendency of B is recovered, both its variance and distribution shape are lost.

In the domain of random numbers, there must be a special method of solving for B when A and C are known called 'deconvolution'. As this numerical example shows, the deconvolution of addition cannot be found by subtraction. This complication occurs for the other arithmetic operators ($-$, $\times$ and $\div$) too. Deconvolutions cannot generally be found by convolutions with the inverse mathematical operator as they can in real arithmetic. It is easy to see why this must be the case by understanding that both addition and subtraction both necessarily widen uncertainty. Although it may seem esoteric, this complication is important for serious applications in risk analysis because the assumptions that correspond to estimating B by $C-A$ are generally hidden within the deterministic model supplied to the Monte Carlo analysis. In the original deterministic model which used real numbers, these assumptions were perfectly valid, and were probably commonly made without much thought. Within the Monte Carlo analysis, however, the assumptions become invalid and lead to incorrect estimation of the results.

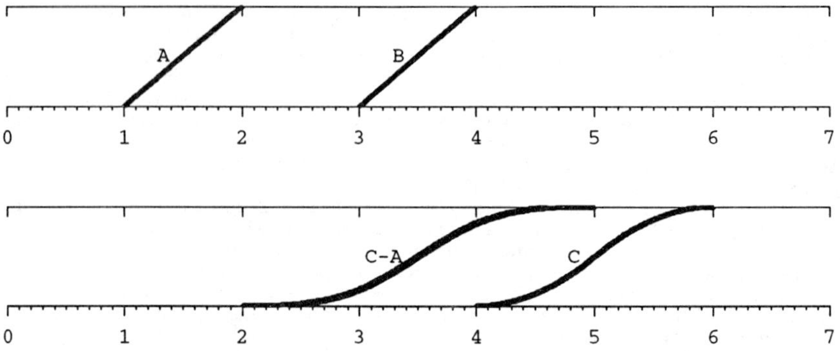

FIG. 1--For random numbers *A*, *B*, and *C* where $A+B=C$, the difference $C-A$ is not equal to *B*. Each random number is shown as a cumulative distribution. (In this discussion, we use the phrase 'random number' to refer to a statistical distribution, rather than the variable in the abstract or a particular value it takes on.)

As an example of when deconvolution ought to be used, consider the estimation of a carcinogenicity potency factor using the defining expression, risk is dose times potency. Suppose the statistical distribution of dose can be directly observed (perhaps via concentrations of urinary metabolites) and that the statistical distribution of risk can be computed (from, say, published mortality data). Because of the nature of mortality data, the measurement of risk cannot be made on particular individual, so we cannot generate pairs of dose and risk for individuals. But if we try to use the Monte Carlo approach and generate deviates from the observed distributions of risk and dose and divide them to estimate deviates for the potency, we will obtain a distribution that is wider than the real distribution of potency in nature.

As might be expected, in practice most every risk analyst using Monte Carlo analysis will estimate a deconvolution by a convolution with the inverse operator. This practice results in overly pessimistic results because the final distribution will be wider (more uncertain) than it would have been had deconvolution operations been used. In this sense, the results will be conservative. Deconvolutions would have dispersion no greater than that of the estimate based on the inverse operator. This means, then, that the analyst can be assured at least that the final result will not underestimate the actual uncertainty.

Of course, it would be false to think that over-optimism of Monte Carlo methods with respect to convolutions and their over-pessimism with respect to deconvolutions would cancel out one another. In an actual risk analysis, there is no way to control how these effects might influence the final result. This means that we cannot state a priori whether any particular result of a risk analysis will be conservative or optimistic. Further, we know of no available procedure to even compute a deconvolution using Monte Carlo methods. And, although the Monte Carlo procedures can be fine-tuned with more empirical information about cross-correlations to correct unwarranted optimism, a considerable amount of data is necessary to do this. In many important applications such detailed data will not be available. In the absence of this detail, a risk analysis involving complex expressions with many variables may yield an answer which is narrower or wider than the actual distribution of risk. There is no way of using standard Monte Carlo methods to make conservative evaluations, because which kind of interdependence among variables gives the most extreme convolution result depends on the particular mathematical operations involved. As a result, a risk analysis based on Monte Carlo methods will have an uncontrolled level of conservativism which may be either too high or too low, but we cannot say which. As a replacement for worst case analysis, it is ironic then that the Monte Carlo approach shares the very property that was considered crippling in the traditional approach.

Human perception of probability is biased.

Another drawback of probabilistic analysis via Monte Carlo methods is related to peculiarities of human perception of probabilities. In many instances, the estimation of probability distributions requires subjective evaluation, which essentially is guessing by informed individuals. Unfortunately, while the axioms of subjective probability (Savage 1954, 1971; Fishburn 1986) are internally consistent, they are not necessarily equivalent to the organization of the human mind. Psychometricians have cataloged a variety of discrepancies (Tversky and Kahneman 1982; Kahneman et al. 1982) between what humans think and what statistics says. In fact, the disparity can be very dramatic. For instance, in predictions of stock market trends (about which considerably more detailed information is known than virtually any ecological process in nature), actual events fall outside of the 1 and 99 percentiles of subjectively assigned probability ranges about 30% of the time! This finding is true both for naive and sophisticated subjects and is insensitive to whether there are monetary incentives for correct estimates. It seems that making overly narrow estimations of probability distributions is somehow a congenital feature of human perception. This tendency translates into an unfounded optimism about the uncertainty of predictions: we are more confident about the prediction than we should be. In a context where such optimism can lead to unpredicted human deaths from environmental toxicants, it may be useful to seek methods which err on the side of conservativism.

DEPENDENCY BOUNDS ANALYSIS

Our primary methodological complaint about using direct convolution or the Monte Carlo techniques to propagate uncertainty through calculations was that they usually assume the several variables involved are mutually independent. Of course, in many and perhaps most situations of interest in risk analysis, this assumption is untenable. Worse yet, data are usually so scarce that estimating the marginal distributions, let alone joint distributions, is very difficult. Therefore, even Monte Carlo methods which could be adapted to incorporate evidence of dependence are helpless if the necessary information is not available. In the remainder of this paper, we review dependency bounds analysis which makes no assumptions about correlations among the variables and therefore should yield conservative results when used in a risk assessment.

If A and B are random variables with known (marginal) distributions, and we want to compute their sum, the result can be formulated in terms of a probability convolution involving their joint distribution. Of course, unless A and B happen to be fairly simple, it can be rather difficult to solve this formulation analytically, which is why Monte Carlo methods were developed. But in cases when the joint distribution is not known, one cannot even formulate the answer even in principle. However, Frank et al. (1987) showed that it is possible to compute *bounds* on the result using only the two marginal distributions and without using any information about their joint distribution. Williamson and Downs (1990) give a numerical method for computing these bounds for a sum and extend the approach to treat subtraction, multiplication and division as well. These algorithms are very general and can be used for practically any distributions (which cannot be said of analytic approaches). Williamson and Downs show the resulting bounds are the pointwise best possible bounds for addition, subtraction, multiplication and division.

Dependency bounds analysis uses lower and upper discrete approximations to the quantile function (the quasi-inverse of the distribution function). The approach kills two birds with one stone in that this single pair of bounds contain both the representation error that accompanies discretization of real functions and "dependency error", i.e., the uncertainty induced by lack of knowledge about statistical dependence among the variates. For instance, when random numbers are added together, the resulting bounds delineate a range of possible distributions that could potentially result from the addition. This approach satisfies the complaints made against Monte Carlo about its loss of conservativism when there are unknown correlations among the variates.

The algorithms used in dependency bounds analysis are rather simple. Perhaps surprisingly, more precise results (smoother curves) can be computed with less computational effort than for comparable Monte Carlo methods. Fig. 2 shows two examples of dependency bounds analysis. In the top panel, *A* and *B* are random numbers depicted as cumulative distributions. Both are normally distributed numbers with specified means and variances. Their sum to the right on the same panel is represented by a pair of cumulative distributions. The curves bound the distributions that could result from the addition, i.e., any distribution that could possibly be the result of adding *A* and *B* will have its cumulative distribution within these bounds. The lower panel depicts the result of multiplying the same two quantities.

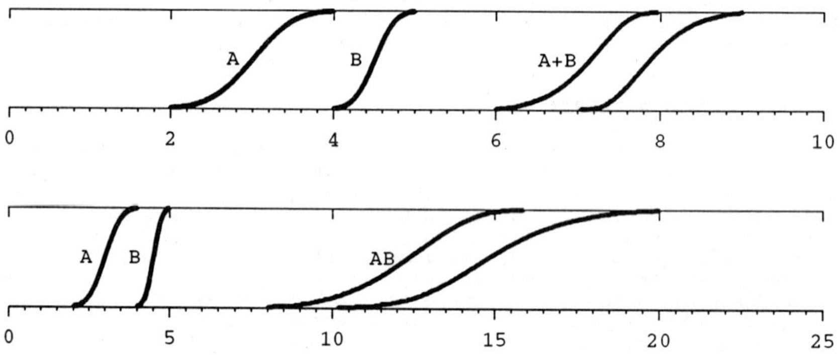

FIG. 2--Normally distributed random numbers *A* (with mean 3.0 and standard deviation 0.4) and *B* (4.5 and 0.2) shown as cumulative distributions. Dependency bounds on their sum (top panel) and product (bottom panel) are expressed as pairs of cumulative probability distributions.

The approach is extendible to other important mathematical functions as well, including minimum, maximum, exponentiation, and taking the logarithm. Bounds on the mean of a bounded distribution and even its variance and higher moments can also be computed from the numerical representation. The variance and especially higher moments can be rather variable within the bounds however, and therefore their bounds often turn out to be uninteresting.

Williamson and Downs (1990) also present a numerical method to convolve distributions when the variables are known to be independent. In this case the result is still represented by two bounding curves which are generally close together but may separate slightly when representation error affects the result. Under the assumption of independence of well defined random numbers, this separation can be made arbitrarily small by increasing the fineness of the discretization. By using the same representation scheme, their method allows calculations that assume independence and calculations that do not to be mixed together in an expression. We note that this numerical method allows more precise estimates of the convolution result than are generally possible with a Monte Carlo approach. That is, to obtain smooth curves describing the calculated distributions with a Monte Carlo approach, one must often make thousands of iterations. With Williamson and Downs' numerical approach the curves can be made arbitrarily smooth.

A NUMERICAL EXAMPLE

To illustrate the application of dependency bounds analysis and explore its differences from standard probabilistic projection, we consider the following example. McKone and Ryan (1989) parameterized a risk analysis model for human exposures to chemicals through food chains. One of the many factors in their analysis was pathway exposure factor for dioxin in the soil through dairy products ingested by human children. To estimate this factor they used the expression

$$I_k\ (I_{sc} + I_{vdc}\ K_{sp})\ f_k\ B_k$$

where I_k is intake of dairy products, I_{sc} is the ingestion rate of soil by cattle, I_{vdc} is the ingestion of pasture grasses by dairy cattle, K_{sp} is a plant/soil partition factor, f_k is the fraction of the population's dairy products that come from a contaminated area, and B_k is the biotransfer factor for cattle intake to dairy products. For these variables they used the following estimated random numbers

I_k ~ lognormal(0.000000174, 0.0000139) kg/kg·sec,
I_{sc} ~ uniform(0.00000116, 0.00000961) kg/sec,
I_{vdc} ~ uniform(0.000127, 0.000266) kg/sec,
K_{sp} ~ lognormal(0.03, 4.0),
f_k ~ constant(1.0), and
B_k ~ lognormal(1700, 260000) sec/kg.

where lognormal(*med*, *gsd*) is a lognormally distributed variable with specified median and geometric standard deviation, uniform(*m*, *M*) is a uniformly distributed random number with the specified range, and constant(*K*) is an invariant distribution of the given value.

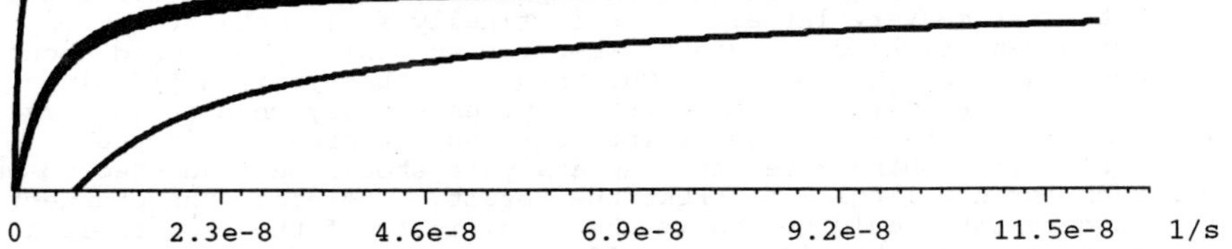

FIG. 3--Dependency bounds (outer lines) on the exposure factor surrounding a Monte Carlo estimate of the exposure factor obtained by assuming zero correlations among the variables (inner line). The abscissa is the exposure factor for dioxin in units of reciprocal seconds. The ordinate is cumulative probability.

Fig. 3 depicts the difference between a Monte Carlo estimation of the exposure factor and the dependency bounds for the quantity. Although not seen in the figure, the support of the Monte Carlo result is the same as the support of the dependency bounds because the two analyses started with the same inputs. This fact suggests that the extreme disparities between other kinds of assumptions (Sielken 1987) made in risk analyses to ensure conservativism will not arise in this context. If the Monte Carlo analysis had assumed some particular covariance structure among the variables other than independence, the resulting curve would be somewhere within the dependency bounds. In general, the range of resulting curves would not be as wide as the dependency bounds themselves, since correlation measures only linear dependencies. More complicated forms of dependency could yield results more extreme than would be possible under an assumption of linear correlation among the variables. However, the dependency bounds are fixed by the distributions of the input variables and the form of the mathematical expression that ties them together. The bounds cannot be made arbitrarily wide, unless, for instance, the calculation divides by a number that could be zero.

CONSERVATIVISM

Correlations among the many variables in a risk analysis can result in the underestimation of uncertainty about risk when using Monte Carlo methods. Since it does not seem reasonable to hold that the many physical and physiological variables involved in a toxicological risk analysis are necessarily independent of one another, and since actually measuring all the relevant correlations is a Herculean if not impossible task, the use of Monte Carlo methods can inadvertently produce estimates of risk that are overly optimistic in terms of their breadths of uncertainty. Thus, Monte Carlo methods may fail to be conservative.

In a probabilistic arithmetic based on dependency bounds analysis, one can explicitly calculate the bounds on the risk distribution, whatever dependencies there may be among the input variables. This makes this approach conservative relative to a method that encourages the assumption of independence. Just because we do not know that variates are correlated, we should not assume they are not. Of course, there are infinitely many ways that variates could fail to be independent. Correlation measures only one particular form of dependence. Thus the problem can be subtle and confounding. The dependency bounds are themselves the best possible bounds in the context of ignorance about the dependency relations.

Are results swamped by uncertainty?

Some analysts worry that a prediction will be overwhelmed by the range of the uncertainty associated with it. Since the range of uncertainty continues to grow in size through the cascade of calculations, it may often become very large. If it is finally so large as to swamp the predicted mean risk, can anything specific be finally concluded about the environmental contaminant? Our answer is that it is decidedly important to be aware of the uncertainty, especially when it is very large so as not to fool oneself into placing any credence in the 'answer'. If nothing more, such an analysis should be conducted to see how much (or how little) to trust the result. Therefore the prospect that uncertainty could overwhelm the specificity of the results is a strong reason to investigate the effect of uncertainty, not a reason to ignore it.

DRAWBACKS OF DEPENDENCY BOUNDS ANALYSIS

There are three properties of dependency bounds analysis that, if ignored, could result in confusion. One obvious drawback to its immediate adoption in risk analysis is that there is no way to draw a probability density function (pdf) that describes the answer (because, of course, there isn't just one). The result must be expressed as a pair of cumulative distributions. Any monotonic curve drawn between these bounds would correspond to a single distribution and could be differentiated to give a possible pdf, but there will generally be an infinite family of such functions between any two dependency bounds. This could be a drawback simply because analysts are accustomed to getting answers as pdfs. This is not a serious problem however, and users can easily adapt to working with cumulative distributions.

Dependency bounds analysis is not as well adapted as Monte Carlo methods are to incorporating information about the correlation structure in those cases when it is available. Although one can freely mix together variables that have unknown correlation with those that have correlation known to be zero in one dependency bounds analysis, the method cannot presently take advantage of empirical correlations that are intermediate between zero and unity. This is a disadvantage compared to Monte Carlo analysis since correlated variables can be simulated by computer in principle (although they rarely are in practice). Future methodological development may allow the method to incorporate such knowledge (Williamson and Downs 1990).

Another drawback to using dependency bounds analysis is that multiple occurrences of a single quantity in an arithmetic expression will yield answers with inflated uncertainty (larger dispersion). The expression should be simplified arithmetically before the dependency bounds analysis is applied, and multiple occurrences of a quantity should be cancelled whenever possible. For instance, consider an estimate of exposure as intake from several pathways, each of which is divided by body weight. The expression

$$I_{\text{air}}/BW \;+\; I_{\text{drinking water}}/BW \;+\; I_{\text{bathing}}/BW \;+\; I_{\text{food}}/BW$$

should be simplified to

$$(I_{\text{air}} + I_{\text{drinking water}} + I_{\text{bathing}} + I_{\text{food}}) \;/\; BW$$

before beginning the analysis. If there remain multiple occurrences of a variable in an expression that cannot be removed by arithmetic cancelling, the fact that they represent the same quantity cannot be accounted for within the analysis. The result will be a conservative approximation, and as such will at least maintain the spirit of the analysis.

The same phenomenon has not been considered a serious problem when it crops up in a step-wise Monte Carlo analysis. For instance, if body weight is used as a divisor in several terms of an expression, an appropriate analysis would use one realization of the variable for all the terms in which it is used. When the terms are estimated separately however, body weight must be simulated several times and doing so incorrectly inserts the uncertainty of body weight into the answer multiple times. The result is conservative, of course, in the sense that the uncertainty is only wider than it would have been had the multiple occurrences of body weight be reduced to a single occurrence. The problem of multiple occurrences is the focus of on-going research (e.g., Neumaier 1990) and may admit solutions or partial solutions in particular cases.

There are several other properties that dependency bounds analysis shares with the Monte Carlo approach that should also be listed as drawbacks to using the analysis. The first is that one must assume distributions have only finite supports. This means that distributions which are theoretically infinite in extent such as the normal curve, must be truncated to finite ranges. This is true for any Monte Carlo implementation as well and has never been considered a serious problem in practical risk analyses.

Secondly, although it seems clear that deconvolutions can be obtained from dependency bounds, the algorithms for computing them have not yet been published. Even if deconvolutions are not used, the estimates based on convolutions with the inverse operator will yield conservative results. That is, if a deconvolution could be found that solves the equation, it would have dispersion no greater than that of the computed difference. This means, then, that risk analysts can be assured at least that they will not underestimate the actual uncertainty and this may be sufficient for practical use.

Finally, like all methods based on probability theory, dependency bounds analysis has no completely satisfactory way to treat non-statistical uncertainty. And insofar as human perception seems to be based on a non-probabilistic schema (Kahneman et al. 1982), dependency bounds analysis will probably fail to be completely intuitive. Thus the practical social problems associated with "risk perception" and "risk communication" are likely to continue under its use. These problems may finally be solved by using yet another approach based on "possibility theory" (Dubois and Prade 1988; Duckstein et al. 1990) and the arithmetic of fuzzy numbers (Ferson and Kuhn 1992).

CONCLUSIONS

Toxicological risk analysis is at a crossroads because the traditional approach which has been widely criticized as pseudo-quantitative and hyperconservative is losing its support in the academic and regulatory communities. The methodology that replaces it should be statistically valid yet also conservative with respect to the public health. The desirability of a method depends on the answers to a variety of questions on issues including appropriateness, simplicity, data requirements, computational efficiency, conservativism, and freedom from assumptions.

Monte Carlo methods almost always are applied with an implicit assumption of independence among the variates. As a result of this assumption, the final answer can have a too narrow variance. This incorrect concentration of the probability density can cause the method to be overly optimistic about uncertainty—which ought to be an anathema to risk analysts (contra Hoerger et al. 1989). The data needed to insure that a Monte Carlo analysis is appropriately conservative can be considerable.

Probabilistic dependency bounds analysis gives conservative answers because it makes no assumption about the dependencies among variables. It therefore expresses the uncertainty in the result arising from ignorance about unmeasured correlations. It is obviously too early to make a general conclusion about the utility of dependency bounds in the practice of risk assessment, although it should be immediately useful in certain circumstances to estimate bounds when unwarranted assumptions about correlations were made out of convenience. The approach is not without it own problems, however, the most important being that multiple occurrences of a variable in an expression that cannot be cancelled algebraically will cause the dispersion in the result to be larger than it should be. In this case, however, the analysis yields answers that are still conservative with respect to uncertainty. Dependency bounds analysis computes formally what worst case analysis tried to estimate informally: a conservative bound on a calculated risk estimate.

ACKNOWLEDGEMENTS

We thank Lev Ginzburg (State University of New York at Stony Brook), Rüdiger Kuhn (Hochschule für Technik und Wirtschaft des Saarlandes), Neal Oden (Applied Biomathematics), Mark Burgman (University of Melbourne), and David Mauriello (Office of Toxic Substances, U.S. Environmental Protection Agency) for helpful discussions.

REFERENCES

Dubois, D. and Prade, H., 1988, Possibility Theory: An Approach to Computerized Processing of Uncertainty, Plenum Press, New York

Duckstein, L. Bardossy, A., Barry, T., and Bogardi, I., 1990, "Health risk assessment under uncertainty: a fuzzy-risk methodology," Risk-Based Decision Making in Water Resources, Haimes, Y.Y. and Stakhiv, E.Z., Eds., American Society of Engineers, New York.

Ferson, S. and Kuhn, R., 1992, "Propagating uncertainty in ecological risk analysis using interval and fuzzy arithmetic," Computer Techniques in Environmental Studies IV, Zannetti, P., Ed., Elsevier Applied Science, London, pp. 387-401.

Finkel, A, 1990, Confronting Uncertainty in Risk Management, Center for Risk Management, Resources for the Future, Washington, D.C.

Fishburn, P.C, 1986, "The axioms of subjective probability," Statistical Science, Vol. 1, pp. 335-358.

Frank, M.J. R.B. Nelson and B. Schweizer, 1987, "Best-possible bounds for the distribution of a sum—a problem of Kolmogorov," Probability Theory and Related Fields, Vol. 74, p. 199-211.

Frome, E.L. and Checkoway, H., 1985, "Use of poisson regression models in estimating incidence rates and ratios," American Journal of Epidemiology, Vol. 121, pp. 309-323.

Hoerger, F.D, Charm, J., Deisler, P.F., Jr., Epstein, M.L., et al., 1989, "Presentation of risk assessments of carcinogens," Report of an ad hoc study group on risk assessment presentation, American Industrial Health Council, Washington, DC.

Kahneman, D., Slovic, P., and Tversky, A., 1982, Judgement Under Uncertainty: Heuristics and Biases, Cambridge University Press, Cambridge.

Karstadt, M., 1988, "Quantitative risk assessment: qualms and questions," Teratogenesis, Carcinogenesis, and Mutagenesis, Vol. 8, pp. 137-152.

McKone, T.E. and Ryan, P.B., 1989, "Human exposures to chemicals through food chains: an uncertainty analysis," Environmental Science and Technology, Vol. 23, pp. 1154-1163.

National Wildlife Federation, 1989, "Lake Michigan sport fish: should you eat your catch?" National Wildlife Federation, Washington, DC.

Neumaier, A., 1990, Interval methods for systems of equations, Cambridge University Press, Cambridge.

Nichols, A.L. and Zeckhauser, R.J., 1988, "The perils of prudence: how conservative risk assessments distort regulation," Regulatory Toxicology and Pharmacology, Vol. 8, pp. 61-75.

Norton, S., McVey, M., Colt, J., Durda, J., and Hegner, R., 1988, Review of Ecological Risk Assessment Methods, EPA/230-10-88-041, Environmental Protection Agency, Office of Policy Analysis, Washington, D.C.

Paustenbach, D.L., 1989, "Health risk assessments: opportunities and pitfalls," Columbia Journal of Environmental Law, Vol. 14, No. 2, pp. 379-410.

Roberts, L., 1990, "Risk assessors taken to task," Science, Vol. 248, p. 1173.

Savage, L.J., 1954, The Foundations of Statistics, Wiley, New York.

Savage, L.J., 1971, "Elicitation of personal probabilities and expectations," Journal of the American Statistical Association, Vol. 66, pp. 783-801.

Sielken, R.L., Jr., 1987, "Cancer dose-response extrapolations," Environmental Science and Technology, Vol 21, No. 11, pp. 1033-1039.

Smith, A.E., Ryan, P.B., and Evans, J.S., 1992, "The effect of neglecting correlations when propagating uncertainty and estimating the population distribution of risk," Risk Analysis, Vol. 12, No. 4, pp. 467-474.

Tversky, A. and Kahneman, D., 1982, "Judgement under uncertainty: heuristics and biases," Judgement Under Uncertainty: Heuristics and Biases, Kahneman, D., Slovic, P., and Tversky, A., Eds., Cambridge University Press, Cambridge, pp. 3-20.

U.S. Environmental Protection Agency, 1987, "Risk assessment guidelines of 1986," Federal Register Vol. 51, No. 185, pp. 33992-34054, U.S. Government Printing Office, Washington, DC.

U.S. Environmental Protection Agency, 1992, "Guidelines for exposure assessment of 1986," Federal Register Vol. 57, No. 104, pp. 22888-22938, U.S. Government Printing Office, Washington, DC.

Williamson, R.C. and Downs, T., 1990, "Probabilistic arithmetic I: numerical methods for calculating convolutions and dependency bounds," International Journal of Approximate Reasoning, Vol. 4, pp. 89-158.

Paul K. Scott[1] and Kim R. Trowbridge[1]

SCREENING-LEVEL VERSUS REFINED MODELING APPROACHES TO ESTIMATING PCB CONCENTRATIONS IN AQUATIC FOOD WEBS: A CASE STUDY OF LAKE ONTARIO

REFERENCE: Scott, P. K., and Trowbridge, K. R., **"Screening-Level Versus Refined Modeling Approaches to Estimating PCB Concentrations in Aquatic Food WEBS: A Case Study of Lake Ontario,"** Environmental Toxicology and Risk Assessment - Third Volume, ASTM STP 1218, Jane S. Hughes, Gregory R. Biddinger, and Eugene Mones, Eds., American Society for Testing and Materials, Philadelphia, 1995.

ABSTRACT: The comparison of a screening-level and a refined food web bioaccumulation model in predicting tissue residues of polychlorinated biphenyls (PCBs) in the salmonid food web of Lake Ontario with measured levels is performed. A screening-level model provided health protective (i.e., conservative) estimates of bioaccumulation for invertebrate and fish species in the Lake Ontario salmonid food web with limited organism and ecosystem specific data. The refined model provided health protective estimates of PCB bioaccumulation for invertebrate and prey fish species. The modeled estimate of PCB bioaccumulation in the highest trophic level species (the salmonids) using the refined model was less conservative and underestimated the measured value. Both approaches provided estimates of PCB bioaccumulation within an order of magnitude and often within 50% of the tissue residue measured in Lake Ontario species. The screening-level model provides excellent bioaccumulation estimates with limited data quality and quantity. The refined model requires a more complete data set for use, however, provides more information regarding key factors in the bioaccumulation process for a particular food web.

KEYWORDS: bioaccumulation, Lake Ontario, PCBs, salmonids, fate and transport modeling, food web

INTRODUCTION

In environmental risk assessments, the use of chemical fate and transport models serves two primary purposes. First, comprehensive characterization of multimedia contamination at any given site is usually unfeasible and cost-prohibitive. Model estimates are therefore used to supplement the inevitable data gaps that exist in any field sampling dataset. Second, sample data from a field investigation provides only a "snapshot" of site conditions as a function of time; usually it is necessary to estimate chemical concentrations so that long-term hazards under future site conditions may be addressed. To date, chemical fate and transport modeling has played a key role in the human health risk assessment process, indeed

[1]ChemRisk®, a division of McLaren/Hart, Cleveland, OH 44122

many regulatory guidance documents have been issued describing appropriate techniques for estimating chemical concentrations at the point of human contact (e.g., via soil vapor emissions into indoor air, particulate emissions from stacks, chemical uptake into edible vegetation, chemical leaching through soil into potable water, etc.) (USEPA 1988; USEPA 1989; SCAQMD 1988). Conversely, the assessment of chemical impacts on wildlife has tended to rely more on organism collection and the analysis of tissue residues in the species of interest. However, as ecotoxicological concerns continue to take a more prominent role in risk assessments of hazardous waste sites, the use of chemical fate and transport models to assess impacts to birds, aquatic species, benthic organisms, etc. will likely increase.

It is important to note that only a few of the chemical migration models typically used in human health risk assessment have actually been verified under field conditions. This is primarily due to the difficulties and costs associated with monitoring (usually low) levels of chemicals in air, groundwater, and subsurface soil. Accordingly, there is a considerable degree of uncertainty associated with the predictions of these models. However, models that predict tissue concentrations in wildlife as a function of exposure to contaminated media provide a unique opportunity for field verification since many species of ecological interest are fairly easy to collect and analyze.

In this report we assess the relative accuracy of two food web bioaccumulation models in predicting tissue concentrations of polychlorinated biphenyls (PCBs) that have been measured in the salmonid food web of Lake Ontario. PCBs are known to be present in the surface water, sediments, and biota of Lake Ontario (Oliver and Niimi 1988). Because of the known toxic effects of PCBs in humans and aquatic species, and the high bioaccumulation potential of PCBs, the presence of PCBs in the Great Lakes salmonid food web is considered to pose serious potential ecological and human health risks. PCBs are one of the most commonly detected contaminants in Great Lakes salmonids (Humphrey 1983). Both planktonic and benthic food webs of Lake Ontario contribute to salmonid PCB bioaccumulation. The planktonic food web evaluated in this study (Figure 1) includes lake water, plankton, mysid (*Mysis relicta*), alewife (*Alosa pseudoharengus*) and smelt (*Osmerus mordax*), coho salmon (*Oncorhynchus velinus namaycush*), lake (*Salvelinus namaycush*), rainbow (*Salmo gairdneri* or *Oncorhynchus mykiss*), and brown (*Salmo trutta*) trout. The benthic food web evaluated includes water, sediment, suspended sediment. amphipod (*Pontoporeia affinis*), oligochaetes (*Tubifex tubifex* and *Limnodrilus hoffmeisteri*), sculpin (*Cottus cognatus*), and salmonids.

Several researchers have evaluated the bioaccumulation of PCBs in Great Lakes aquatic food webs using modeling and direct measurement approaches (Oliver and Niimi 1985, 1988; Barber et al. 1991; Niimi and Oliver 1983, 1988; Borgmann and Whittle 1992; Niimi 1981; Rasmussen et al. 1990; Ankley et al 1992; Oliver 1984). However, very few studies have attempted to compare bioaccumulation model predictions with actual data, or critically evaluate the appropriateness of such models for different risk assessment applications (Gobas 1992; Thomann et al 1992a, 1992b; Connolly 1991).

In this analysis, bioaccumulation of total PCBs due to surface water, sediment and food web exposure in Lake Ontario is evaluated using a screening-level (Gobas 1992) and a refined (Thomann et al. 1992) food web bioaccumulation model. The results of these two modeling approaches are compared to measured total PCB tissue residue data from the salmonid food web of Lake Ontario as reported by Oliver and Niimi (1988). The Oliver and Niimi (1988) data were chosen as a

Figure 1
Lake Ontario Food Web

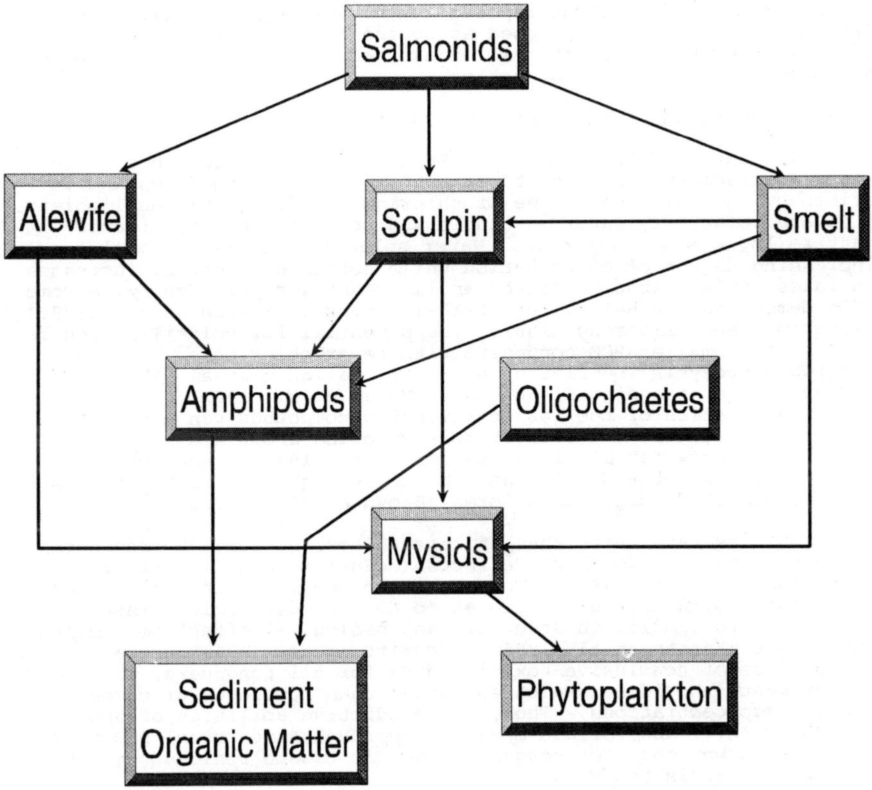

result of their complete characterization of PCB tissue residue in the Lake Ontario salmonid food web and because both modeling approaches have previously been calibrated to the Great Lakes ecosystem. The relative accuracy, sensitivity, and theoretical uncertainty associated with the predictions of both models are also evaluated. The purpose of these comparisons is to: 1) determine whether either modeling approach yields reasonable accurate estimates of measured data, and 2) assess whether the more refined modeling approach provides any significant increase in predictive ability.

METHODS

In this section, the total PCB concentrations in Lake Ontario surface water and sediment reported by Oliver and Niimi (1988) are presented. These data are used as source terms for the models. The criteria used to select the two models, and a full description of each are also presented in this section.

PCBs in Water and Sediment of Lake Ontario

The fate and transport of PCBs and their behavior in surface water and sediment dictates their availability to organisms and is driven by the relative degree of chlorination of the biphenyl moiety. PCBs are relatively water insoluble and sorb strongly to organic matter (log K_{ow}s = 4.0 - 8.5). Water solubility decreases with increasing degree of chlorination while sorption potential increases. In lakes, volatilization can be an important loss process, with some PCBs demonstrating half-lives of 10-12 hours (Callahan et al. 1979; Swackhamer and Armstrong 1986). The potential for volatilization is greater for smaller PCB congeners with fewer chlorines. PCBs can undergo photolysis (Leifler et al. 1983; Callahan et al. 1979) but do not hydrolyze at a significant rate (Mabey et al. 1982). Biotransformation of the less chlorinated compounds can occur; however, molecules with four or more chlorine atoms are considered persistent (Brown et al. 1987; Leifer et al. 1983). Anaerobic conditions allow the dechlorination of the highly chlorinated PCBs to less chlorinated, degradable forms (Brown et al. 1987).

Studies have shown that at least 18 of the 209 PCB congeners have the potential for toxic effects (McFarland and Clark 1989; Tanabe 1988; Tanabe et al. 1987). The non-ortho and mono-ortho chlorine substituted compounds are believed to be the most toxic. These compounds are similar in structure and biological effect to dioxins and furans (Kannan et al. 1988). Schmitt et al. (1985) argue that in the absence of conclusive toxicity data for all congeners, total PCB measurements should be evaluated rather than homologue or congener specific concentrations. Thus, the predictive abilities of the screening-level and refined modeling approaches for total PCB tissue residues rather than for congener-specific tissue residues will be evaluated in this study.

PCB concentrations in water and suspended sediments in Lake Ontario were reported by Oliver and Niimi (1988) for a variety of PCB congeners. They reported concentrations of PCBs from samples collected from a variety of sample matrices (surface water, sediment, and biota) in Lake Ontario over a five year period. The samples were collected from numerous sites encompassing all of Lake Ontario, and the data were collected for use in evaluating bioaccumulation modeling estimates for Lake Ontario (Gobas 1992; Thomann et al. 1992a, 1992b, Barber et al, 1991). Total PCB concentrations are used as the source terms for the two bioaccumulation models evaluated in this analysis. The arithmetic mean concentrations of total PCBs in bottom sediments and for water are 570 ng/g (dry weight) and 1 100 pg/l, respectively

(Oliver and Niimi 1988).

In addition to the reported sediment concentrations, total PCB concentrations in interstitial pore water and sediment organic carbon are also needed as source terms. For this analysis, the concentrations of total PCBs in interstitial water were estimated using a linear equilibrium partitioning approach presented by Jury et al. (1983) for saturated soils and by Connolly et al (1987) for sediments. This approach assumes that chemicals in sediment exist in two phases: aqueous, or liquid phase and a solid, or sorbed phase. The concentration of total PCBs sorbed to sediment organic carbon was estimated using an equation presented in Thomann et al. (1992a). The estimated total PCB concentration in interstitial pore water is 0.019 μg/l. The estimated total PCB concentration sorbed to sediment organic matter is 14 300 ng/g.

Bioaccumulation Model Selection

There are two levels of modeling analysis that can be used to estimate chemical concentrations in aquatic food webs. The most basic level of modeling analysis is the screening-level model, which is characterized by low data requirements and the use of conservative assumptions. Because of these characteristics screening-level models are particularly useful for initial assessments when availability of site-specific data is low. Conservative assumptions regarding parameter values and estimation methods are used to ensure that the screening-level model will consistently overestimate chemical concentrations in the organisms of interest. The screening-level model is typically used to identify whether potential hazards exist under "worst-case" assumptions and whether a more detailed assessment is necessary. The next level of sophistication is the refined model which uses a more detailed quantitative approach to estimate chemical concentrations. Most refined approaches need to be calibrated or validated for each different application in order to ensure the most accurate predictions possible.

Several models were reviewed for use as either the screening-level or refined model in this analysis. The screening level model had to meet two basic criteria. First, the approach had to have very limited site-specific data requirements for use. Next, previous applications of the model should be reasonably close to observed data, if possible overestimating the observed values by no greater than an order of magnitude. The refined model had to be biologically-based and focus on the specific exposure processes that are most important for the bioaccumulation of PCBs in the salmonid food web, specifically dietary exposures. If the refined model had been previously applied to a Great Lakes food web similar to the Lake Ontario salmonid food web, it was preferred over approaches which had not. This ensured that any parameters of the model that should be calibrated using site-specific data could be estimated with little effect on model predictions.

Selection of the screening-level model-- Two basic types of screening-level approaches exist for use in evaluating the food web bioaccumulation of PCBs. The simplest approach is to use laboratory derived bioconcentration factors (BCFs) to predict biota concentrations from surface water concentrations (Rand and Petrocelli 1985; Oliver and Niimi 1985; MacKay 1982). The second approach is to use chemical equilibrium partitioning to evaluate concentrations in lower trophic levels (phytoplankton, zooplankton, and benthic invertebrates) and a more detailed analysis for the upper trophic levels such as forage and piscivorous fish. An example of this type of approach is the model presented by Gobas (1992). BCFs of the PCB congeners range from 26 000 to 660 000 and increase with increasing degree of chlorination (Leifer et al. 1983). However, it is known that laboratory-derived BCFs consistently underestimate PCB levels in the salmonids by a factor of at least five and often as much as an order of magnitude (Oliver and Niimi 1985; 1988). This is because consumption of contaminated food, which is not accounted for in laboratory studies of bioconcentration, is apparently the major source of fish exposure to PCBs (Oliver and Niimi 1985). Accordingly, any screening-level model used to estimate PCB bioaccumulation should consider dietary exposures. The model developed by Gobas (1992) considers dietary exposure and thus was used in this evaluation.

Selection of the refined model-- Several refined models exist for estimating food web bioaccumulation (Connolly 1991; Connolly et al. 1987; Connolly and Tonelli 1985; Barber et al. 1991; Thomann et al. 1992a, 1992b; Thomann 1981, 1989; Thomann and Connolly 1984; Borgmann and Whittle 1992). However, most approaches focus exclusively on upper trophic levels (e.g., forage and piscivorous fish) (Barber et al. 1991; Borgmann and Whittle 1992). Also, many of the approaches are identical or simple refinements of one another (Connolly 1991; Connolly et al. 1987; Connolly and Tonelli 1985; Thomann et al. 1992a, 1992b; Thomann 1981; 1989, Thomann and Connolly 1984). Since the accuracy of model predictions is dependent on the accuracy of the input parameters used, a model that has been either designed or previously used to quantify chemical levels in a Great Lakes food web was preferred for this analysis. The Food and Gill Exchange of Toxic Substances model (FGETS) (Barber et al. 1988; 1991) was not used here because it considers only exposures to fish. Use of FGETS would require use of additional methods to estimate concentrations in zooplankton and benthic invertebrates. Of the models reviewed, the approach of Thomann et al. (1992a, 1992b) was used in this evaluation because it utilized refined approaches for all food web compartments and had originally been designed for a Great Lakes food web (Thomann and Connolly 1984). Also, the Thomann et al. approach has been calibrated for a more simplified version of the Lake Ontario food web which included sediment interactions (Thomann et al. 1992b).

Screening-level Modeling Approach

The Gobas (1992) food web bioaccumulation model is made up of five major compartments: phytoplankton, zooplankton, benthic organisms, forage fish, and piscivorous fish. Chemical concentrations in the phytoplankton, zooplankton, and benthic organism compartments are estimated using chemical equilibrium partitioning from water and sediment to biota, while concentrations in the forage fish and piscivorous fish compartments are estimated using mass-transfer coefficients that characterize organism uptake of water, ingestion of lower trophic levels, excretion, and growth. For this evaluation, each organism of interest in the salmonid food chain was placed in the appropriate compartment and concentrations for each were estimated, as described below.

Phytoplankton and Zooplankton compartments-- Various studies have shown that the uptake and bioaccumulation of chemicals in phytoplankton are largely controlled by chemical exchange between the organism and the water (Geyer et al. 1984; Mallhot 1987; Gobas et al. 1991). Due to their small size and large area/volume ratio, the uptake and bioaccumulation of organic chemicals in zooplankton are also predominantly due to chemical exchange between the organism and the water (Clayton et al. 1977). Since lipids are usually the predominant site for bioaccumulation of hydrophobic substances, the chemical concentration can be satisfactorily approximated by using a function of the chemical octanol-water partition coefficient, K_{ow}:

$$C_{A,Z} = L_{A,Z} * K_{ow} * C_w \tag{1}$$

where:

$C_{A,Z}$ = Concentration of PCB in phytoplankton or zooplankton (μg/kg wet);
C_w = Concentration of PCB in water (μg/l);
$L_{A,Z}$ = Lipid content of phytoplankton or zooplankton;
K_{ow} = Octanol-water partition coefficient (ml/g).

Benthic Compartment-- Two species of benthic invertebrates were evaluated for the benthic compartment: amphipods (*Pontoporeia affinis*) and oligochaetes (*Tubifex tubifex*). The approach used in the Gobas (1992) model to estimate chemical concentrations was applied to both species, but using different species-specific parameter values. This screening-level food web model views the uptake and bioaccumulation of organic chemicals in benthic organisms as the result of an equilibrium partitioning of the chemical between the lipids of the organism, the organic carbon fraction of the sediment, and the interstitial water (Shea 1988; Gobas et al. 1989b). The equation for the concentration of total PCBs in benthic organisms is:

$$C_B = \frac{L_B * d_{oc} * C_s}{d_l * X_{oc}} \tag{2}$$

where:

C_B = Concentration of PCBs in the benthic organism (μg/kg wet);
C_s = Concentration of PCBs in the bottom sediments (μg/kg dry);
L_B = Lipid fraction of the benthic organism (kg lipid/kg organism);
d_l = Density of lipids in the benthic organism (kg/l);
d_{oc} = Density of organic carbon in sediments (kg/l);
X_{oc} = Fraction of organic carbon in sediment (kg oc/kg sediment).

The values used for the phytoplankton, zooplankton, and benthic organism compartments (Table 1) are those used by Gobas in his application of the model to a similar Lake Ontario food web (Gobas 1992).

TABLE 1 -- Model parameters used in the screening-level model for phytoplankton, zooplankton, and benthic organisms[a]

Parameter	Value
Lipid content of phytoplankton (%):	0.5
Lipid content of zooplankton (%):	5.0
Total PCB octanol-water partition coefficient, K_{ow} (ml/g):	4.0 x 10^{-6}
Sediment organic carbon fraction (%):	2.0
Density of organic carbon (kg/l):	0.9
lipid density of benthic organisms (kg/l):	0.9
Lipid content of amphipods (%):	3.0
Lipid content of oligochaetes (%):	1.0

[a] - All values from Gobas (1992)

Forage and Piscivorous Fish compartments-- Fish adsorb chemicals directly from water via gill exchange and through the consumption of food (Bruggeman et al. 1981). Chemical loss or elimination can occur via the gills to water, via egestion of fecal matter or as the result of metabolic transformation (Gobas 1992). Also, fish growth can have a considerable effect on the bioaccumulation of hydrophobic chemicals in fish, particularly for chemicals with high log K_{ow}s (Thomann and Connolly 1984; Clark et al. 1990). The following steady-state equation for the concentration of PCBs in forage and piscivorous fish utilizes rate constants to account for the various uptake and loss processes:

$$C_F = \left(\frac{k_1}{k_2 + k_E + k_M + k_G}\right) * C_w + \left(\frac{k_D}{k_2 + k_E + k_M + k_G}\right) * C_D \qquad (3)$$

where:
C_F = Concentration of PCBs in forage fish (μg/kg wet);
C_w = Concentration of PCBs in overlying water (μg/kg wet);
C_D = Concentration of PCBs in diet (μg/kg wet);
k_1 = Gill uptake coefficient (l/kg-day);
k_2 = Gill elimination coefficient (day^{-1});
k_E = Fecal egestion elimination coefficient (day^{-1});
k_M = Metabolic transformation coefficient (day^{-1});
k_G = Fish growth rate coefficient (day^{-1});
k_D = Chemical uptake from food coefficient (day^{-1}).

This equation was used to estimate total PCB levels for the salmonids and the three primary forage fish in the food web: the smelt, the sculpin, and the alewife (Oliver and Niimi 1988). These parameter values (Table 2) are the same values that were used by Gobas (1992) in his application of the model to a similar Lake Ontario food web.

The mass-transfer coefficient values used for the sculpin, alewife, smelt, and salmonids were estimated using methods presented in Gobas (1992) (Table 2). These methods are based on empirical relationships between organism weight, organism lipid content, and diet percentage of the prey items for each of the forage and piscivorous fish (Gobas 1992). However, since there are few models or methods which can be used to estimate the metabolic transfer coefficient for organic substances in fish or other organisms, it was conservatively assumed for this analysis that no PCBs were lost due to metabolic transformation, i.e. $k_M = 0$. This assumption is consistent with past applications of the model (Gobas 1992).

Refined Modeling Approach

In Thomann et al. (1992a, 1992b) a five compartment model is presented which models bioaccumulation from surface water and sediments in a basic aquatic food web consisting of phytoplankton, zooplankton, benthic organisms, forage fish, and piscivorous fish. This modeling approach avoids the use of simple chemical equilibrium relationships to determine the concentrations of PCBs in zooplankton and benthic organisms. Concentrations for all members of the food web except phytoplankton are assumed to come from both direct exposure to PCBs dissolved in water and/or sorbed to sediment and from indirect exposures through the ingestion of PCBs accumulated in prey. For this evaluation the zooplankton compartment consists solely of mysids, the benthic compartment consists of both amphipods and oligochaetes, the forage fish compartment consists of sculpin, alewife, and smelt, and the piscivorous fish compartment consists of the salmonids such as coho salmon, lake trout, rainbow trout, and brown trout.

TABLE 2 -- Model parameters and estimated mass-transfer coefficients used in the screening-level model for the forage and piscivorous fish[a]

Parameter or Coefficient	Sculpin	Alewife	Smelt	Salmonid
Weight (g):	5.4	32	16	2 150
Lipid Content (%):	8.0	7.0	4.0	16
Diet				
%zooplankton:	18	60	54	---
%amphipods:	82	40	21	---
%sculpin:	---	---	25	10
%alewife:	---	---	---	50
%smelt:	---	---	---	40
Gill Uptake Rate, k_1 (L/kg-day):	1.8×10^{-6}	8.8×10^{-7}	1.2×10^{-6}	1.6×10^{-7}
Gill Elimination Rate, k_2 (day^{-1}):	2.2×10^{-3}	1.3×10^{-3}	2.9×10^{-3}	4.1×10^{-4}
Dietary Uptake Rate, k_D (kg/kg-day):	3.6×10^{-2}	2.8×10^{-2}	3.1×10^{-2}	1.5×10^{-7}
Excretion Rate, k_E (day^{-1}):	7.2×10^{-3}	5.5×10^{-3}	6.2×10^{-3}	3.0×10^{-3}
Metabolism Rate, k_M (day^{-1}):	0	0	0	0
Growth Rate, k_G (day^{-1}):	4.7×10^{-3}	3.3×10^{-3}	3.8×10^{-3}	1.4×10^{-3}

a - All parameter values from Gobas (1992) or estimated using methods in Gobas (1992)

--- - Parameter not applicable to compartment

The refined model evaluate chemical concentrations on a lipid basis rather than a wet weight basis for the various compartments of the salmonid food web. In order to allow for comparison of the refined model with the screening-level model and the Oliver and Niimi (1988) data, total PCB concentrations in each compartment reported on a lipid basis (ng PCB/ g lipid) were converted to a wet-weight basis (ng PCB/ g wet) using the following equation:

$$C_i = V_i * L_i \quad \textbf{(4)}$$

where:

C_i = Concentration of PCBs in the ith organism on wet-weight basis (ng/g wet);

V_i = Concentration of PCBs in the ith organism on a lipid basis (ng/g lipid);

L_i = Fraction of lipids in ith organism (kg lipid/kg wet).

The equations for estimating total PCB concentrations in all compartments except for phytoplankton are presented on a lipid weight basis. However, since the measured and screening-level estimated concentrations are presented on a wet-weight basis, the results of the refined model are also presented on a wet-weight basis.

General Model Equation-- The accumulation of PCBs by the various members of the food web can be characterized by the following equation (Connolly 1991; Thomann and Connolly 1984; Thomann et al. 1992a, 1992b):

$$V_i = \frac{(k_{ui} * C_w) + \sum (p_{ij} * \alpha * I_{ij} * V_j)}{K_i + G_i} \quad (5)$$

where:

V_i = Concentration of PCBs in the ith organism on a lipid basis (ng/g lipid);

k_{ui} = Chemical uptake rate across the gill for the ith organism (L/g-day);

C_w = Concentration of PCBs in overlying water (μg/L);

p_{ij} = Percentage of the ith organism's diet consisting of the jth organism;

α = Chemical assimilation efficiency;

I_{ij} = The ingestion rate of the ith organism on the jth organism (g/g-day);

V_j = Concentration of PCBs in the jth organism on a lipid basis (ng/g lipid);

K_i = Chemical excretion rate constant for the ith organism (day^{-1});

G_i = Growth rate constant for the ith organism (day^{-1}).

The first term in the numerator of the equation ($k_{ui}*C_w$) represents the direct uptake of PCBs by the organism from water. The second term of the equation (Σ ($p_{ij}*\alpha*I_{ij}*V_j$)) represents the contribution of diet to PCB body burden. The two terms in the denominator, excretion (K_i) and growth rate (G_i), represent the major loss or dilution pathways for PCBs. The major inputs to this equation are the concentrations of PCBs dissolved in Lake Ontario waters. However, for the benthic organism exposures to PCBs dissolved in interstitial pore water and sorbed to sediment organic matter are also considered. The concentration of PCBs in phytoplankton are estimated for the refined approach using the same relationship described for the screening-level approach. The concentrations for all other compartments of the food web were estimated using the preceding equation. All of the parameters in the general equation were estimated for each organism in the food web using the physiologically based relationships presented by Thomann et al (1992a, 1992b) and Connolly (1991). The estimates for each of these parameters are presented in Tables 3 and 4.

Phytoplankton compartment-- As stated earlier, various studies have shown that uptake and bioaccumulation of chemicals in phytoplankton are largely controlled by chemical exchange between the organism and the water (Geyer et al. 1984; Malhot 1987; Gobas 1991). Because of these results the same approach that was used in the screening-level approach to estimate total PCB concentrations in phytoplankton was used for the refined approach. In order to estimate the ingestion rate of phytoplankton for higher trophic levels of the food web, the wet-dry ratio of phytoplankton must be determined. A value of 10 was used for phytoplankton (Thomann et al. 1992a, 1992b).

Zooplankton compartment-- Bioaccumulation of PCBs in zooplankton is due to either direct exposure to water or from the ingestion of exposed phytoplankton. Thus, PCB levels in zooplankton can be characterized by the following equation:

$$V_z = \frac{(k_{uz} * C_w) + (\alpha * I_{za} * V_a)}{K_z + G_z} \tag{6}$$

Wherever applicable the same parameter values that were used for the screening-level model were used for the refined model (Table 3).

Benthic compartment-- Benthic organisms in Lake Ontario are directly exposed to PCBs in the overlying water and in the sediment interstitial pore water as well as indirectly via the ingestion of PCBs in sediment organic matter and in phytoplankton. The PCB body burden in amphipods and oligochaetes inhabiting Lake Ontario sediments can be related to sediment and phytoplankton PCB levels by the following equation (Thomann et al. 1992a, 1992b):

$$V_b = \frac{[k_{ub} * (b_{bs} * C_{iw} + b_{bw} * C_w)] + [(p_{bs} * \alpha * I_{bs} * r_s) + (p_{ba} * \alpha * I_{ba} * V_a)]}{K_b + G_b} \tag{7}$$

The terms b_{bs} and b_{bw} represent the fraction of exposure the benthic organism has to either interstitial pore water (C_{iw}) or the overlying lake water (C_w). Because the amphipods and oligochaetes are known to spend most of their time buried in sediments (Wetzel, 1983), both the amphipods and the oligochaetes were assumed to spend 100% of their time exposed to interstitial water. Also, the diets of both amphipods and oligochaetes consisted entirely (100%) of sediment organic matter (Thomann et al. 1992b), and phytoplankton ingestion was, therefore, not evaluated.

TABLE 3 -- Model parameters used in the refined model for the phytoplankton, zooplankton, and benthic organism compartments

Parameter	Phyto plankton	Zoo plankton	Amphipod	Oligochaete
Weight (g)[a]:	---	0.01	0.002	0.002
Lipid content (%)[a]:	0.5	5.0	3.0	3.0
Wet-dry ratio[b]:	10	5	7	7
Food assimilation efficiency[b]:	---	0.3	0.2	0.2
Gill uptake rate (l/kg-day)[c]:	---	0.0078	0.013	0.038
Excretion rate (day^{-1})[c]:	---	0.0056	0.012	0.035
Growth rate (day^{-1})[c]:	---	0.0041	0.0056	0.0056
PCB assimilation efficiency (g/g)[b]:	---	0.7	0.7	0.7
Consumption rate (g/g-day)[c]				
phytoplankton:	---	0.023	---	---
sediment:	---	---	0.14	0.14

[a] - Value same as that used for screening-level model (Gobas 1992)

[b] - Value same as one used by Thomann et al. (1991)
[c] - Value calculated using estimation methods presented in Thomann et al. (1991)
--- - Parameter not applicable to compartment

Forage and Piscivorous Fish compartment-- The body burden of PCBs in the forage fish (sculpin, alewife, and smelt) and piscivorous fish (salmonids) inhabiting Lake Ontario are due to exposure from water and from the ingestion of exposed prey (zooplankton or amphipods). The equations used to estimate PCB concentrations for each of the four fish are similar yet because of differences in diet they vary slightly. The following equations were used to estimate total PCB concentrations in the various fish:

For sculpins:

$$V_{sc} = \frac{(k_{usc} * C_w) + (p_{scb} * \alpha * I_{scb} * V_b) + (p_{scz} * \alpha * I_{scz} * V_z)}{K_{sc} + G_{sc}} \tag{8}$$

For alewife:

$$V_{al} = \frac{(k_{ual} * C_w) + (p_{alb} * \alpha * I_{alb} * V_b) + (p_{alz} * \alpha * I_{alz} * V_z)}{K_{al} + G_{al}} \tag{9}$$

For smelt:

$$V_{sm} = \frac{(k_{usm} * C_w) + (p_{smb} * \alpha * I_{smb} * V_b) + (p_{smz} * \alpha * I_{smz} * V_z) + (p_{smsc} * \alpha * I_{smsc} * V_{sc})}{K_{sm} + G_{sm}} \tag{10}$$

For salmonids:

$$V_{sal} = \frac{(k_{usal} * C_w) + (p_{salsc} * \alpha * I_{salsc} * V_{sc}) + (p_{salal} * \alpha * I_{salal} * V_{al}) + (p_{salsm} * \alpha * I_{salsm} * V_{sm})}{K_{sal} + G_{sal}} \tag{11}$$

Similarly to the phytoplankton, zooplankton, and benthic organism compartments, all of the applicable parameter values that were used for the screening-level model were used in the refined model (Table 4).

RESULTS

The results of the screening-level and refined models were compared to measured total PCB tissue residues in each organism (Table 5). Overall, the screening-level estimates for total PCBs tissue residues are very close to measured concentrations. The estimates for the benthic, forage fish, and salmonids are only slightly overestimated and, in the case of the alewife, the predicted concentrations are equal to the measured concentrations. A model is typically considered accurate if the ratios of the estimated value to the observed value are between 0.5 and 2 (Cox 1988). For the screening-level model these ratios range from 0.4 to 1.6 with a ratio of 1.2 for the salmonids (Figure 2). This indicates that the screening-level model can give fairly accurate results compared to the amount of data that are needed to calculate them. With estimated-observed ratios ranging from 0.4 to 2.6, the refined model estimates were consistent with the screening-level model (Figure 2). For the forage and piscivorous fish the ratios ranged from 0.9 for salmonids to 1.7 for smelt. The only estimate with a ratio greater than 2 was that for the oligochaetes. This overestimation is most likely due to the use of compartment-specific rather than species-specific values for weight, wet-dry ratio, and food assimilation efficiency.

TABLE 4 -- Model parameters used in the refined model for the forage and piscivorous fish compartments

Parameter	Sculpin	Alewife	Smelt	Salmonids
Weight (g)[a]:	5.4	32	16	2 150
Lipid content (%)[a]:	8.0	7.0	4.0	16
Wet-dry ratio[b]:	4	4	4	4
Food assimilation efficiency[b]:	0.8	0.8	0.8	0.8
Gill uptake rate (l/kg-d)[c]:	0.0017	0.0011	0.0025	0.00023
Excretion rate (day^{-1})[c]:	0.0021	0.0014	0.0025	0.00047
Growth rate (day^{-1})[c]:	0.0017	0.00081	0.00093	0.00035
PCB assimilation efficiency (g/g)[b]:	0.7	0.7	0.7	0.7
Consumption rate (g/g-day)[c]				
zooplankton:	0.0097	0.0068	0.016	---
amphipods:	0.008	0.0057	0.013	---
sculpin:	---	---	0.0025	0.0019
alewife:	---	---	---	0.0019
smelts:	---	---	---	0.001
Percent of diet[a]				
zooplankton:	18	60	54	---
amphipods:	82	40	21	---
sculpin:	---	---	25	10
alewife:	---	---	---	50
smelts:	---	---	---	40

a - Value same as that used for screening-level model (Gobas 1992)
b - Value same as one used by Thomann et al. (1991)
c - Value calculated using estimation methods presented in Thomann et al. (1991)
--- - Parameter not applicable to compartment

To properly compare the results of the two modeling approaches to one another, a necessary first step to understanding how changes in the parameterization of the model affect the estimated concentrations of PCBs in the salmonids is to identify the food web compartment that has the greatest influence on salmonid PCB concentrations. For this evaluation, a simplistic sensitivity analysis of concentration effects was performed by doubling the concentrations of each input (sediment and water) and compartment (phytoplankton, mysids, amphipods, etc.) in turn and observing the resultant change in estimated salmonid concentration. Also, the relative contributions of PCBs from water and from each salmonid prey item (sculpin, alewife, and smelt) were calculated to evaluate the contribution of each exposure route to the overall total PCB body burden in the salmonids. Both of these analyses were performed for the screening-level and refined modeling approaches.

TABLE 5 -- Comparison of estimated total PCB concentrations in each organism of the Lake Ontario salmonid food web with observed concentrations

Organism	Concentrations (ng/g wet) Observed Values[a]	Screening-level Model Estimates	Refined Model Estimates
Phytoplankton	50	22	22
Mysids	330	220	360
Amphipods	790	860	560
Oligochaetes	180	290	480
Sculpin	1 600	1 890	2 400
Alewife	1 300	1 300	1 650
Smelt	1 010	1 850	1 740
Salmonids	4 300	5 210	3 970

[a] - Reported by Oliver and Niimi (1988)

Concentration Changes

To characterize how changes in concentration of the water and sediment inputs and lower compartments affect estimated salmonid PCB levels for each model, a simple sensitivity analysis was performed by doubling the concentrations of each compartment in turn and observing the resultant change in estimated salmonid concentration (USEPA 1992). By identifying how changes in concentration in a lower compartment affect salmonid PCB concentrations, a more detailed sensitivity analysis of the parameters of that compartment can then be performed to determine the exact parameters (weight, lipid content, etc.) to which the model is most sensitive. For example, the total PCB sediment concentration was doubled, and the new salmonid concentrations for both the screening-level and refined model were recorded and compared to the original estimate. The original total PCB concentrations for the screening-level and refined models were 5 210 and 3 970 ng/g wet, respectively. The resulting new PCB concentrations for these two models were 9 070 and 5 850 respectively. In other words, doubling the sediment concentration changed the predicted salmonid total PCB concentration for the screening-level model by a factor of 1.79 and for the refined model by a factor of 1.48. As a point of comparison, if doubling sediment concentration had no effect the factor would be 1; if sediment and salmonid concentrations were linearly related the factor would be 2.

Each input (water and sediment) and food web compartment concentration except for oligochaetes was doubled and the relative change in salmonid concentration for each is presented (Figure 3). For the screening-level model, the doubling of the total PCB concentration in sediment and amphipods had the greatest effect on salmonid concentration. The doubling of the levels in these compartments increased levels in the salmonid compartment by a factor of 1.79. Concentration changes in water and mysid compartments had

Figure 2
Comparison of Estimated Total PCB Levels in Each Food Web Compartment with Observed Levels in Lake Ontario as Reported by Oliver and Niimi (1988)

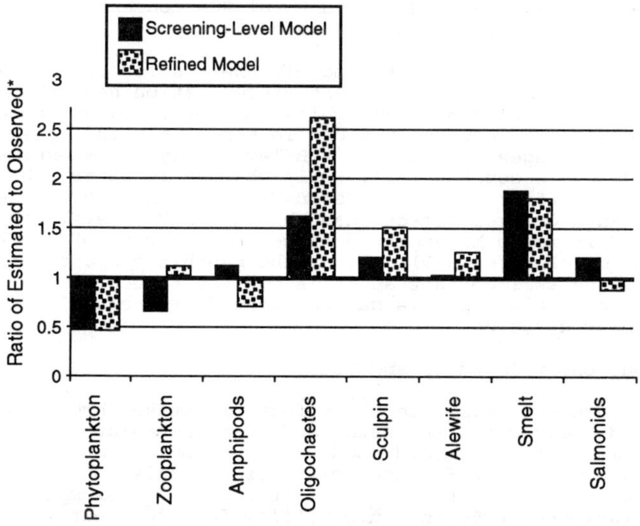

* The ratio of estimated to observed concentration is equal to [model estimate / observed value]

Figure 3
The Effect of Concentration Changes in Each Organism of the Lake Ontario Food Web on the Salmonid Total PCB Concentrations Estimated by Both the Screening-Level and Refined Model

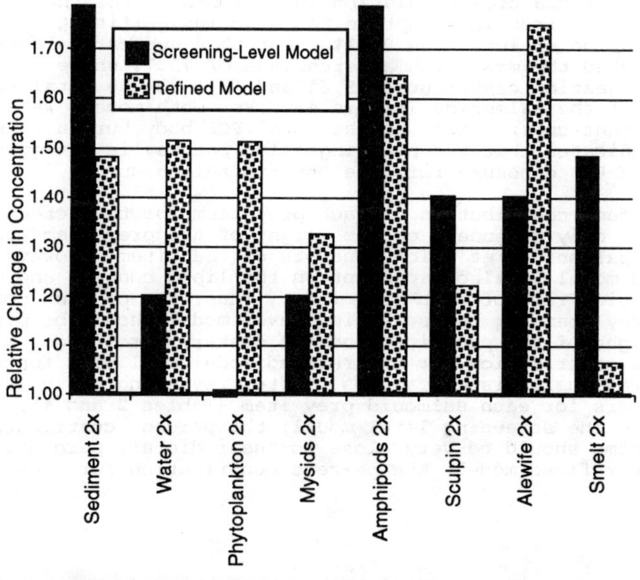

the least effect on PCB levels in salmonids; doubling caused a change of only a factor of 1.2. For the refined model, the doubling of PCB levels in the alewife had the greatest effect on salmonid PCB levels causing them to increase by a factor of 1.74. Changes in amphipod levels had the next highest effect causing an increase in salmonid levels of 1.66. Changes in smelt and sculpin PCB levels had the least effect on the estimated salmonid total PCB concentration causing increases of only 1.07 and 1.23 respectively.

For the screening-level model, the results of this analysis indicate that changes in sediment concentration have the greatest effect on salmonid PCB levels while changes in water concentration have the smallest effect on those levels. This indicates that for this model changes in sediment PCB levels may alter estimates of salmonid levels substantially while changes in water PCB levels will have little effect. For the refined model, changes in alewife PCB levels had a greater effect than changes in PCB levels in sculpin and smelt. This is to be expected since the majority of the salmonid diet consists of alewife (50%). Also, the benthic compartment of this model may be as important as it is for the screening-level model since changes in amphipod levels had the second greatest effect on salmonid tissue concentration.

<u>Contributions from Water and Diet</u>

In order to evaluate the effect of uptake through gill exchange of PCBs dissolved in lake water and PCBs accumulated in the primary prey items of the salmonid food web, the concentrations of PCBs in water, sculpin, alewife, and smelt were "toggled on" individually and all other concentrations were set at zero. For example, the concentration of PCBs in sculpin, alewife, and smelt were set at zero for each modeling approach and only the concentration of total PCBs in salmonids due to uptake of water was evaluated. This process was continued for each prey item in turn and the resulting total PCB salmonid body burdens were recorded.

For the screening level model, the uptake of water contributed less than 0.01% to the estimated total PCB body burden of the salmonids while sculpin, alewife, and smelt contributed 11.9%, 41.3%, and 46.8% respectively (Figure 4). Obviously for this model, gill exchange of PCBs dissolved in water is an insignificant exposure pathway for PCB bioaccumulation in salmonids. For the refined model, contribution from water uptake was also insignificant with a percent contribution of less than 0.01%. For this approach alewife ingestion contributed the most with a percentage of 73.7% while sculpin and smelt ingestion contributed 19.6% and 6.7% to the total PCB body burden of the salmonids (Figure 4). For both models water made no significant contribution to the total PCB body burden in salmonids. This indicates that the prey ingestion pathway is the most important route of PCB exposure for Lake Ontario salmonids.

The percent contribution of each prey item for the screening level model is only dependent on the weight of the prey item and the percent of the salmonid diet which consists of that item. However, the refined model is also dependent on the lipid content and salmonid consumption rate of each prey item. Thus, the percent contribution of each prey item for the screening level model should be proportional to the weight of the prey item and its dietary percentage, while the percent contribution for the refined model will be a function of the four previously listed factors. After reviewing the values for these parameters for each salmonid prey item (Tables 2 and 4), it is clear that for the screening level model, the percent contribution for all prey items should be very close to their dietary percentages, while for the refined model, the percent contribution for alewife should be

Figure 4
Percent Contribution of Each Prey Item on the Estimated Salmonid Toyal PCB Body Burden

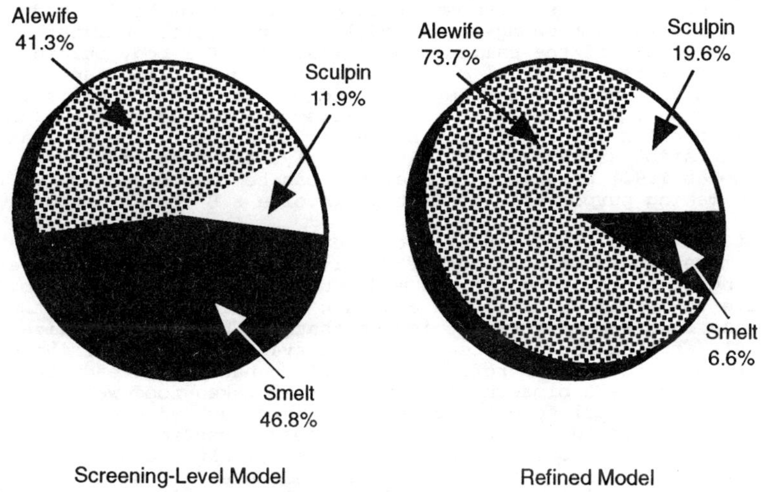

much greater than the percent contributions for sculpin and smelt.

DISCUSSION

One of the primary purposes of this evaluation was to evaluate whether the predictions of screening-level models were accurate enough for use in initial assessments of ecological risk. In this analysis, the estimated total PCB levels in the various compartments of the Lake Ontario salmonid food web using the screening-level model are very close to the measured levels reported by Oliver and Niimi (1988). Accordingly, while the screening-level model does not provide the level of detail the refined model does, it still gives quality information about the bioaccumulation potential in a food web of interest. For example, the refined model identifies salmonid ingestion of alewife as the most critical contributor to PCB body burden, while the screening-level model does not differentiate the importance of any of the salmonid prey items for PCB body burden. However, the screening-level model does indicate the importance of diet over direct uptake of PCBs dissolved in water as the primary source of PCBs for salmonids. Considering how little food web and chemical specific information is needed by this model, the estimates of concentration are excellent. Accordingly, the screening-level model (Gobas 1992) used in this analysis can be considered useful for decision making purposes in areas that involve PCB contamination.

Of additional importance in this evaluation was whether the refined model would be more cost-effective than comprehensive direct monitoring of biota. The refined model data requirements are too extensive to make it a desirable approach for initial assessments unless the food web of interest is one that has been characterized previously at a different site. For this evaluation it would have been difficult to use the refined model if it had not already been used to evaluate PCB bioaccumulation in Great Lakes food webs. If organism and chemical specific data parameters such as chemical assimilation efficiency, wet-dry ratios, food ingestion efficiency, and weights for the lower trophic levels (zooplankton and benthic invertebrates) are not readily available in the existing literature, model predictions will have a high degree of uncertainty. This is also why it is important to calibrate the model with measured biota data when using this model for detailed assessments of ecological risk. Since the data required for the appropriate use of the refined model are high and the accuracy of its estimates is not significantly greater than that of the screening-level model, this model is recommended primarily for use in more detailed ecological risk assessments. The refined model is appropriate for addressing specific questions regarding the contributors to higher trophic level bioaccumulation and for making predictions regarding future risks of bioaccumulation in a particular food web.

REFERENCES

Ankley, G.T., P.M. Cook, A.R. Carlson, D.J. Call, J.A. Swenson, H.F. Corcoran, and R.A. Hoke., 1992, "Bioaccumulation of PCBs from Sediments by Oligochaetes and Fishes: Comparison of Laboratory and Field Studies," Canadian Journal of Fishery and Aquatic Science, 49:2080-2085.

Barber, M.C., L.A. Suarez, R.R. Lassiter, 1991, "Modelling bioaccumulation of organic pollutants in fish with an application to PCBs in Lake Ontario salmonids," Canadian Journal of Fishery and Aquatic Science, 48:318-337.

Borgmann, U., and D.M. Whittle, 1992, "Bioenergetics and PCB, DDE, and Mercury Dynamics in Lake Ontario Lake Trout (*Salvelinus namaycush*): A Model based on Surveillance Data," Canadian Journal of Fishery and Aquatic Science, 49:1086-1096.

Bruggeman, W.A., L.B.J.M. Matron, D. Kooiman and O. Huntzinger, 1981, "Accumulation and Elimination Kinetics of Di-, Tri-, and Tetra Chlorobiphenyls by Goldfish after Dietary and Aqueous Exposure," Chemosphere, 10:811-832

Brown, J.F., Jr., B.L. Bedard, M.J. Brennan, J.C. Carnahan, H. Feng, and R.E. Wagner, 1987, "Polychlorinated Biphenyl Dechlorination in Aquatic Sediments," Science, 236:709-712.

Callahan, M.A., M.W. Slimak, N.W. Gabel, I.P. May, C.F. Fowler, J.R. Freed, P. Jennings, R.L. Durfee, F.C. Whitmore, B. Maestri, W.R. Mabey, B.R. Holt, and C. Gould, 1979, "Water-Related Environmental Fate of 129 Priority Pollutants, Vol. I," U.S. Environmental Protection Agency, Office of Water Planning and Standards, Washington, D.C. EPA-440/4-79-029a.

Clark, K.E., F.A.P.C. Gobas, and D. Mackay, 1990, "Model of Organic Chemical Uptake and Clearance by Fish from Food and Water," Environmental Science and Technology, 24: 1203-1213.

Clayton, J.R., S.P. Pavlou, and N.F. Breitner, 1977, "Polychlorinated Biphenyls in Coastal Marine Zooplankton," Environmental Science and Technology 18: 676-682.

Connolly, J.P., 1991, "Application of a Food Chain Model to Polychlorinated Biphenyl Contamination of the Lobster and Winter Flounder Food Chains in New Bedford Harbor," Environmental Science and Technology 25:760-770.

Connolly, J.P., and R. Tonelli, 1985, "Modelling Kepone in the Striped Bass Food Chain of the James River Estuary," Estuarine, Coastal Shelf Science, 20: 349-366.

Connolly, J.P., D.M. DiToro, C.J. Pedersen, and J.R. Newton, 1987, "A Model of PCB in the Water, Bed, and Food Chain of Lake Ontario," USEPA report, Region V, Chicago, IL, part of the International Joint Commission Task Force on Chemical Loading.

Cox, W.M., 1988, "Protocol for Determining the Best Performing Model," U.S. Environmental Protection Agency (USEPA) Report, August.

Geyer, H., G. Politizki, and D. Freitag, 1984, "Prediction of Ecotoxicological Behaviour of Chemicals: Relationship Between n-Octanol-Water Partition Coefficient and Bioaccumulation of Organic Chemicals by Alga Chlorella," Chemosphere, 13: 269-284.

Gobas, F.A.P.C., 1992, "Modeling the Accumulation and Toxicity of Organic Chemicals in Aquatic Food Chains," Chemical Dynamics in Fresh Water Ecosystems, edited by F.A.P.C. Gobas and J.A. McCorquodale, Lewis Publishers, Ann Arbor, MI.

Gobas, F.A.P.C. and D. Mackay, 1987, "Dynamics of Hydrophobic Organic Chemical Bioconcentration in Fish," Environmental Toxicology and Chemistry, 6: 495-504.

Gobas, F.A.P.C., D.C. Bedard, J.J.H. Ciborowski and G.D. Haffner, 1989, "Bioaccumulation of Chlorinated Hydrocarbons by the Mayfly *Hexagenia Limbata* in Lake St. Clair," Journal of Great Lakes Research, 15: 581-588.

Humphrey, H.E.B., 1983, "Evaluation of Humans Exposed to Water Borne Chemicals in the Great lakes. Final Report to the Environmental Protection Agency," Cooperative Agreement CR-807192. USEPA, Washington, D.C.

Jury, W.A., Spencer, W.F. and Farmer, W.J, 1983, "Behavior assessment model for trace organics in soil: I. model description," Journal of Environmental Quality, 12(4):558-564.

Kannan, N., S. Tanabe, R. Tatsukawa, 1988, "Potentially hazardous residues of non-orthochlorine substituted coplanar PCBs in human adipose tissue," Archives of Environmental Health, 43:11-14.

Leifer, A., R.H. Brink, G.C. Thom, K.G. Partymiller, 1983, "Environmental Transport and Transformation of Polychlorinated Biphenyls," U.S. Environmental Protection Agency, Washington, D.C. EPA-560/5-83-025.

Mabey, W.R., J.H. Smith, R.T. Podoll, H.L. Johnson, T. Mill, T.W. Chou, J. Gates, I.W. Partridge, H. Jaber, and D. Vandenberg, 1982, Aquatic Fate Process Data for Organic Priority Pollutants. SRI International. EPA 440-4-81-014.

MacKay, D., 1982, "Correlation of Bioconcentration Factors," Environmental Science and Technology, 16:274-278.

Malhot, H., 1987, "Prediction of Algal Bioaccumulation and Uptake Rate of Nine Organic Compounds by Ten Physicochemical Properties," Environmental Science and Technology, 21: 1009-1013.

McFarland, V.A., and J.U. Clark, 1989, "Environmental occurrence, abundance, and potential toxicity of polychlorinated biphenyl congeners: considerations for a congener-specific analysis," Environmental Health Perspectives, 81:225-239.

Niimi, A.J. 1981, "Gross Growth Efficiency of Fish (K_1) Based on Field Observations of Annual Growth and Kinetics of Persistent Environmental Contaminants," Canadian Journal of Fishery and Aquatic Science, 38:250-253.

Niimi, A.J., and B.G. Oliver, 1983, "Biological Half-Lives of Polychlorinated Biphenyl (PCB) Congeners in Whole Fish and Muscle of Rainbow Trout (*Salmo gairdneri*)," Canadian Journal of Fishery and Aquatic Science, 40:1388-1394.

Niimi, A.J., and B.G. Oliver, 1988, "Influence of Molecular Weight and Molecular Volume on Dietary Absorption Efficiency of Chemicals by Fishes," Canadian Journal of Fishery and Aquatic Science, 45:222-227.

Norstrom, R.J., A.E. McKinnon, and A.S.W. De Freitas, 1976, "A

Bioenergetics-Based Model for Pollutant Accumulation by Fish. Simulation of PCB and Methylmercury Levels in Ottawa River Yellow Perch (*Perca flavescen*)," Journal of Fishery Resources Board Canada, 33: 248-367.

Oliver, B.G., 1984, "Uptake of Chlorinated Organics from Anthropogenically Contaminated Sediments by Oligochaete Worms," Canadian Journal of Fishery and Aquatic Science, 41: 878-883.

Oliver, B.G., and A.J. Niimi, 1985, "Bioconcentration Factors of Some Halogenated Organics for Rainbow Trout Limitations in Their Use for Prediction of Environmental Residues," Environmental Science and Technology, 19: 842-849.

Oliver, B.G, and A.J. Niimi, 1988, "Trophodynamic Analysis of Polychlorinated Biphenyl Congeners and Other Chlorinated Hydrocarbons in the Lake Ontario Ecosystem," Environmental Science and Technology 22:388-397.

Rand, G.M., and Sam R. Petrocelli. 1985. Fundamentals of Aquatic Toxicology. Hemisphere Publishing Company, New York. 666 pp.

Rasmussen, J.B., D.J., Rowan, D.R.S., Lean, and J.H., Carey, 1990, "Food Chain Structure in Ontario Lakes Determines PCB Levels in Lake Trout (*Salvelinus namaycush*) and Other Pelagic Fish," Canadian Journal of Fishery and Aquatic Science, 47:2030-2038.

South Coast Air Quality Management District (SCAQMD). 1988. "Multi-Pathway Health Risk Assessment Input Parameters Guidance Document". Prepared for SCAQMD by Clement Associates, Inc.

Schmitt, C.J., J.L. Zajicek, and M.A. Ribick, 1985, "National Pesticide Monitoring Program: Residues of Organochlorine Chemicals in Freshwater Fish, 1980-81," Archives of Environmental Contaminant Toxicology, 14:225-260.

Shea, D., 1988, "Developing National Sediment Quality Criteria," Environmental Science and Technology, 22: 388-397.

Swackhamer, D.L., and D.E. Armstrong, 1986, "Estimation of the Atmospheric and Nonatmospheric Contributions and Losses of Polychlorinated Biphenyls for Lake Michigan on the Basis of Sediment Records of Remote Lakes," Environmental Science and Technology, 20(9):879-883.

Tanabe S. 1988, "PCB problems in the future: foresight from current knowledge," Environmental Pollution, 50:5-28.

Tanabe, S., N. Kannan., A. Subramanian, S. Watanabe, R. Tatsukawa, 1987, "Highly toxic coplaner PCBs: occurrence, source, persistency and toxic implications to wildlife and humans," Environmental Pollution, 47:147-163.

Thomann, R.V., 1981, "Equilibrium Model of Fate of Microcontaminants in Diverse Aquatic Food Chains," Canadian Journal of Fishery and Aquatic Science, 38: 280-296.

Thomann, R.V., 1989, "Bioaccumulation Model of Organic Chemical Distribution in Aquatic Food Chains," Environmental Science and Technology, 23: 699-707.

Thomann, R.V., and J.P. Connolly, 1984, "Model of PCB in the Lake Michigan Lake Trout Food Chain," Environmental Science and Technology, 18:65-71.

Thomman, R.V., J.P. Connolly, T. Parkerton, 1992a, "Modeling the Accumulation of Organic Chemicals in Aquatic Food Webs," Chemical Dynamics in Fresh Water Ecosystems, edited by F.A.P.C. Gobas and J.A. McCorquodale, Lewis Publishers, Ann Arbor, MI.

Thomann, R.V., J.P. Connolly, and T.F. Parkerton. 1992b. "An Equilibrium Model of Organic Chemical Accumulation in Aquatic Food Webs with Sediment Interaction," Environmental Toxicology and Chemistry, 11:615-629.

U.S. Environmental Protection Agency (USEPA), 1988, "Superfund Exposure Assessment Manual," EPA/540/1-88/001. Office of Remedial Response.

U.S. Environmental Protection Agency (USEPA), 1989, "Risk Assessment Guidance for Superfund: Volume I Human Health Evaluation Manual (Part A)," EPA/540/1-89/002. Office of Emergency and Remedial Response.

U.S. Environmental Protection Agency (USEPA), 1992, "Guidance for Exposure Assessment," Federal Register 59(104)22888-22936. March 29, 1992.

Wetzel, R.G., 1983, Limnology, 2nd Edition, Saunders College Publishing, Philadelphia.

Wayne G. Landis[1], Robin A. Matthews[1], April J. Markiewicz[1] and Geoffrey B. Matthews[2].

Non-linear Oscillations Detected By Multivariate Analysis in Microcosm Toxicity Tests: Implications for Risk Assessment and Biomonitoring.

REFERENCE: Landis, W. G., Matthews, R. A., Markiewicz, A. J., and Matthews, G. B., **"Non-linear Oscillations Detected by Multivariate Analysis in Microcosm Toxicity Tests: Implications for Risk Assessment and Biomonitoring,"** Environmental Toxicology and Risk Assessment - Third Volume, ASTM STP 1218, Jane S. Hughes, Gregory R. Biddinger, and Eugene Mones, Eds., American Society for Testing and Materials, Philadelphia, 1995.

ABSTRACT: This study compares the dynamics of the effects of the water soluble fraction (WSF) of both Jet-A and JP-4 using the Standard Aquatic Microcosm (SAM) using several types of multivariate analysis. In these studies we investigate the common assumption in environmental toxicology, that after the initial stress, ecosystems recover to resemble the control or reference state. This assumption may be based more on our inability to observe an ecosystem with sufficient resolution to detect differences, than reality. Among the more interesting effects observed in both studies were the shifts in time of population peaks and some other variables compared to non-dosed microcosms. In both experiments, multivariate analysis was able to differentiate oscillations that separate the treatments from the reference group, followed by what would normally appear as recovery, followed by another separation into treatment groups as distinct from the reference treatment. These patterns generally were not detected by conventional analysis.

Two sets of related explanations exist for the observed phenomenon. First, the addition of the toxicant initiates an alteration in the community so that the quality of the food resources for the later successional stages is significantly different from the control. This difference in resource quality and quantity leads to the repeated and replicated oscillations. The second explanation is that the oscillations are the result of the intrinsic complex and perhaps even chaotic behavior of population interactions. The initial impact of the toxicant re-set the dosed communities into different regions of the n-dimensional space where recovery may be an illusion due to the incidental overlap of the trajectories of the systems occurring along a few axes. Some of the implications of complex or chaotic dynamics upon the prediction of ecological risk and in biomonitoring are discussed.

KEYWORDS: Standardized Aquatic Microcosm, jet fuel, non-linear dynamics, nonmetric clustering and association analysis, risk assessment

[1]Institute of Environmental Toxicology and Chemistry, Huxley College of Environmental Studies and
[2]Computer Science Department, Western Washington University, Bellingham, WA 98225.

INTRODUCTION

Distinguishing toxicant effects from other community-level changes has become one of the most critical obstacles to the interpretation of multispecies data sets. Over the last 15 years a variety of multispecies toxicity tests have been developed with the hope that in doing so, the increased complexity of the test would result in a more realistic comparison to community-level responses to the toxicant. However, the addition of more than one species, and the generally longer time periods associated with these multispecies tests, also result in much more complex data sets.

Multispecies toxicity tests are usually referred to as microcosms or mesocosms, although a clear definition of the size or complexity to distinguish these terms has not been put forth. In the Standardized Aquatic Microcosm (SAM) developed by Taub and colleagues (Taub 1969, 1976, 1988, 1989, Taub and Crow 1978, Crow and Taub 1979, Taub et al. 1980, 1987, 1988, Kindig et al. 1983, Conquest and Taub 1989) the physical, chemical, and biological components are defined as to species, media and substrate. The SAM system has undergone round robin testing (Conquest and Taub 1989) and has been used with a variety of toxicants and degradative organisms (Landis et al. 1989, 1993).

One of the major difficulties in the evaluation of multispecies toxicity tests has been the difficulty in the analysis of the large data set on a level consistent with the goals of the toxicity test. Typically, the goals of the multispecies toxicity test are twofold:

- to detect changes in the population dynamics of the individual taxa that would not be apparent in single species tests; and,

- to detect structural and functional community-level differences that are correlated with treatment groups thereby representing a deviation from the control group.

A number of methods have been developed in an attempt to satisfy the goals of multispecies toxicity testing. Analysis of variance (ANOVA) is the classical method to examine single variable differences from the control group. However, because multispecies toxicity tests generally run for weeks or even months, there are problems with using conventional ANOVA. These include the increasing likelihood of introducing a Type II error (accepting a false null-hypothesis), temporal dependence of the variables, and the difficulty of graphically representing the data set. Conquest and Taub (1989) developed a method to overcome some of the problems by using intervals of non-significant difference (IND). This method corrects for the likelihood of Type II errors and produces intervals that are easily graphed, facilitating further analysis. The method is routinely used to examine data from SAM toxicity tests, and it is applicable to other multivariate toxicity tests. The major drawback of the IND is the limitation of examining one variable at a time over the course of the experiment. While this method addresses the first goal in multispecies toxicity testing, listed above, it ignores the analysis of directly examining the interactions important at the community level and must rely on summations or indexes that reduce the interactions to a one dimensional metric. In many instances, community-level responses are not as straightforward as the classical predator/prey or nutrient limitation dynamics, that are usually selected as examples of single-species responses representing complex interactions.

Multivariate methods have proved promising as a method of evaluating the entire dimensionality of the systems under study. One of the first methods used in toxicity testing was the calculation of ecosystem strain as developed by Kersting (1984, 1985, 1988) for a three compartment microcosm. This method has the advantage of incorporating all of the parameters measured by the investigator to search for treatment-related differences. Concurrently and independently, Johnson (1988a, 1988b) developed a multivariate algorithm using the n-dimensional coordinates of a multivariate data set and the distances between these coordinates as a measure of divergence between treatment groups. Both of these methods have the advantage of examining the ecosystem as a whole rather than by single variables, and can track such processes as succession, recovery and the deviation of a system due to an anthropogenic input.

However, a major disadvantage of both these methods, and of many conventional multivariate methods, is that all of the data are often incorporated without regard to the units of measurement, or to the appropriateness of including all variables in the analysis. Random variables indiscriminately incorporated into the analysis, may contribute so much noise that they overshadow variables that do show treatment-related effects. The use of Mahalanobis distances does reduce the impact of noisy variables, but the measure can still be overwhelmed.

Recently developed for the analysis of ecological data, nonmetric clustering and association analysis is a multivariate derivative of artificial intelligence research, that satisfies all these criteria and has the potential of circumventing many of the problems of conventional multivariate analysis (Matthews et al, 1994). Initially, clusters are searched for without prior knowledge of treatment using a conceptual clustering algorithm incorporated in the program Riffle. As clusters are identified an association analysis is performed to examine the relationship of the identified clusters to the treatment groups. This clustering methodology has a number of advantages over traditional methods:

- It does not combine counts from dissimilar taxa or other variable classifications by means of sums of squares, or other *ad hoc* mathematical techniques.

- It does not require transformations of the data, such as normalizing the variance.

- It will work without modification on incomplete data sets. Since attributes are not combined, missing values do not hamper the evaluation of the other attributes.

- It will work without further assumptions on different data types (*e.g.*, numeric, categorical, species counts, presence/absence data, *etc.*).

- Significance of a variable to the analysis is not dependent on the absolute size of its count, so that taxa having a small total variance, i.e. rare taxa, can compete in importance with common taxa, and taxa with a large, random variance will not automatically be selected, to the exclusion of others.

- It will provide an integral measure of the quality of the analysis, i.e. whether the data set differs from a random collection of points.

- It will, in some cases, identify a subset of the variables that serve as reliable indicators of the physical and biological environment.

The major disadvantage of nonmetric clustering and association analysis is that, in order to find a clustering of the data points with the desirable qualities listed above, a massive search through thousands of potential clustering candidates is made before settling the "right" one. Even after an extensive search, there is no guarantee that the optimal clustering has been found. However, in the broad variety of the field and laboratory research conducted to date, Riffle does find an excellent clustering in a reasonable amount of time.

In this paper, we use three multivariate techniques to compare patterns in the data sets from two SAM toxicity tests using turbine fuels. The multivariate techniques include two conventional tests based on the ratio of multivariate metric distances (Euclidean distance and cosine of the vector distance), and one relatively new program, Riffle, which employs nonmetric clustering and association analysis (Matthews and Hearne 1991). All three of the multivariate techniques have proven useful in analyzing complex ecological data sets (Matthews et al. 1991a, 1991b). The use of these techniques enable us to observe repeated oscillations in the treatment groups relative to treatment 1, the non-dosed replicates. We define oscillation as repeated deviation from a reference state without regard to periodicity or magnitude. These observations and the patterns of the oscillations have led us to adopt a new approach to the evaluation of toxicant impacts upon ecological systems. In addition we have begun to strongly question the use of indices and metaphors such as ecosystem health.

EXPERIMENTAL METHODS

Reagents

All chemicals used in the culture of the organisms and in the formulation of the microcosm media were reagent grade or as specified by the ASTM method.

Jet-A was provided by Fliteline Services of Bellingham, Washington and was refined by Chevron. The sample was obtained from the sample valve used for quality control. The shipment lot was recorded and is on file. JP-4 was supplied by the U. S. Air Force Toxicology Laboratory at Wright Patterson, AFB, Ohio.

Water Soluble Fractions

The water soluble fraction was prepared in glassware washed in nonphosphate soap, rinsed, then soaked in 2N HCl for at least one hour, rinsed ten times with distilled water, dried and finally autoclaved for 30 minutes. Microcosm medium, T82MV, acted as the diluent for the water fraction of the WSF.

Twenty five mL of fuel is added to one liter of T82MV in a one liter separatory funnel, and is agitated as follows: [1] shake separatory funnel for five minutes, releasing built up pressure as necessary; [2] allow funnel contents to remain undisturbed for 15 minutes; [3] shake contents for five minutes, allow to stand 15 minutes; [4] continue same pattern for a total time of one hour; and finally [5] allow separatory funnel contents to remain undisturbed for eight hours. Globules are then broken up and mixed using a sterile glass rod. At the end of this procedure, usually completed in the afternoon, the mixture was allowed to stand overnight, for a minimum of 12 hours. The next day all but 100 mL of T82MV/water soluble fraction of jet fuel mixture is drained from the separatory funnel (leaving the lighter, insoluble fuel mixture in the flask) was drained into a cleaned, sterile 1 liter amber glass bottle and capped with a Teflon-lined screw cap. The WSF was used within

24 hours or stored at 4°C for no longer than 48 hours before use as the toxicant mixture.

Gas Chromatography of WSF

This protocol utilizes a Tekmar LSC 2000 Purge and Trap (P&T) concentrator system in tandem with a Hewlett Packard 5890A Gas Chromatograph with a Flame Ionization Detector (FID)(ASTM D3710, D2887, Westendorf 1986). Instrument blanks and deionized distilled water blanks are used to verify the P&T and GC columns cleanliness prior to analysis of samples. A five mL sample is injected into a five milliliter sparger, purged with pre-purified nitrogen gas for eleven minutes and dry purged for four minutes. Volatile hydrocarbons, purged from the sample and collected on the Tenax/Silica Gel column, are desorbed at 180°C directly onto the gas chromatograph SPB-5, 30m x 0.53 mm ID 1.5μm film, fused silica capillary column. The column, at 35°C, is held at that temperature for two minutes, increased to 225°C at 12°C/min. and held at that temperature for five minutes. A Spectra-Physics 4290 Integrator records the FID signal output of the volatile hydrocarbons that have been separated and eluted from the column by molecular weight. A comparison is then made of the sample chromatograph to n-paraffin and n-naphtha chromatograph standards for sample concentration determinations.

Identification and Quantification of GC Fractions

Qualitative identification of some components in the WSF were determined using a Simulated Distillation (SIMDIS) Calibration Mixture. The ASTM Method D3710 Qualitative Calibration Mixture is the standard test method for determining the Boiling Range Distribution of Gasoline and Gasoline Fractions by Gas Chromatography. This mixture was used as a calibration standard to determine the retention times for each known component in the mixture against which unknown components, in the WSF of the fuel mixture, were compared and identified.

SAM Protocol

The 64-day SAM-protocol previously has been described (ASTM E1366). Briefly, the microcosms were prepared by the introduction of ten algal, four invertebrate, and one bacterial species into 3L of sterile defined medium. An artificial sediment consisting of 200 g acid washed silica sand, 0.5 g cellulose and 0.5 g of ground chitin and 3 L of T82MV media are placed in 4 L glass jars. The test containers are autoclaved for 1 h; immersed in a water bath to a point above the level of the sediment during sterilization to prevent breakage.

Numbers of organisms, dissolved oxygen (DO) and pH were determined twice weekly. Room temperature was 20°C ± 2°. Illumination was 80.0 μEm^{-2} sec^{-1} PhAR with a range of 78.6-80.4 and a 12/12 day/night cycle.

Two major modifications were made to the SAM protocol. The first was the means of toxicant delivery. Test material was added on day 7 by stirring each microcosm, removing 450 mL from each container and then adding appropriate amounts of the WSF to produce concentrations of 0, 1, 5 and 15 percent WSF. After toxicant addition, the final volume was adjusted to 3L. A 250 mesh Nitex filter was used to retain the larger invertebrates within the SAM system during the removal of the media. All graphs and statistical analysis start with the next sampling day, day 11. The second modification was the substitution, in the JP-4 experiment, of *Tetrahymena thermophila* BIV for the hypotrichous ciliate. The hypotrichous ciliate was becoming increasingly difficult to culture, very likely due to the age of the clone. The results of the JP-4 study demonstrated the suitability of the Tetrahymena for inclusion in the protocol.

Data Analysis

All data were recorded onto standard computer entry forms and checked for accuracy. Parameters calculated included the concentrations of each of the species, DO, DO gain and loss, net photosynthesis/respiration ratio (P/R), pH, algal species diversity, algal biovolume, and biovolume of available algae. The statistical significance of these parameters, compared to the controls, was also computed for each sampling day using the IND plots developed by Conquest. The net photosynthesis/respiration ratio is not derived using ^{14}C methods but by comparing oxygen concentrations before lights on, at the end of the photosynthetic period just before lights off, and then at the next morning, as specified in the standard protocol.

The multivariate methods used in the analysis include cosine and vector distances and nonmetric clustering. All of these methods have been previously described (Matthews et al. 1991b, Landis et al. 1993) and are reviewed in this volume (Matthews et al 1994). Variables used in the multivariate analysis are presented in Table 1.

The nonmetric clustering is performed by the program Riffle as developed by G. Matthews. Using a blind search algorithm, Riffle examines the data and assembles the best clusters as determined by similarity in characteristics, not proximity in n-dimensional space. The variables that contribute characteristics statistically important to the determination of the clusters are ranked in importance. The clusters are then compared to the treatment groups using a goodness of fit test to test the correspondence of the clusters to treatment.

RESULTS

Persistence of the fuels. In the case of both WSFs, within three weeks after dosing the majority of the original material had been volitilized or degraded. In the case of JP-4, benzene, 2,4-dimethylpentane, ethylbenzene, 2-methylpentane, 2-methylpropane, o-xylene and toluene, persisted in the media, but may be degradation products.

TABLE 1. Biotic parameters used in the multivariate statistical tests. Biotic variables such as diversity, available biovolume, and total algal biovolume are not used since they are derived from and therefore not independent of the variables listed below.

Jet-A	**JP-4**
Anabaena	Anabaena
Ankistrodesmus	Ankistrodesmus
Chlamydomonas	Chlamydomonas
Chlorella	Chlorella
Daphnia	Daphnia
Ephipia	Ephipia
Small Daphnia	Small Daphnia
Medium Daphnia	Medium Daphnia
Large Daphnia	Large Daphnia
Hypotricha	Tetrahymena
Lyngbya	Lyngbya
Miscellaneous sp.	Miscellaneous sp.
Ostracod (Cyprinotus)	Ostracod (Cyprinotus)
Philodina (Rotifer)	Philodina (Rotifer)

Scenedesmus	Scenedesmus
Selenastrum	Selenastrum
Stigeoclonium	Stigeoclonium
Ulothrix	Ulothrix

Comparison of Algal Population Dynamics-Highest Treatment. These area graphs (Fig. 1) show the contribution of each algal species to the algal assemblage for the highest treatment concentration for each experiment. In the Jet-A treatment the algal populations were highest, reflecting the increased toxicity of the Jet-A to the daphnid populations. In both experiments however, an algal bloom was observed during the first 30 days of the experiment. At the end of the experiment the numbers and composition of the algal assemblage were similar, although the proportions of the species making up the assemblage had some differences. Chlorella seemed to be a greater constituent of the community in the JP-4 experiment. A more detailed description of the dynamics can be found in Landis et al. (1993a, 1993b)

Daphnid Population Dynamics. The most direct effect of the jet fuel upon the population dynamics of the daphnid populations was the delay in daphnid reproduction (Fig. 2). Peaks were delayed in the Treatment 4 microcosms in both instances. Using nonmetric clustering, daphnids were very statistically important as determined by the Riffle program, in distinguishing the clusters in the early part of each experiment but were not as important later. In both experiments two peaks of daphnid populations are observed. The first reflects the presence of the toxicant, the second occurs in both the dosed and not dosed systems. Error bars are not shown for clarity.

Ostracod Population Dynamics. Ostracod populations did not increase until late in each experiment (Fig. 3). In the Jet-A experiment (Fig. 3A), the numbers started an increase between days 40 and 45. The experiment using JP-4 as a toxicant (Fig. 3B) did not see the increase in ostracods until between days 50-55, approximately ten days later. Consequently, the total numbers of ostracods observed were not as high in the JP-4 microcosms. Note that the order of densities in the Jet-A experiment followed a dose response pattern, as did the JP-4 experiment, even with the lower total numbers. Conventional analysis did not demonstrate significance, however non-metric clustering did indicate the importance of the ostracods in determining clusters in both sets of microcosm experiments.

Philodina Population Dynamics. Philodina did not become prevalent in the microcosms until the second half of the experiment. One of the major problems was the inherent variability in the sampling and in the replicates. Organisms that reproduce rapidly can show large differences in population sizes during the course of a sampling day. Although, in the later stages of the microcosm experiments the dosed systems had a generally larger number of the rotifers, the results were not statistically significant using conventional IND plots. However, using cluster analysis, Philodina were also determined to be a statistically important variable as defined by Riffle in defining clusters. This held true for both the Jet-A and JP-4 experiments.

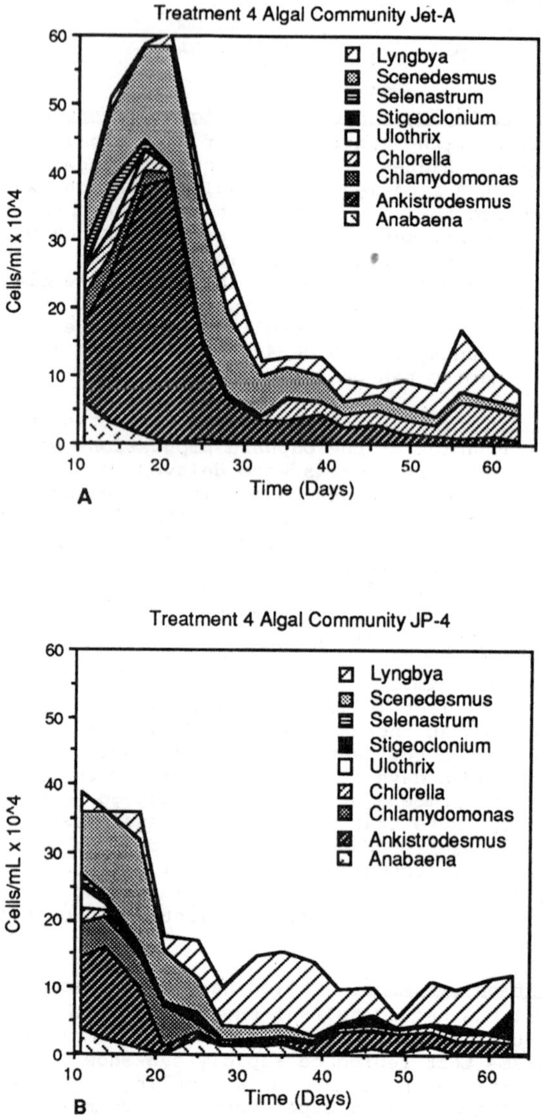

FIG. 1--Comparison of algal population dynamics-highest treatment using an area graph. The values used are means for each algal species. Area graphs are particular useful in observing patterns of abundance as well as counts of total algae.

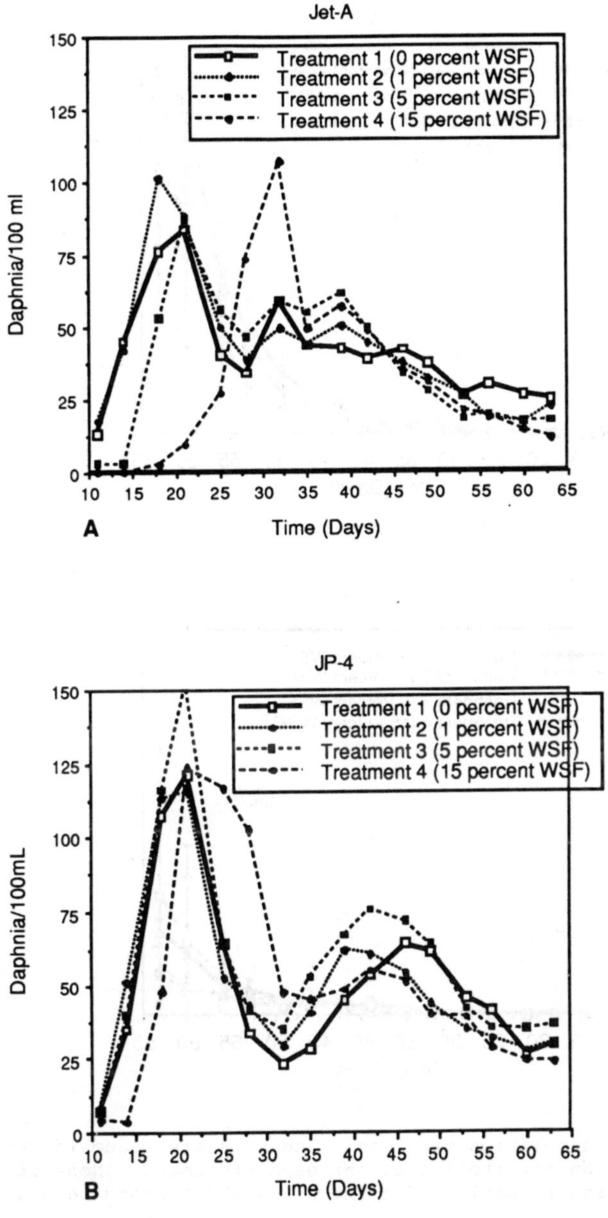

FIG. 2--Daphnid population dynamics. In the Jet-A experiment (FIG 2a) the daphnia peak is delayed in Treatment 4, the highest concentration. A similar delay is not apparent in the JP-4 experiment (FIG 2b).

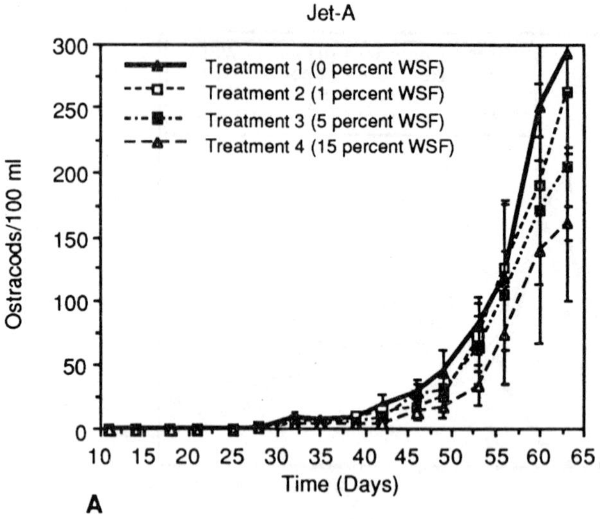

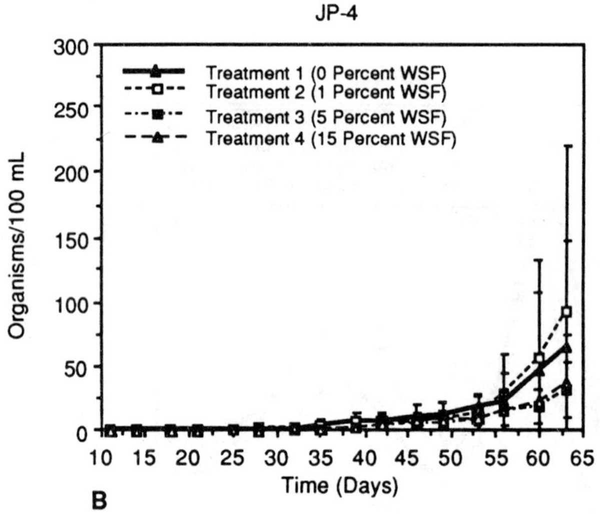

FIG. 3--Ostracod population dynamics. The bars are standard deviations of the means of the six replicates for each treatment. None of the treatments are significantly different using ANOVA based techniques such as the IND.

Comparisons of pH dynamics of the Jet-A and JP-4 Experiments. Unlike the biotic variables, pH did reflect some of the oscillations detected by the cluster analysis (Fig. 4). In both the Jet-A and the JP-4 experiments the highest concentrations demonstrated a statistically significant difference, determined by the interval of non-significant difference during the first 30 days of the experiment. The second oscillation, between days 45 and 50, is not as clear since only one sampling date demonstrated the statistically significant difference using IND. Type II error becomes a concern with so many comparisons, even with the corrections incorporated into the IND plots.

Photosynthesis/Respiration Ratio. The photosynthesis/respiration ratio reflects the oscillations seen in pH and the clustering analysis for the first 30 days and then only for the Jet-A water soluble fraction. In the Jet-A experiment, a second deviation from the IND plot was noted in the period corresponding to the second oscillation, but the result is difficult to distinguish from a type II error. In the JP-4 experiment, the IND plots are large, reflecting the variance in those sampling days. As an "emergent property", it is not clear if the P/R ratio provides any more information in this experiment than the clustering based upon the biotic components.

Oscillations in Community Trajectories Observed in both the Jet-A and the JP-4 Experiments. The Jet-A and the JP-4 SAM experiments both displayed a series of oscillations; revealed by the three clustering techniques employed in the analysis (Fig. 5). The first oscillation, as defined by Cosine Distance common to each experiment, is due to the interaction of the daphnid population and the algae. The result is statistically significant, as determined by the goodness-of-fit confidence level, graphed by day in Fig. 6. Figure 6 provides the significance level for each of the methods used, cosine, vector distance and nonmetric clustering. In both experiments, the oscillation is within the first 30 days of the SAM time-line. Interestingly, the magnitude of the first oscillation, as determined by Cosine Distance, is less in the JP-4 experiment, possibly reflecting the reduced acute and chronic toxicity of the mixture.

A second series of divergences from treatment 1, as measured by Cosine Distance, occur in the last thirty days of each experiment. Again the deviations from treatment 1 (0 percent WSF) are statistically significant.

The participants in the community that contribute to these deviations are different judging by the table of statistically important variables (Table 2) determined by nonmetric clustering. Unfortunately, the length of the SAM protocol is not sufficient to conduct an analysis of the period and amplitude of the oscillations. Another complication in interpreting the results is the difficulty in making direct comparisons between experiments. Although the Cosine Distance may be the same, the orientation of the angle can be quite different. Two objects may have very different spatial coordinates, yet have the same relative angle compared to a third or reference system.

Table 3 does compare the frequency of variables ranked important for the two microcosm experiments. A Daphnia variable, Chlorella and Ankistrodesmus were the top three in occurrence in both the Jet-A and JP-4 experiments. Ostracods and Philodina were also similar in frequency of importance in the two experiments, both becoming critical after day 28 of the experiments (see Table 2 for JP-4 data).

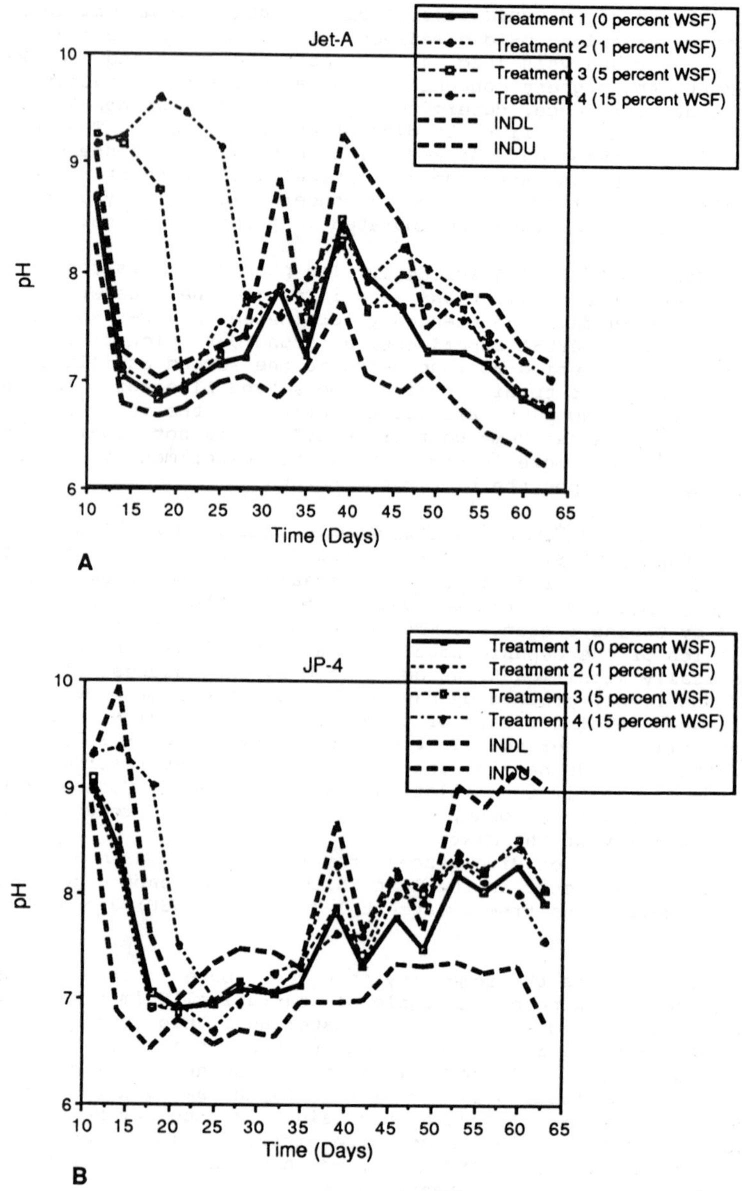

FIG. 4--Comparisons of pH during the SAM studies. In both experiments the pH demonstrated an early and late significant difference from the control as demonstrated by the IND plots (arrows).

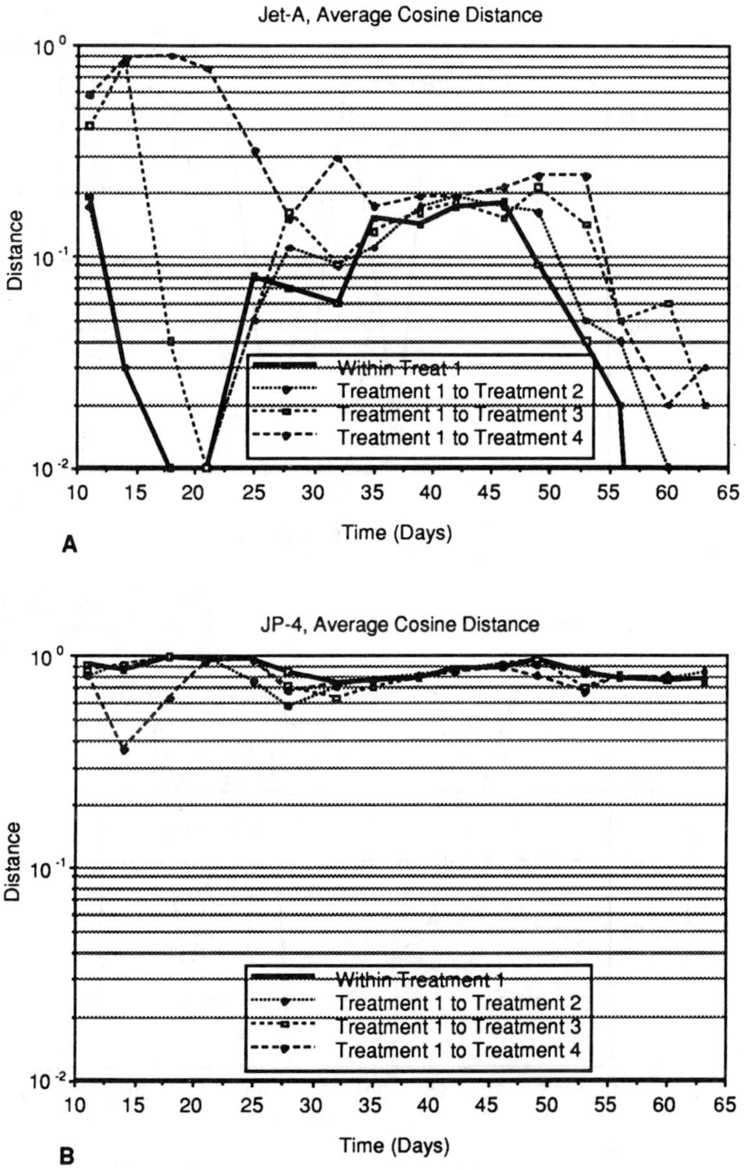

FIG. 5--Cosine Distances of the Treatment 1 to the dosed treatments in the Jet-A and the JP-4 SAMs.

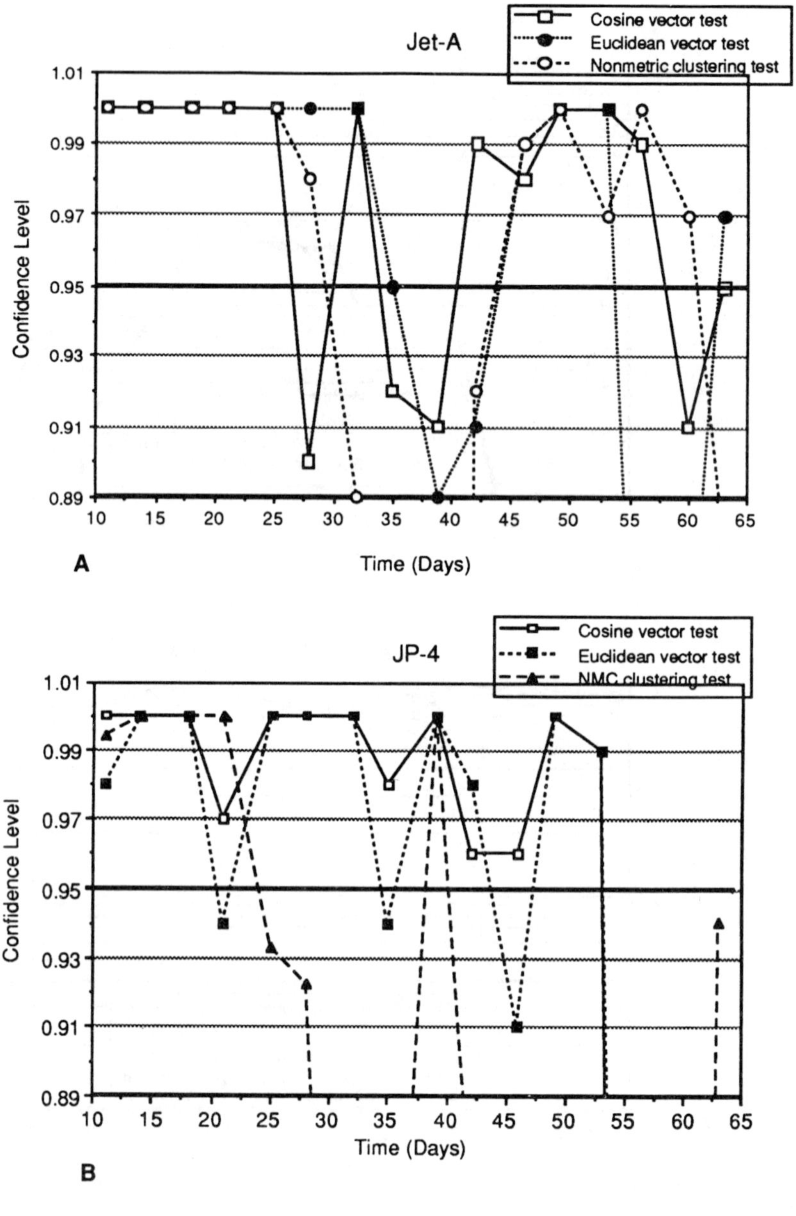

FIG. 6--Significance of the association analysis of the 4 Treatments in the Jet-A and the JP-4 SAMs.

TABLE 2. Important variables as determined by nonmetric clustering ranked according to contribution for each sampling day for JP-4. Some variables such as Ankistrodesmus were important in determining group clusters in the first half of the experiment. Some of the variables such as **Ostracod** and Philodina were more important in the latter stages of the experiment. Note that the order of importance of even the more common contributors often changed from sampling day to sampling day, with no one variable being consistently ranked, *Chlorella* and S. Daphnia being the closest.

Day	Important Variables in Determining Clusters in Rank Order
11	Selenastrum, M. Daphnia, *Chlorella*, Ankistrodesmus
14	Selenastrum, S. Daphnia, M. Daphnia-Ankistrodesmus[1], L. Daphnia-Stigeoclonium
18	Scenedesmus, Selenastrum, Ankistrodesmus, S. Daphnia, *Chlorella*, L. Daphnia
21	Scenedesmus, Ankistrodesmus, Chlamydomonas
25	*Chlorella*, S. Daphnia
28	*Chlorella*, Ankistrodesmus-Lyngbya, Philodina
32	**Ostracod**
35	**Ostracod**, Philodina, Scenedesmus
39	Scenedesmus, S. Daphnia
42	Lyngbya, S. Daphnia, Philodina, Ankistrodesmus
46	M. Daphnia
49	Scenedesmus, Chlorella, Philodina
53	*Chlorella*, Philodina
56	M. Daphnia-S. Daphnia
60	S. Daphnia, **Ostracod**, Lyngbya
63	*Chlorella*, S. Daphnia, M. Daphnia, Lyngbya

[1] Hyphen between variables denotes equal rank

TABLE 3. Variable ranking by success in determining clusters as defined by nonmetric clustering. Nonmetric clustering produces a ranking of the importance of the variables in determining the clusters for each sampling day. Variables such as Ankistrodesmus and the Daphnia classes ranked highly in the course of this study. However, reliance on any particular organism or a small combination of variables would inadequately describe the dynamics of the system.

Jet-A Variable	Ranked	**JP-4** Variable	Ranked
Ankistrodesmus	12	Chlorella	8
M. Daphnia	11	S. Daphnia	8
Chlorella	9	Ankistrodesmus	6
Scenedesmus	7	Scenedesmus	5
S. Daphnia	6	Philodina	5
L. Daphnia	5	M. Daphnia	4
Ostracod	4	Lyngbya	4
Philodina	4	L. Daphnia	3
Selenastrum	4	Ostracod	3
Lyngbya	3	Selenastrum	3
Ulothrix	1		

DISCUSSION

Microcosm Dynamics and Interpretation

The examination of individual parameters provided only a limited view of the dynamic responses of the SAM system to Jet-A and JP-4. In the case of the both experiments, the univariate data did show that there were some significant responses to the toxicant as determined by the daphnid and algal data as well as the chemistry.

The biological responses that were most evident were of only dramatic impacts, such as the increase in the algal populations due to the inhibitory effect of the Jet-A and JP-4 upon the grazer populations. Axiomatically, an inhibition of the predominant grazer in the early stages of the microcosm, the Daphnia, is going to result in an algal bloom. These types of responses do not provide a depth of understanding of the function and structure of the artificial ecosystem. In contrast to the biological data, pH did demonstrate some statistically significant differences using the IND methodology that hinted at an early major impact in treatment 4 and a later divergence for both experimental systems. It is likely that pH is measuring an alteration in the metabolism of the system and therefore a change in the functionality, but without structural differences it is difficult to attribute the functional differences to structural alterations.

The multivariate analyses of the structural data revealed patterns not observed using the univariate analysis of the biotic data. The Jet-A experiment demonstrated at least two major divergences from the non-dosed treatment as measured by all three methods. In the JP-4 experiment, three oscillations from the non-dosed treatment 1 could be observed that were statistically significant. Two of these oscillations correspond well to the divergences seen in the pH analysis. However in the divergences seen between days 25-30 and 50-55 (Figures 5 and 6), suggestions of a dose-response can be seen that are not apparent in the pH data. These oscillations were observed after the demise of the original WSF mixture.

Changes in the structural composition of the systems did occur repeatedly during the course of the experiments even in these relatively simple systems. These oscillations, repeated divergence, convergence and redivergence events, point to effects not readily observed or predicted by single species systems. The repeated divergence of the dosed systems from the reference systems may be accounted for in two ways:

- It may reflect the functioning of the community in terms of parameters not directly sampled by the SAM protocol.

- It may be a persistent fluctuation in the community structure initiated by the initial stress, but is only periodically visible, as if it were an incompletely dampened nonlinear oscillation in the systems' inherent dynamics.

If you kill or restrict the reproduction of most of the Daphnia, the next microcosm response is likely an algal bloom. This result could easily have been predicted by the short term toxicity tests and was expected. However, recent modeling efforts by Taub et al. (submitted) suggest that the dynamics of these interactions and the resulting magnitudes of the algal blooms are highly dependent upon the timing of the stressor event. Measuring these types of gross responses to the toxicant do not provide much more insight into impact of the toxicant in the ecosystem than do the short-term single-species tests. The absolute magnitude of the disturbance and the period of recovery can be obtained from the microcosm experiment, in the sense of a classical predator prey interaction. However, the multivariate analysis reveals a more interesting dynamic.

The multivariate patterns suggest a much more complex pattern of multiple divergences and convergences in the similarities between treatment groups. Much as an ecosystem could be expected to display the rise and fall of species assemblages, the SAM microcosms appear to indicate that the first divergence is only the beginning of a series of responses.

Using nonmetric clustering, we can list the variables that were the most important for separating the treatment group clusters for each day that measurements were collected (Table 2). The list of variables suggests that the first divergence, which occurred from about day 11 through day 25, results from predator/prey interactions between primary producers (algae) and first order consumers (daphnia). This divergence should be characterized by the following properties:

- The divergence will be fast, because the algae and daphnia populations are introduced into the microcosm after being cultured in optimal laboratory conditions and then placed into cultures with high available nutrient concentrations. Predation, or the lack of predation, or other limiting factors will cause rapid changes in the algal and herbivore populations.

- The divergence will be short-lived, because the populations are unstable in the nutrient rich early successional microcosm. There will be a tendency for the microcosms to drift away from the early "treatment" effect into a more typical community based on both algae and detritus as the food source for the secondary consumers. Initially, this drift may mask treatment effects and be interpreted as recovery of the system.

The first divergence is the only type of response that is normally searched for in microcosm tests using conventional statistics. This response is typical of many reported SAM experiments (Taub et al., 1988; Taub, 1988; Haley et al., 1988; Landis et al., 1989).

The additional divergences occurred from between days 25-30 and 50-55 in the SAMs. During this time, Daphnia and some of the algal taxa were often still important in the cluster development; however, other secondary consumers (Ostracods and Philodina) entered the list. The second divergence may represent the long-term effects of the initial toxicant on a more successionally mature community that is fueled by both algal productivity and detritus. If so, the resulting divergences should have the following characteristics:

- It should be strongly influenced by detritus quality. Detritus is conditioned by bacteria and fungi, which are highly sensitive to toxicants but are unmeasured in the microcosm. Also, detritus that has passed through the gut of a consumer (e.g., consumed algae) is different from detritus that originates directly from dead algae (unconsumed). Therefore, the quality of the detritus may be highly affected by the treatment, but none of the factors influencing the effects will be measured directly.

- Secondary consumers of detritus and bacteria are no less affected by the quality of their food source than algal consumers, so the treatment-related alterations of the quality of detritus and bacteria will cause differences in the secondary consumer populations.

Therefore, the series of divergences following the initial algal-daphnid interaction may still represent a direct response to the initial treatment effects, but because it occurs late in the microcosm experiment, it is easily misinterpreted as noisy or the effects of a degradation product. An inclusion of measures of detritus quality and microbial metabolism may answer these questions and such studies are currently being incorporated into our series of microcosm experiments.

However, invoking unseen properties of an ecosystem or other mechanistic explanations may not be needed to explain the pattern of divergence, convergence and subsequent redivergence from a non-dosed reference system. An alternative and complimentary explanation is available that perhaps describes the dynamics of multispecies systems at a more fundamental level.

First, the apparent recovery or movement of the dosed systems towards the reference or treatment 1 case may be an artifact of our measurement systems that allow the n-dimensional data to be represented in a two dimensional system. In an n-dimensional sense, the systems may be moving in opposite directions and simply pass by similar coordinates during certain time intervals. Positions may be similar but the n-dimensional vectors describing the movements of the systems can be very different. A representation of these dynamics is presented in Fig. 7. The two systems intersect, although the vectors are quite different.

The apparent recoveries and divergences may also be artifacts of our attempt to choose the best means of collapsing and representing n-dimensional data into a two or three dimensional representation. In order to represent such data it is necessary to project n-dimensional data into three or less dimensions. As information is lost as the shadow from a cube is projected upon a two dimensional screen, a similar loss of information can occur in our attempt to represent n-dimensional data. Not every divergence from the reference treatment may have a cause directly related to it in time. Differentiating those events from those due to degradation products or other perturbations will be challenging. However, the phenomena observed in the SAM systems can be placed in a broader and more universal context.

Complexity and Chaotic Dynamics in Model Ecosystems

Not only may system recovery be an illusion, but there are strong theoretical reasons that seem to indicate that recovery to a reference system may be impossible or at least unlikely. In fact, systems that differ only marginally in their initial conditions and at levels probably impossible to measure are likely to diverge in unpredictable manners. May and Oster (1978) in a particularly seminal paper investigated the likelihood that many of the dynamics seen in ecosystems that are generally attributed as chance or stochastic events are in fact deterministic. In fact, simple deterministic models of populations can give rise to complex dynamics. Using equations resembling those used in population biology, bifurcations occur resulting in several distinct outcomes. Eventually, given the proper parameters, the system appears chaotic in nature although the underlying mechanisms are completely deterministic. Obviously, biological systems have limits, extinction being perhaps the most obvious and best recorded. Another ramification is that the noise in ecosystems and in sampling may not be the result of stochastic processes but are the result of underlying deterministic and chaotic relationships.

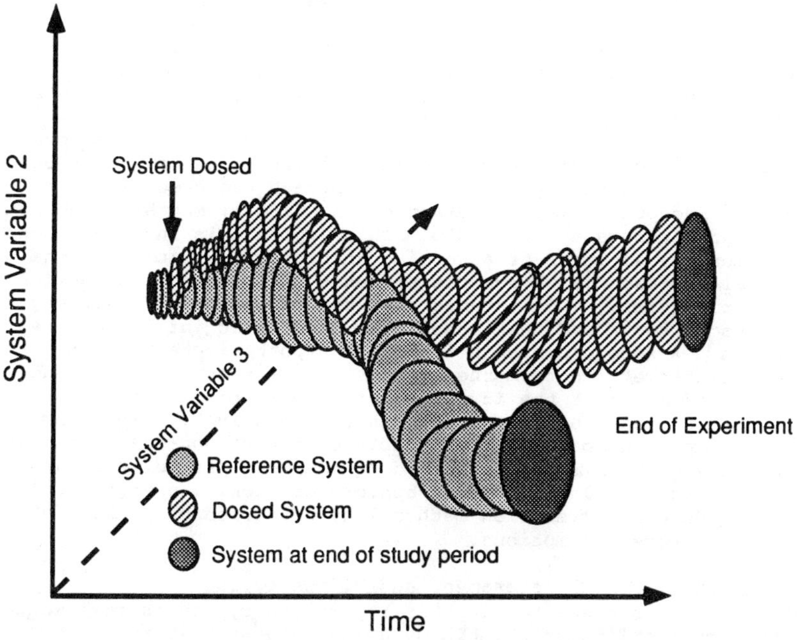

FIG. 7--Visualization of hypothetical ecosystem dynamics to reflect transitory convergence of two systems, a possible interpretation of the relative dynamics of the dosed systems and the non dosed systems using jet fuels.

These principals also apply to spatial distributions of populations as recently reported by Hassell et al. (1991). In a study using host-parasite interactions, a variety of spatial patterns were generated, ranging from static 'crystal lattice' patterns, spiral waves, chaotic variation, or extinction with the appropriate alteration of only three parameters within the same set of equations. The deterministically related patterns could be extremely complex and not distinguishable from stochastic environmental changes.

Given the perhaps chaotic nature of populations it may not be possible to predict accurately species presence, population interactions, or structural and functional attributes. Kratz *et al.* (1987) examined the spatial and temporal variability in zooplankton data from a series of five lakes in North America. Much of the analysis used the limnological data collected by Birge and Juday from 1925 to 1942. Copepods and cladocera, except *Bosmina*, exhibited larger variability between lakes than between years in the same lake. Some taxa showed consistent patterns among the study lakes. They concluded that the controlling factors for these taxa operated uniformly in each of the study sites. However, in regards to the depth of maximal abundance for calanoid copepods and Bosmina, the data obtained from one lake had little predictive power for application to other lakes. Part of this uncertainty was attributed to the intrinsic rate of increase of the invertebrates with the variability increasing with a corresponding increase in r_{max}. A high r_{max} should enable the populations to accurately track changes in the environment. Kratz et al. suggest that these taxa be used to track changes in the environment. Unfortunately, in the context of environmental toxicology, the inability to use one "reference" lake to predict the non-dosed population dynamics of these organisms in another eliminates comparisons of the two systems as measures of anthropogenic impacts.

A better strategy may be to let the data and a clustering protocol identify the important parameters in determining the dynamics of and impacts to ecological systems. This approach has been recently suggested independently by Dickson et al. (1992), Matthews and Matthews (1991) and Matthews et al. 1991b. This approach is in direct contrast to the more usual means of assessing anthropogenic impacts. One classical approach is to use the presence or absence of so called indicator species. This assumes that the tolerance to a variety of toxicants is known and that chaotic or stochastic influences are minimized. A second approach is to use hypothesis testing to differentiate metrics from the systems in question. This second approach assumes that the investigators know *a priori* the important parameters to measure. Given that in our relatively simple SAM systems that the important parameters in differentiating non-dosed from dosed systems change from sampling period to sampling period, this assumption can not be made. Classification approaches such as nonmetric clustering or the canonical correlation methodology developed by Dickson et al, eliminates these assumptions.

<u>Implications for Risk Assessment and Biomonitoring</u>

These results presented in this report and by others reviewed above and the implications of chaotic dynamics suggest that reliance upon any one variable or an index of variables may be an operational convenience that may provide a misleading representation of pollutant effects and associated risks (Landis et al., 1994). The use of indices such as diversity and the Index of Biological Integrity have the effect of collapsing the dimensions of the descriptive hypervolume. Just as the shadow of a cube is only two dimensional and must loose information, the use of an index may also collapse variables in arbitrary ways and also loose vital information content. Indices, since they are composited variables, are not true measurement endpoints. The collapse of the dimensions that are composited tends to eliminate crucial information, such as the variability in the importance of variables. The mere presence or absence and the frequency of these events can be analyzed using techniques such as nonmetric clustering that preserve the nature of the dataset. A useful function was certainly served by the application of indices, but the new methods of data compilation, analysis and representation derived from the Artificial Intelligence tradition and more traditional statistical procedures can now replace these approaches and illuminate the underlying structure and dynamic nature of ecological systems.

The implications are important. Currently, only small sections of ecosystems are monitored or a heavy reliance is placed upon so called indicator species. These data suggest that to do so is dangerous, and may produce misleading interpretations resulting in costly error in management and regulatory judgments. Much larger toxicological test systems are currently analyzed using conventional statistical methods on the limit of acceptable statistical power. Interpretation of the results has proven to be difficult, if not confusing. Application of the approach and tools that proved successful in revealing the complex dynamics of these small microcosms should prove useful in analyzing larger toxicological test systems and field research.

CONCLUSIONS

(1) In both of the experiments, multiple oscillations of the dosed treatment groups away from the reference treatment were observed using multivariate statistics. The first oscillation is due to the differential impact of the WSF of the jet fuels to the algae-daphnid population dynamics. The cause of the following oscillations, although statistically significant and seen in both experiments, is not as clear cut.

The divergence of the second and perhaps subsequent oscillations may be due to two separate mechanisms.

(a) A fluctuation due to the initial stress has occurred, but in such a fashion that an incompletely dampened oscillation repeats. There has been no fundamental alteration in the functioning of the ecosystem, and the oscillations are a result of the inherent time lags and stochastic factors governing the dynamics of the system.

(b) A fundamental aspect of the ecosystem has been altered so that the repeated oscillations reflect the persistence of the impact in a cascade of indirect effects. An alteration in the detritus quality or in the community involved in the recycling of detritus may have long term impacts as other nutrients become limiting in the systems. Analysis of these reactions to stressors using complexity theory or chaos mathematics has proven illuminating.

(2) Although simple systems, the SAM experiments exhibits complex dynamics and behaviors. The protocol results in a persistent system with good replicability within an experiment, even with complex species interactions.

(3) Techniques that allow the reduction and visualization of even these relatively simple multispecies toxicity tests should contribute to our understanding of system dynamics and improve hazard and risk assessment. The use of indices and other summary statistics should be closely examined.

ACKNOWLEDGMENTS

This research was funded by United States Air Force Office of Scientific Research Grant No. AFOSR-91-0291 DEF.

REFERENCES

ASTM D2887. Standard Test Method for Boiling Range Distribution of Petroleum Fractions by Gas Chromatography, 1988 Annual book of ASTM Standards, Vol. 5.02, pp 506-513. American Society for Testing and Materials, Philadelphia.

ASTM D3710. Standard Test Method for Boiling Range Distribution of Gasoline and Gasoline Fractions by Gas Chromatography, 1988 Annual Book of ASTM Standards, Vol. 5.03, pp 78-88. American Society for Testing and Materials, Philadelphia.

ASTM E 1366-91. 1991. Standard Practice for the standardized aquatic microcosm: fresh water, Vol. 11.04. pp 1017-1051. American Society for Testing and Materials, Philadelphia.

Conquest, L.L. and Taub, F.B. 1989. Repeatability and reproducibility of the Standard Aquatic Microcosm: Statistical properties. In

U.M. Cowgill and L.R. Williams, eds., *Aquatic Toxicology and Hazard Assessment: 12th Volume, ASTM STP 1027.* American Society for Testing and Materials, Philadelphia, PA, pp. 159-177.

Crow, M.E. and Taub, F.B. 1979. Designing a microcosm bioassay to detect ecosystem level effects. *Intern. J. Environmental Studies.* 141-147.

Dickson, K.L., Waller, W.T., Kennedy, J.H. and Ammann, L.P. 1992. Assessing the relationship between ambient toxicity and instream biological response. *Env. Tox. Chem.* 11:1307-1322.

Hassell, M.P.H, Comins, N. and May, R.M. 1991. Spatial structure and chaos in insect population dynamics. *Nature* 353:255-258.

Haley, M.V., Johnson, D.W., Muse, Jr., W.T. and Landis, W.G. 1988. The Aquatic Toxicity and Fate of Brass Dust. *Aquatic Toxicology and Hazard Assessment: 10th Volume, ASTM STP 971*, W.J. Adams, G.A. Chapman, and W.G. Landis, Eds., American Society for Testing and Materials, Philadelphia, pp. 468-479.

Johnson, A.R. 1988a. Evaluating ecosystem response to toxicant stress: a state space approach. *Aquatic Toxicology and Hazard Assessment: 10th Volume, ASTM STP* 971, W.J. Adams, G.A. Chapman and W.G. Landis Eds., American Society for Testing and Materials, Philadelphia, pp. 275-285.

Johnson, A.R. 1988b. Diagnostic variables as predictors of ecological risk. *Environmental Management* 12:515-523.

Kratz, T.K., Frost, T.M. and Magnuson, J.J. 1987. Inferences from spatial and temporal variability in ecosystems: Long-term zooplankton data from lakes. *Amer. Nat.* 129:830-846.

Kersting, K. 1984. Development and use of an aquatic micro-ecosystem as a test system for toxic substances. Properties of an aquatic micro-ecosystem IV. *Int. Revue ges. Hydrobiol.* 69:567-607.

Kersting, K. 1985. Properties of an aquatic micro-ecosystem V. Ten years of observations of the prototype. *Verh. Internat. Verein. Limnol.* 22:3040- 3045.

Kersting, K. 1988. Normalized ecosystem strain in micro-ecosystems using different sets of state variables. *Verh. Internat. Verein. Limnol.* 23:1641-1646.

Kindig, A.C., Loveday, L.C. and Taub, F.B. 1983. Differential sensitivity of new versus mature synthetic microcosms to streptomycin sulfate treatment. *Aquatic Toxicology and Hazard Assessment: Sixth Symposium, ASTM 802.* W.E. Bishop, R.D. Cardwell and B.B. Heidolph Eds. American Society for Testing and Materials, Philadelphia, pp. 192-203.

Landis, W.G., Chester, N.A., Haley, M.V., Johnson, D.W., Muse, Jr., W.T. and Tauber, R.M. 1989. Utility of the Standardized Aquatic Microcosm as a Standard Method for Ecotoxicological Evaluation. *Aquatic Toxicology and Environmental Fate: Eleventh Volume, ASTM STP*

1007, G.W. Suter II and M.A. Lewis, Eds., American Society for Testing and Materials, Philadelphia, pp. 353-367.

Landis, W.G., Chester, N.A., and Haley, M.V. 1993. Evaluation of the Ability of *Alcaligenes denitrificans denitrificans* CR-1 to Degrade the Riot Control Agent CR Using the Standardized Aquatic Microcosm. *Environmental Toxicology and Risk Assessment, ASTM STP 1179*, Wayne G. Landis, Jane S. Hughes, and Michael A. Lewis, Eds., American Society for Testing and Materials, Philadelphia, pp. 159-177.

Landis, W.G., Haley, M.V. and Chester, N.A. 1993a. The use of the standardized aquatic microcosm in the evaluation of degradative bacteria in reducing impacts to aquatic ecosystems. In W.G. Landis, J. Hughes and M. Lewis., eds., *In press, Environmental Toxicology and Risk Assessment: First Volume, ASTM STP -1179*. American Society for Testing and Materials, Philadelphia, PA.

Landis, W.G., Matthews, R.A., Markiewicz, A.J., Shough, N.J. and Matthews, G.B. 1993b. Multivariate analysis of the impacts of turbine fuel using a standard aquatic microcosm toxicity test. *J. Env. Sci.* In Press.

Landis, W. G., Matthews, G. B., Matthews, R. A. and Sergeant, A. 1994. Application of multivariate techniques to endpoint determination, selection and evaluation in ecological risk assessment. *Environ. Toxicol. Chem.* In Press.

Matthews, G.B. and Hearne, J. 1991. Clustering without a metric. IEEE *Transactions on Pattern Analysis and Machine Intelligence*, 13:175-184.

Matthews, G.B. and Matthews, R.A. 1991. A model for describing community change. In *Pesticides in Natural Systems: How Can Their Effects Be Monitored? Proceeding of the Conference*, Environmental Research Laboratory/ORD, Corvallis, OR, EPA 9109/9-91/011.

Matthews, G. B., Landis, W. G. and Matthews, R. A. 1994. Nonmetric clustering and association analysis: implications for the evaluation of multispecies toxicity tests and field monitoring. Environmental *Toxicology and Risk Assessment-Third Volume, ASTM 1218*, Jane S. Hughes, Gregory R. Biddinger, and Eugene Mones, Eds., American Society for Testing and Materials, Philadelphia.

Matthews, R.A., Matthews, G.B. and Ehinger, W.J. 1991a. Classification and ordination of limnological data: a comparison of analytical tools. *Ecological Modeling*. 53:167-187.

Matthews, G.B., Matthews, R.A. and Hachmoller, B. 1991b. Mathematical analysis of temporal and spatial trends in the benthic macroinvertebrate communities of a small stream. *Canadian Journal of Fisheries and Aquatic Sciences*. 48:2184-2190.

May, R.M. and Oster, G.F. 1978. Bifurcations and dynamical complexity in simple ecological models. *Amer. Nat*. 110:573-599.

Taub, F.B. 1969. Gnotobiotic models of freshwater communities. Verh *Internat. Verein. Limnol.* 17, 485-496.

Taub, F.B. 1976. Demonstration of pollution effects in aquatic microcosms. *Intern J. Environmental Studies.* 10, 23-33.

Taub, F.B. 1988. Standardized aquatic microcosm - development and testing. Aquatic *Ecotoxicology* II.

Taub, F.B. 1989. Standardized aquatic microcosms. *Environm. Sci. Technol.* 23:1064-1066.

Taub, F.B., Kindig, A.C. and Conquest, L.L. 1987. Interlaboratory testing of a standardized aquatic microcosm. In W.J. Adams, G.A. Chapman and W.G. Landis, eds., *Aquatic Toxicology and Hazard Assessment: 10th Volume, ASTM STP 971.* American Society for Testing and Materials, Philadelphia, PA, pp. 385-405.

Taub, F.B., Kindig, A.C., Conquest, L.L. and Meador, J.P. 1988. Results of the interlaboratory testing of the Standardized Aquatic Microcosm protocol. In G. Suter and M. Lewis, eds., *Aquatic Toxicology and Hazard Assessment: Eleventh Symposium, ASTM.* American Society for Testing and Materials, Philadelphia, PA.

Taub, F.B. and Crow, M.E. 1978. Loss of a critical species in a model (laboratory) ecosystem. *Verh. Internat. Verein. Limnol.* 1270-1276.

Taub, F.B. , Crow, M.E. and Hartmann, H.J. 1980. Responses of aquatic microcosms to acute mortality. *Microcosms in Ecological Research.* Giesy, J.P. Jr. Technical Information Center, U. S. Department of Energy. Washington, D.C., 513-535.

Taub, F.B., Rose, K.A., Swartzman, G.L. and Taub, J.H. Submitted. Translating population toxicity to community effects. *Env. Tox. Chem.*

Westendorf, R.G. 1986. Performance aspects of volatile organics analysis by purge and trap capillary column gas chromatography with flame ionization detectors. Tekmar Technical Papers, Tekmar Company, Cincinnati, Ohio.

Joanna S. Jaworska,[1] Thomas G. Hallam,[2] Shandelle M. Henson,[3] William R. McKinney,[4] and Ray R. Lassiter[5]

ECOTOXICOLOGY OF PREDATOR - PREY COMMUNITIES: AN INDIVIDUAL - BASED MODELING APPROACH

REFERENCE: Jaworska, J. S., Hallam, T. G., Henson, S. M., McKinney, W. R., and Lassiter, R. R., "**Ecotoxicology of Predator - Prey Communities: An Individual - Based Modeling Approach**"Environmental Toxicology and Risk Assessment - Third Volume, ASTM STP 1218, Jane S. Hughes, Gregory R. Biddinger, and Eugene Mones, Eds., American Society for Testing and Materials, Philadelphia, 1995.

ABSTRACT: Physiologically structured population models are used to study the effects of nonpolar narcotic chemicals on two predator-prey community models. The biological focus is on the individual, which allows a discussion of exposure and effects, two necessary attributes of ecological risk assessment. Exposure is represented here by an exchange model between the environment and the organism with two possible routes - food and environment. Quantitative structure activity relationships (QSARs) are used to assess both lethality and chronic effects such as reduction in growth. Densities of lipid, carbohydrate and structure, variables used to describe an individual, are compiled to describe population dynamics. Variation among individuals is entirely responsible for the response of the population to toxic stress. Direct and indirect effects of stress on the community level of organization are observed for two model predator-prey systems:

[1]Graduate Research Associate, Environmental Toxicology Program, University of Tennessee, Knoxville, TN 37996-1300

[2] Professor, Department of Mathematics and Graduate Program in Ecology, University of Tennessee, Knoxville, TN 37996-1300

[3]Graduate Research Associate, Department of Mathematics, University of Tennessee, Knoxville, TN 37996-1300

[4]Assistant Professor, Department of Mathematics, North Carolina State University, Raleigh, NC 27695-8205

[5]Research Ecologist, Biology Branch, Environmental Research Laboratory, Environmental Protection Agency, Athens, GA 30613

rainbow trout *(Oncorhynchus mykiss)* - *Daphnia* and *Tetrahymena pyriformis* - *Escherichia coli.* The direct effects include changes in the lipid, structure, age and size distributions of individuals in the populations. An example of an indirect effect is starvation of predators caused by death of prey in particular size classes.

KEY WORDS: aquatic toxicology, community models, ecological risk assessment, individual - based models, *Daphnia magna, Oncorhynchus mykiss, Tetrahymena pyriformis, Escherichia coli*

INTRODUCTION

Risk assessment at the community or ecosystem level is in a rudimentary state of development. Many approaches for investigating the dynamics of higher ecological organizational levels employ highly aggregated models that focus on average properties of individuals in the populations. Recent efforts to represent populations by utilizing an individual - based approach have led to new dynamic perspectives that reflect realistic individual variation in populations and allow chemical exposure to be adequately treated (Hallam et al. 1990a). Implementing extensions of these ideas at the community level results in a physiologically oriented, mechanistic approach to community risk assessment.

The basis of community dynamics is contained in the individuals that compose the community and the interactions of these individuals. When the feeding mechanism of an individual predator on a prey population is prescribed, growth of the individual predator is determined by the predator individual model and mortality caused by this predator on the prey population can be assessed. With the information coupling the predator and prey organisms, it is possible to construct a predator - prey community from population formulations for the prey and predator.

A general methodology for studying a stressed and an unstressed individual - based community requires development of the following components:

1. Formulation of an individual model for each species in the community.
2. Development of a toxicant exposure model and an effect model as well as linking them to the individual model.
3. Formulation of the population models incorporating a diverse group of individuals.
4. Coupling population models into a community model.

We now indicate how each part of the protocol is modeled for community risk assessment purposes.

ECOLOGICAL RISK ASSESSMENT MODULES

Individual Models

The individual model incorporates biological information in order to describe the physiology of the organism and toxicological stress in a realistic and mechanistic way. Physiological variables that are crucial for describing dynamics of growth and reproduction of an single organism, those which might get affected during stress and those that determine toxicant distribution in the body need to be included in the model. Here, the individual models utilize energy budget techniques much like those suggested by Kooijman and Metz (1984) and Kooijman (1986).

We focus on two individual - based predator - prey models, a microbial *Tetrahymena p.* - *E.coli* system and a *Daphnia* - rainbow trout *(Oncorhynchus mykiss)* system, and illustrate some effects of exposure to nonpolar narcotics. Individual models of *Daphnia* and fish have been described previously in detail (Hallam et al. 1990b; Lassiter et al. 1993) and the reader is referred to those articles for details. The models for trout and *Daphnia* are systems of ordinary differential equations that describe the dynamics of the physiological components. However, developments for the microbial system are new (Jaworska 1993) and are individually - oriented in that they are rule based. We briefly indicate the life history utilized in the microbial system models.

The Life History Model of an Individual Tetrahymenid

The tetrahymenid model is related to the individual daphnid model (Hallam et al. 1990b) in that it represents *lipid* and *structure* (all nonlipid, noncarbohydrate dry mass, including protein and nucleic acids) dynamics but differs in several assumptions, some specific to the biology of the modeled organisms. In particular, due to importance of glycogen as a storage compartment, carbohydrate dynamics are also followed. Conversions between compartments are possible (i.e protein can be converted to lipid or carbohydrate). Ingested resource (carbohydrate, lipid, protein) is not necessarily assimilated to the corresponding compartment of the consumer or in special cases may not be assimilated at all. Feeding and reproduction are assumed to occur on discrete scales, while other processes like digestion and assimilation operate in a continuous manner. Energy requirements are computed based on the allometric relationship between the volume and the oxygen consumption of the individual. Amounts of lipid,carbohydrate and protein not used for energy purposes are assimilated. It is assumed that the growth of the protein compartment must be accompanied by proportional growth of the polar lipid compartment. Lipid not used to build structure is assimilated to the storage lipid compartment. Assimilation of carbohydrate is decoupled from lipid and protein assimilation in that it can only be assimilated to the carbohydrate compartment. The storage compartments, i.e neutral lipids and glycogen, also grow independently from each other but their growth is limited by the total mass of the organism.

Cell division into two identical daughter cells occurs in the model when the following three conditions are met simultaneously. First, the cell size is bigger than the reproductive size for a given food density; the reproductive size is a prescribed hyperbolic function of the food density. Second, the cell protein compartment is greater than a minimum size. Third, the nutritional status of the organism has to be sufficient to meet all energetic needs without utilization of the structure components, during the nonfeeding period prior to division. When all these conditions are met, the cell enters the reproductive mode. While in this mode, the organism does not feed but still can assimilate nutrients available in the storage vacuoles.

Sexual reproduction does not occur in cells such as *Tetrahymena p.* that have a micronucleus.

The Life History Model of Individual Bacterium, *E.coli*

The model is based on the developments of the biochemically structured model for *E.coli* formulated by Shuler and Domach (1983) and later simplified by Joshi and Palsson (1988). It expands the capabilities of their model by adding the process of starvation and a modification of the reproduction process. An individual bacterium is described by three pools: nucleic acids, proteins and cell envelop. Nucleic acids and protein form the proteinous part of the organism. The cell wall is composed of approximately 50% lipids and 50% complex carbohydrates. Cell geometry governs reproduction. The cell is cylindrical in shape with closed hemispherical ends. It grows in length and width in the cell cycle according to the growth of the pools. The reproduction process is initialized when the length of the organism reaches the reproductive length set by a hyperbolic function of the resource. From that time until division the cell does not elongate, rather it widens and builds a septum wall. At the moment when the length of the septum wall is equal to the diameter of the cell, separation of two daughter cells takes place.

Exposure Model

The exposure model coupled with the individual model is a modification of FGETS (Barber et al. 1988). This model, based upon a thermodynamic potential, represents the chemical exchange between an individual fish and its aqueous environment. This model assumes passive diffusion across gill membranes and across gut walls from ingestion of contaminated food. The model depends upon the total toxicant concentration in the organism, in the environment, and in the food and assumes immediate partitioning between the lipid, protein and aqueous phases of the organism. Internal instantaneous equilibration provides the worst case scenario for the chemical uptake because no more chemical can be allocated to compartments; however, it elicits a minimal depuration time (Lassiter and Hallam 1990).

Effects of Chemicals on Individuals

The basic ideas employed to assess the effects of chemicals on an individual and on a static population are given in (Hallam et al. 1990a; Lassiter and Hallam 1990). Quantitative structure activity relationships (QSARs) are used to assess acute effects such as mortality for fish (Veith et al. 1983) and *Daphnia* (Hermens et al. 1985) and chronic effects such as reduction in growth for *Tetrahymena* (Schultz et al. 1990) and *E.coli* (Jaworska and Schultz 1993). An effect is assumed to occur at the characteristic concentration in the reference phase, the aqueous portion of the organism (Lassiter and Hallam 1990). This representation allows for incorporation of both lethal and sublethal effects at the individual level. It is assumed that all individuals who reach a designated effect level, (for example, EC50 - the concentration where growth is reduced by 50%) in the reference phase, respond in an identical way as dictated by that effect. Morphology and body composition modify time to reach the threshold so that some individuals respond more quickly while others may escape the effect completely. The growth effects syndrome, when completely implemented, assumes that sublethal effects occur on a continuous scale and range from the no effect concentration through reduction in growth to the LC50 (the concentration that kills 50% of the exposed organisms) where mortality is assumed to occur. For narcosis effects, Lassiter (1991) indicates that r, the fractional reduction of enzyme sites that occurs through competitive inhibition, is a hyperbolic function in effect concentration and that the intercept of the quantitative dose-response representation is a continuous function of the reduction fraction r. This hyperbolic representation incorporates discrete empirical data such as the no observable effect, growth reduction, and mortality as depicted in Figure 1 for *Daphnia* in a continuous manner (Hallam et al. 1993) for a specific form of this hyperbolic function).

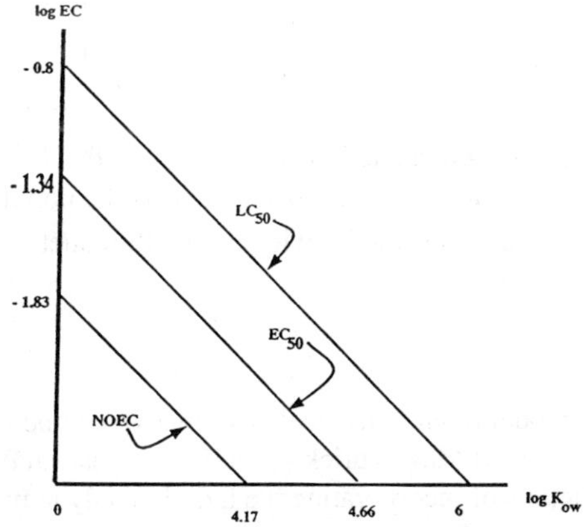

Figure 1. QSARs for 3 endpoints: LC50, the concentration that kills 50% of the exposed individuals; EC50, the 50% growth reduction concentration; NOEC, the no observed effect concentration. All bioassays are for *Daphnia magna*. The horizontal axis is the logarithm of the 1-octanol/ water partition coefficient. The vertical axis is the effect concentration in the environment (Lassiter and Hallam 1990). Data from Hermens et al. (1985).

If the time of exposure is equal to or less than a generation time then fractional reduction in growth of the population is equivalent to the same fractional reduction of growth of individuals in this population. However , the QSARs used in the microbial model study employ multigeneration endpoint, such as 48-h 50% growth inhibition for *Tetrahymena* or 10-h 50% growth inhibition for bacteria. In order to determine how growth of the average individual is reduced to produce known reduction in the population biomass, we have simulated both populations separately by reducing the food uptake function. We found an interesting nonlinear relationship between population and individual effects, which is best described by Figure 2.

The choice of the uptake function as the one reduced in the model is arbitrary. We reduced other physiological variables (e. g. assimilation rate) and obtained a similar effect.

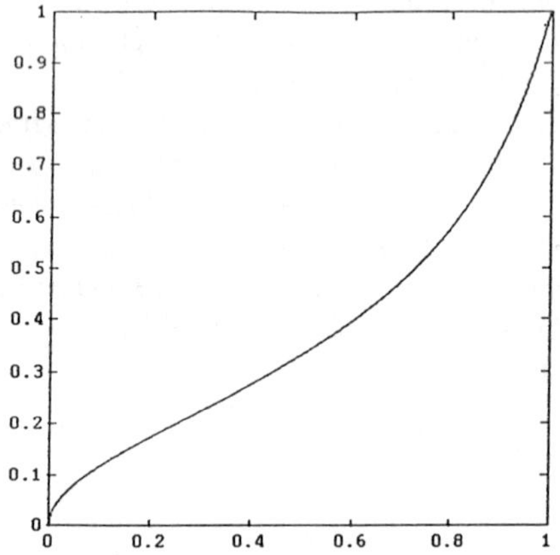

Figure 2. The relationship between reduction in biomass of the *E. coli* population and reduction in growth of the individuals. The horizontal axis is the population biomass reduction effect and the vertical axis is the individual growth reduction effect.

Population Model

Once the dynamic model of an individual is known, it can be incorporated into a population model via an extended McKendrick - von Foerster partial differential equation (Hallam et al. 1993); the details of incorporating the individual dynamics into a population are indicated in (Hallam et al. 1990a). This equation represents transport processes based upon a conservation law and is a hyperbolic partial differential equation of the form

$$\rho_t + \rho_a + \Sigma_i (\rho g_i)_{m_i} = - \mu\rho \qquad (1)$$

where the subscripts t, a, and m_i indicate partial derivatives with respect to that subscripted variable. In (1) , t represents time, a represents age, and m_i represents the physiological variables used to describe the individual. The sum in (1) ranges from i= 1, 2,...,n where n is the number of physiological variables used to structure the model of the individual. The physiological variables, m_i, are often determined by the particular problem being investigated. Two natural candidates for these variables in almost any population modeling endeavor are some measure of size and lipid. Size is a determining factor for some physiological processes such as ingestion and maintenance. Size of individuals is important at the community level because prey selection by a predator is often size dependent and the size of the predator determines the size of prey it can eat. Lipid is important for many aspects of energetics and reproduction. Our original interest in these variational structured problems was from the ecotoxicological perspective where many toxicological effects relate to the fraction of lipid present in the chemically stressed organism. The function g_i is the growth rate of the physiological variable m_i in a model that represents the individual organism. The dependent variable $\rho = \rho(t,a,m_1,m_2,...,m_n)$ is the population density function, and μ represents the mortality rate function of the population.

In order for the problem to make sense biologically and for the mathematical problem to be well posed, it is necessary to prescribe initial and boundary conditions for the population. The initial distribution

$$\rho(0,a,m_1,m_2,...,m_n) = \varphi(a,m_1,m_2,...m_n)$$

describes the population at time $t = 0$. A boundary condition, often called the renewal equation, indicates the birth process of the population. In structured models this can have numerous forms. For example, one form is

$$\rho(t,0,m_1(0),m_2(0),...,m_n(0)) =$$

$$\int...\int\beta(t,a,m_{10},m_{20},...,m_{n0},m_1,m_2,...,m_n)\rho(t,a,m_1,m_2,...,m_n)da\,dm_1dm_2...dm_n,$$

where β is the fertility rate function that describes the number of eggs with the initial physiological dimensions $m_{i0} = m_i(0),\ i = 1,2,...,n$ produced by a organism of age a and physiological state $m_1,...,m_n$ at time t. The function β is determined by the individual model in that the allocation to eggs must be represented at the times of reproduction for each organism.

For fish and *Daphnia* the boundary condition is required to describe the birth process. The functions g_i describe the individual dynamics of the lipid and protein compartments.The equations for *Tetrahymena* and *E.coli* dynamics do not require a boundary condition due to the reproductive scheme of these organisms (Metz and Diekmann 1986; Sinko and Streifer, 1971). This modeling approach together with the technique for solving it (the method of characteristics) is advantageous because it allows for incorporation of both individual and toxicant dynamics at the population level.

The Predator - Prey Model

To create a community from the population approach described above we first consider a trout - *Daphnia* example. We need only specify how each of the individuals in the fish population feeds upon the *Daphnia* population and how subsequent mortality due to predation is assessed in the *Daphnia* population. An individual fish has a prey window, a range in the size of prey that it can eat, whose boundaries are determined by linear functions of the predator length. The individual fish is assumed to have access to the entire prey population (to minimize computations, the prey population is scaled for a particular subset of the lake) and, according to the density of daphnids it encounters, captures, and grows from the daphnids in its prey window.

In the microbial food chain model, ciliates feed on bacteria without size selection and have access to the entire prey population. In addition, *Tetrahymena* excrete by-products, called autochtonous substances, of metabolism which are excellent nutrients for bacteria (Sambanis 1985). Their exact composition is not known but included are amino acids and carbohydrates. The model assumes that the amount of these substances generated is proportional to the biomass of tetrahymenids with the carbohydrates to amino acids amount always being in a fixed ratio. This creates an interesting feedback in the system.

The two communities, trout - *Daphnia* and *Tetrahymena - E.coli* have different resource dynamics. The first is a continuous culture with constant concentrations of algae serving as a sources of food for different ecotypes of *Daphnia.* The second is a batch setting where nutrients are depleted. Both models focus on physiological processes and reference fixed nominal environmental conditions.

RESULTS AND DISCUSSION

Both predator - prey systems are investigated numerically with the nominal, unstressed simulations compared to simulations with toxicant stress. We report results of two toxicant releases. The first stress is near the starting time of the simulation when the community is not well organized. The second is in the middle of the simulation, after the community was given more time to organize. The relationship between toxic stress and extinction is also discussed.

There are conclusions drawn from the analysis of the individual - based predator - prey system that agree with conclusions obtained from classical predator - prey models. There is a community threshold of persistence; when the mortality scale factor is below this threshold, there is ultimate extinction of the fish population. This extinction can occur through two obvious avenues. One is that the fish are not the appropriate size to eat available daphnids. In this case they can find nothing to eat, the fish population starves and goes to extinction, and the *Daphnia* population survives. A second extinction behavior is that the fish eat all available daphnids, the *Daphnia* population crashes, the fish population then goes to extinction and, consequently, the complete community goes to extinction. The threshold is clearly a function of the scale factors associated with each of the populations and the physiological size structures in the population.

Figure 3 consists of graphs representing the age structures of the *Daphnia* and trout populations in a stressed simulation of the dynamical community model. The simulation is initiated by putting the two populations together and letting the predators initiate feeding on the prey. There is an organizational period for the community, followed by the dynamics of the mature community. Here, the chemical stressor is applied after the community is organized. Young fish with small lipid storages are affected. The stressed *Daphnia* population becomes more diverse in age than occurs in the nominal run, probably due to a release in predation pressure coupled with the toxic effects. This diversity in age structure has also been observed for the *Daphnia* population under chronic, sublethal stress but without predation (Hallam et al. 1993). As illustrated in Figure 3, the diversity in age is even more than in the healthy community. The undisturbed portion of this figure before the toxic stress occurs may be used for comparison with the dynamics of Figure 4 where the effects of the nonpolar narcotic chemical release occurs early in the community organizational stage. The most prominent effects are on the younger fish and as well as the entire *Daphnia* population where community organization is delayed.

This structured predator - prey system allows investigation of the processes and mechanisms of interactions between two populations. We tend to look for features of the system that are fundamental to the understanding of the nature of predation. This requires finding basic attributes of populations and determining what changes ensue when the two populations involved in the predator - prey interaction are coupled. The intrinsic oscillatory frequencies present in population dynamics represent population markers that might be affected by coupling the populations. There are longer term *Daphnia* frequencies (50 - 250 days) that are of a similar order as the reproductive frequency of the fish (1 year). Consequently, it might be expected that these frequencies could be modified by the interactions of individuals. We have found this to be the case. Different numerical simulations show that the long term frequency of the prey, *Daphnia,* and the reproductive period of the predator, trout, can be altered through community interactions. Other changes due to community interactions and perturbations caused by toxicant stress are currently under investigation.

Because of the second model's totally different resource setting - a batch culture - in which environmental conditions constantly change, it is important to follow the amount of organic material circulating in the environment such as dead organisms and feces. As time progresses more and more toxicant is bound to this organic material, thus providing a buffer of protection for the living species. During mild stress, it is possible that toxicant is not available in sufficient concentration at the end of the simulation to cause any adverse effect although initially there were effects. The dynamics of such a community is generally only slightly perturbed, in that it takes longer for the community to organize, compared to the nominal behavior. With initial predation at low levels, the bacterial population is not depleted as fast as in the nominal run and the massive death of ciliates occurs later. This causes the shift of the ciliate "dip" in time (Figure 5). Figure 5 demonstrates the effects of a toxic chemical on the *Tetrahymena - E.coli* community. Here, the dynamic lipid

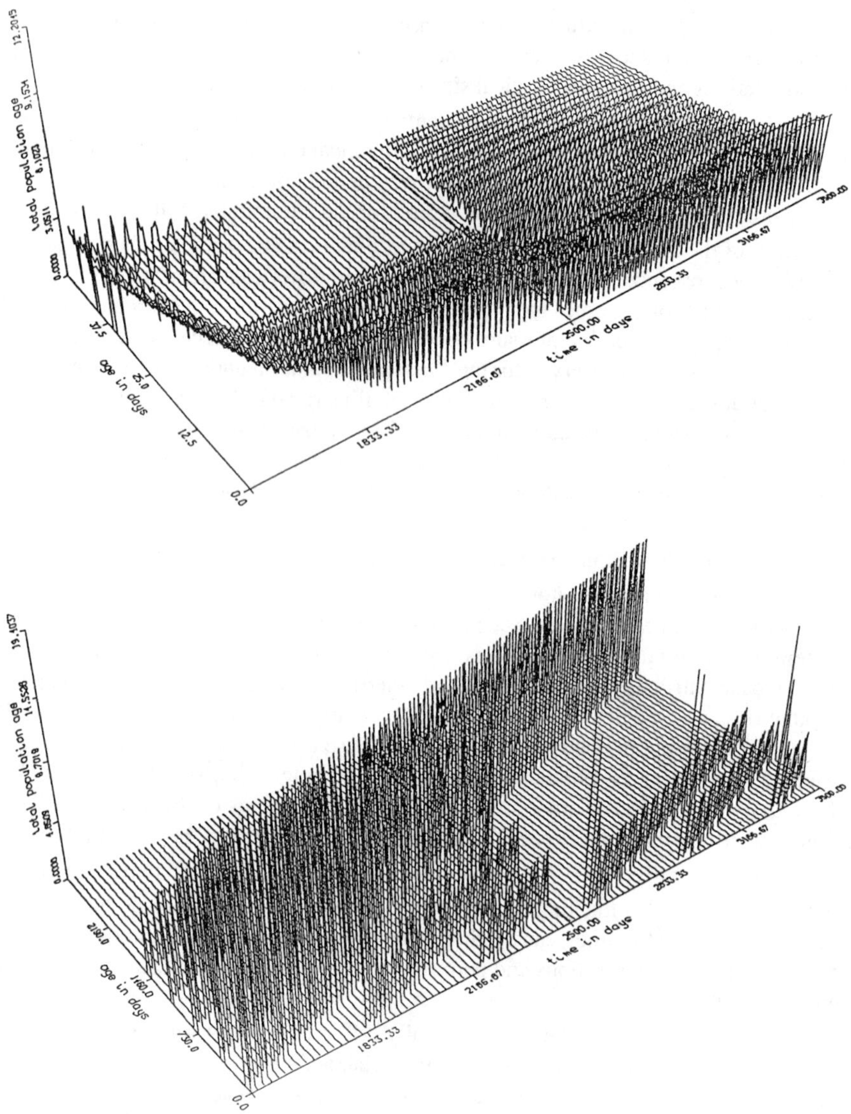

Figure 3. The distribution of age in the *Daphnia* and trout populations as a function of time. The graphs of the simulation are for 1500 - 3500 days and the community was exposed to a toxicant from 2503 - 2505.3 days. The right horizontal axis is the time axis. The left horizontal axis is the age of the individual. The vertical axis is the log of the number of individuals with a given age. Top: *Daphnia magna*; Bottom: *Oncorhynchus mykiss*.

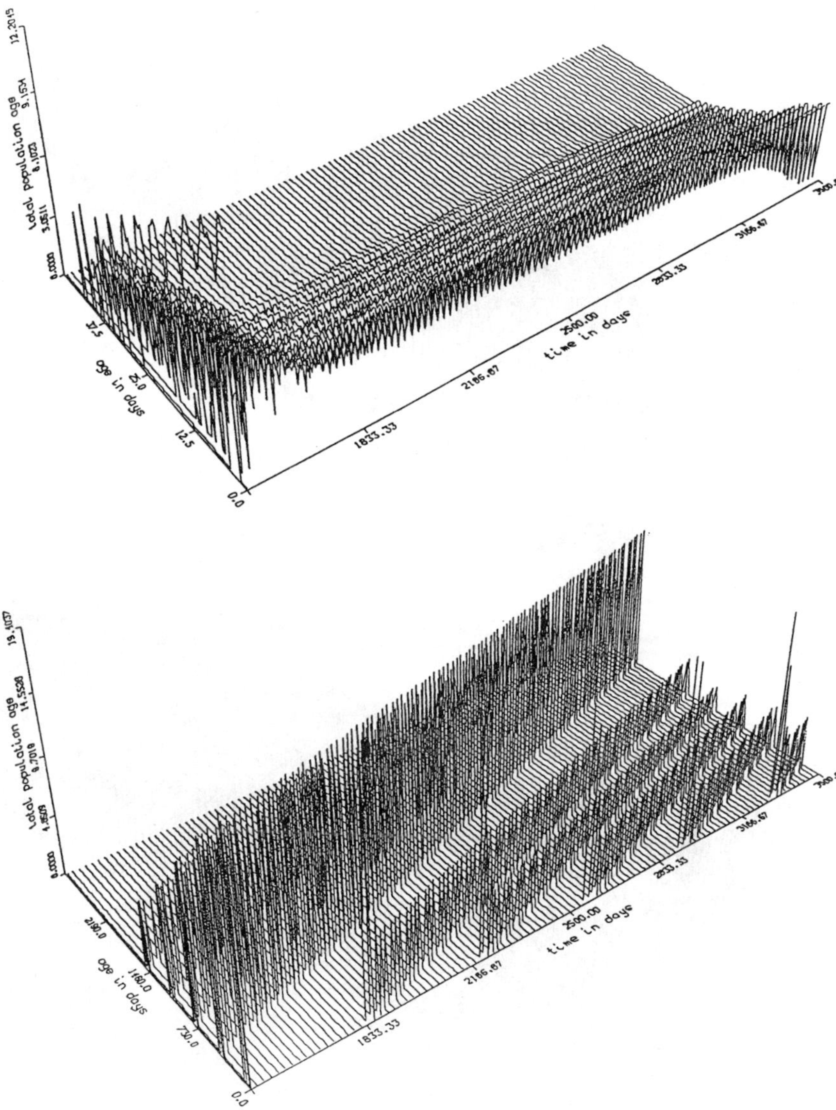

Figure 4. The distribution of age in the *Daphnia* and trout populations as a function of time. The graphs of the simulation are for 1500 - 3500 days and the community was exposed to a toxicant from 1503 - 1505.3 days. The right horizontal axis is the time axis. The left horizontal axis is the age of the individual. The vertical axis is the log of the number of individuals with a given age. Top: *Daphnia magna*; Bottom: *Oncorhynchus mykiss*.

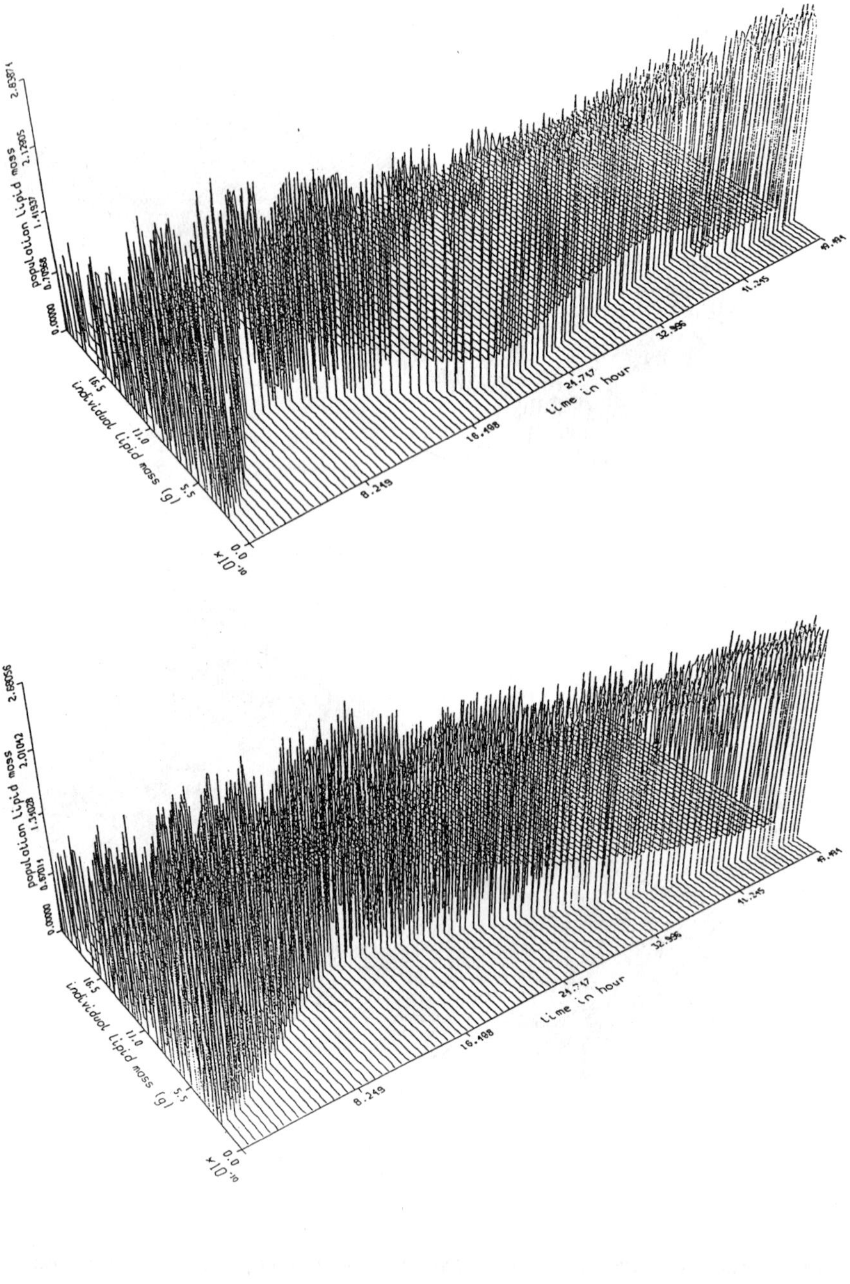

Figure 5. The distribution of lipid in the *Tetrahymena pyriformis* population as a function of time. The graphs of the simulation are for 0 to 50 hours. The right horizontal axis is the time axis. The left horizontal axis is the lipid content of the individual. The vertical axis is the log of the number of individuals with a given lipid content. Top: Unstressed simulation. Bottom: The community was exposed to a toxicant from 0 - 50 hours.

distribution is shown for the stressed and unstressed *Tetrahymena* population. Lipid distributions are examined because of their importance during toxic stress by lipophilic chemicals. Note the delay in development that is expected because the growth rate of the tetrahymenids is reduced by the stressor.

Another important feature of this community is that ciliates and bacteria are not equally susceptible to the toxicant. This becomes apparent under severe stress. Based on QSARs analysis, bacteria are less sensitive than ciliates. Therefore, it is common to observe that only one population - the ciliates - is adversely affected. This lowers the predation pressure on the bacteria population which escape the control and, subsequently, bloom. The exploding bacteria population provides excellent food conditions for the ciliates. However, the remaining predators are unable to fully utilize the resource because of toxic stress reflected as reduced food uptake, cessation of growth, or ultimately, starvation. If the decreased uptake of food does not meet energy requirements, tetrahymenids have to utilize their storage. In the situation where this continues for a sufficiently long period, starvation ensues. Such behavior of bacterial dominance is well documented in the wastewater literature. Depending on the water quality, different organisms dominate, with bacteria surviving in the most contaminated waters.

When both populations are affected, there are two types of outcomes. First, the stress has to be very toxic to the ciliate population in order to have an impact on the bacterial population. Then, the ciliates die off quickly, the bacteria are released from predation but do not bloom as before because their growth is reduced by toxicant stress. The case when both populations die off is the least interesting; here, extinction of ciliates proceeds extinction of bacteria.

Comparison of toxicant response to both systems reveals that despite dramatic differences such as continuous versus batch culture, acute versus sublethal stress, temporary presence of the toxicant versus continuous presence we can find some commonalities. In particular, stress in the middle of the simulation produces different effects in both communities than stress during the community organizational period. It is hypothesized that as communities evolve over time and ultimately reach a more organized state where initial transient behavior has damped, certain toxic stresses have less disrupting effects. In the *Daphnia* and fish population models, as time progresses, there is an ecotype that dominates population dynamics, a behavior called "survival of the fittest". In both predator - prey models, reduction in diversity from the initial distribution is noted in the predator population. Relatively small size individuals predominate in stressed environments. On the other hand, initial diversity of prey population tends to remain.

ACKNOWLEDGMENT. This research was supported in part by the U. S. Environmental Protection Agency through Cooperative Agreements CR 816081 and XE 819569.

REFERENCES

Barber, M. C., Suarez, L. A., and Lassiter, R. R., 1988, "Kinetic Exchange of Nonpolar Organic Pollutants by Fish," Environmental Toxicology and Chemistry, Vol. 7, pp. 545-558.

Hallam, T. G., Lassiter, R. R., Li, J., and McKinney, W., 1990a, "Toxicant Induced Mortality in Models of *Daphnia* Populations," Environmental Toxicology and Chemistry, Vol.9, pp. 597- 621.

Hallam, T. G., Lassiter R. R., Li J. and Suarez L.A., 1990b, "Modelling Individuals Employing an Integrated Energy Response: Application to *Daphnia,*" Ecology, Vol. 71, pp. 938-954.

Hallam, T. G., Canziani, G. A., and Lassiter, R. R., 1993, "Sublethal Narcosis and Population Persistence: A Modeling Study on Growth Effects," Environmental Toxicology and Chemistry, Vol. 12., pp. 947 - 954.

Hermens, J., Broekhuyzen, E., Canton, H. and Wegman, R., 1985, "QSARs and Mixture Toxicity Studies of Alcohols and Chlorohydrocarbons: Effects on Growth of *Daphnia magna*". Aquatic Toxicology, Vol. 6, pp. 209-217.

Jaworska, J. S., 1993, "The Ecology and Toxicology of a Predator - Prey System: *Tetrahymena pyriformis - E. coli*: A Modelling Study with an Individual - Based Approach," Ph.D. dissertation, University of Tennessee, Knoxville.

Jaworska , J.S. and Schultz, T.W., 1993, "Mechanism - Based Comparisons of Toxicities Elicited by Industrial Chemicals in Procariotic and Eucariotic Systems, " (submitted).

Joshi,A. and Palsson, B. O., 1988, "*Escherichia coli* Growth Dynamics: A Three - Pool Biochemically Based Description," Biotechnology and .Bioengineering, Vol. 31, pp. 102-116.

Kooijman, S. A. L. M., and Metz J. A. J., 1984, "On the Dynamics of Chemically Stressed Populations: The Deduction of Consequences from Effects on Individuals," Ecotoxicology and Environmental Safety, Vol.8, pp. 254-274.

Koojiman, S. A. L. M., 1986, "Population Dynamics on the Basis of Budgets," In J.A.J. Metz and O.Diekmann, eds., The Dynamics of Physiologically Structured Populations, Lecture Notes in Biomathematics, Vol. 68, Springer -Verlag,

Berlin, pp. 266-297.

Lassiter, R. R., 1991, "A Theoretical Basis for Predicting Sublethal Effects of Toxic Chemicals," Research Report, U.S. Environmental Protection Agency, Environmental Research Laboratory - Athens, GA.

Lassiter, R. R. and Hallam, T. G., 1990, "Survival of the Fattest:: Implications for Acute Effects of Lipophilic Chemicals on Populations," Environmental Toxicology and Chemistry, Vol .9, pp. 585-595.

Lassiter, R. R., Hallam, T. G., and Henson, S. M., 1993, " Modelling fish population dynamics: A physiologically based perspective," (to appear).

Metz, J.A.J and Diekmann, O., 1986, The Dynamics of Physiologically Structured Populations, Lecture Notes in Biomathematics, Vol. 68, Springer-Verlag, Berlin, Germany.

Sambanis , S. 1985, "Experimental and Modelling Studies on the Dynamics of Cultures of the Ciliate *Tetrahymena pyriformis* Grown on Several Bacterial Species," Ph.D dissertation, University of Minnesota.

Schultz, T.W., Wyatt N.L., and Lin D.T., 1990, "Structure-Toxicity Relationships for Nonpolar Narcotics: A Comparison of Data from the *Tetrahymena*, Photobacterium and *Pimephales* Systems ", Bulletin of Environmental Contamination and Toxicology, Vol.44, pp. 67-72.

Shuler, M. L. and Domach, M. M., 1983, "Mathematical Models of the Growth of Individual Cells: Tools for Testing Biochemical Mechanisms," In Foundations of Biochemical Engineering, Kinetics and Thermodynamics in Biological Systems, ACS Symposium Series, Vol. 207, pp. 93-134.

Sinko , J.W. and Streifer W., 1971, "A Model for Populations Reproducing By Binary Fission," Ecology, Vol. 52, pp. 330-335.

Veith,G.D., Call D.J. and Brooke L.T., 1983, "Structure-Toxicity Relationships for the Fathead Minnow, *Pimephales promelas*: Narcotic Industrial Chemicals," Canadian Journal of Fisheries and Aquatic Sciences, Vol.40, pp. 743-748.

T. Wayne Schultz,[1] Joanna S. Jaworska,[2] and Robert S. Hunter[3]

VOLUME FRACTION ANALYSES FOR SELECTED MECHANISMS OF TOXIC ACTION

REFERENCE: Schultz, T. W., Jaworska, J. S., and Hunter, R. S., **"Volume Fraction Analyses for Selected Mechanisms of Toxic Action,"** Environmental Toxicology and Risk Assessment - Third Volume, ASTM STP 1218, Jane S. Hughes, Gregory R. Biddinger, and Eugene Mones, Eds., American Society for Testing and Materials, Philadelphia, 1995.

ABSTRACT: Recently, it was demonstrated, using nonpolar and polar narcotics, that volume fraction analyses can be used as a tool for distinguishing different mechanisms of action. The present study expanded upon this thesis by evaluating chemicals thought to act through the weak acid respiratory uncoupler and primary amine narcosis mechanisms. Toxicity data used in these evaluations were the 96-hour flow through 50 percent mortality for the fathead minnow *Pimephales promelas* and the 48-hour static 50 percent inhibitory growth concentration data for axenic cultures of the ciliate *Tetrahymena pyriformis*. The target/water partition coefficients (K_{tw}) were analyzed and assumed to be a power function of K_{ow} ($K_{tw} = K_{ow}^{(1-a)}$) where "a" describes hydrophobicity of the target site and assumed to be constant for a given mechanism of action. The "a" values and the mean volume fraction (MVF) for fish and ciliates, were determined for each mechanism of action. The results suggests volume fraction analyses can be used to distinguish different mechanisms of action by meeting one of the following criteria: 1) if "a" values are different, MVF values do not matter; 2) if "a" values are the same, MVF values must be different.

KEY WORDS: narcosis, respiratory uncoupling, volume fraction analyses, *Tetrahymena pyriformis*, *Pimephales promelas*

The "critical volume" hypothesis states that reversible, physical toxic responses occur when the toxicant occupies a specific amount of space at the molecular target site. This concept first proposed by Overton (See Lipnick 1991) has been examined in the studies of Mullins

[1]Professor, College of Veterinary Medicine, [2]Graduate Student, Environmental Toxicology Program, The University of Tennessee, P.O. Box 1071, Knoxville, TN 37901-1071 USA.

[3]Supervisory Application Programmer, Natural Resources Research Institute, University of Minnesota-Duluth, 3151 Miller Trunk Highway, Duluth, MN 55811 USA.

(1954) and Seeman (1972). More recently, this hypothesis has been reviewed by Abernethy et al. (1988).

Abernethy and Mackay (1987) proposed the use of the volume fraction (V_f) correlation as a means of quantitatively examining the "critical volume" hypothesis. In their paper, they provided theoretical grounds and methodology for calculations. Additionally, they tested the hypothesis of a constant V_f for the narcosis mode of action with the analyses of data for 113 chemicals and 4 test systems. Although they performed just one analysis, the result supported the idea of a constant V_f. Drummond and Russom (1991) noted the difference between mode and mechanism of toxic action. Mode refers to what happens at the organismal level whereas, mechanism refers to what happens at the biochemical level. More recently, Jaworska and Schultz (1993) demonstrated that V_f analyses can be used to distinguish mechanisms of toxic action using classical nonpolar and polar narcotics. They observed that the relative toxicity of both nonpolar and polar narcotics, measured in both the fathead minnow lethality assay and the *Tetrahymena* population growth assay was linear to the 1-octanol/water partition coefficient (log K_{ow}). Analyses of target hydrophobicity by determination of "a" indicated the hydrophobicity of the molecular site of action was constant for chemicals eliciting the same mechanism of action but distinct for a given test system. Previously, mean volume fraction analyses indicated that the V_f in the target phase was constant for each mechanism of action regardless of test system and protocol.

The present investigation expands this thesis by evaluating weak acid respiratory uncouplers and amine narcotics, two other groups of non-reactive chemicals thought to act through distinct mechanisms of toxic action. Additionally, the present study compares the results of volume fraction analyses for the four toxic mechanisms.

MATERIALS AND METHODS

Toxicity Data

The toxicity data used in these computations were from two test systems, 96-h flow-through 50% mortality (LC_{50}) assay for the fathead minnow *Pimephales promelas* and 48-h static 50% inhibitory growth concentration (IGC_{50}) assay for axenic cultures of the ciliate *Tetrahymena pyriformis*. Fathead minnow data was from the literature (Center for Lake Superior Environmental Studies, 1984; 1985; 1986; 1988; 1990). Ciliate data was from Schultz et al. (1991a; 1991b) or experimentally determined following the procedure outlined by Schultz et al. (1990a).

Chemicals

Chemicals selected for these analyses included weak acid respiratory uncouplers, [divided into a training set (n = 12) evaluated in both test systems and validation set (n = 13) evaluated only in the *Tetrahymena* system] and amine narcotics, i.e., alkyl- and/or aryl-substituted primary amines, [similarly, divided into a training set (n = 17) and validation set (n = 17)].

1-octanol/water partition coefficient, pK_a, and molar volume determinations

Log K_{ow} values were computer estimated by MEDCHEM CLOGP version 3.53 (Leo and Weininger 1988) or retrieved as measured values from the same program. Each pK_a value (data not shown) was calculated using the computer-assisted version (Hunter 1988) of the Perrin method (Perrin et al. 1981). For molar volume calculation, the SMILES string (Anderson et al. 1987) was converted to three-dimensional coordinates via CONCORD version 2.9.1. The MAXMIN2 module of SYBYL version 5.41C was used in a minimization procedure and the local minimal energy configuration determined. The molar volume values were calculated from the Van der Waals surface of this configuration.

QSAR Analyses

Fathead minnow LC_{50} and *Tetrahymena* IGC_{50} values were converted to log inverse mmol/L and used as dependent variables. Log K_{ow} values were used as the independent variable. For QSAR development, the least-squares method of the General Linear Model (GLM) routine of Statistical Analysis System (SAS) software (SAS Institute Inc. 1989) was employed.

Volume Fraction Analyses

Based on the assumption that the toxicant reaches thermodynamic equilibrium in the tested system, Abernethy and Mackay (1987) presented a means of computing V_f of a chemical in the target phase. This work has been reviewed by Jaworska and Schultz (1993) and provides a working thesis for this investigation. Briefly,

$$V_f = C_w \cdot MV \cdot K_{tw} \quad (1)$$

where C_w is the toxicant concentration in water required to elicit a 50% biological response, MV is the molar volume and, K_{tw} is the target/water partition coefficient. In this study, C_w values were given in mmol/L and MV in ml/mole. A correction factor of 10^{-6} was used to account for the differences in units. V_f is dimensionless. Abernethy et al. (1988) postulated that K_{tw} could be estimated by using K_{ow} to the power of (1 - a), i.e., $K_{tw} = K_{ow}^{(1 - a)}$. Substitution into Eq. (1) results in Eq. (2):

$$V_f = 10^{-6} \cdot C_w \cdot MV \cdot K_{ow}^{(1-a)} \quad (2)$$

with rearrangement leading to Eq. (3):

$$\log V_f + a \log (K_{ow}) = \log (10^{-6} \cdot C_w \cdot MV \cdot K_{ow}). \quad (3)$$

A plot of log $(10^{-6} \cdot C_w \cdot MV \cdot K_{ow})$ versus log K_{ow} gives a line where the slope is an estimate of "a" and the intercept an estimate of log V_f. While "a" was computed using simple regression analysis of log $(10^{-6} \cdot C_w \cdot MV \cdot K_{ow})$ versus log K_{ow}, MVF was computed as the average of the individual V_f's determined by the previous equation. The latter method was chosen because it allowed for the detection of possible outliers. Regression analyses were conducted using the GLM routine of SAS.

RESULTS

Structure-Toxicity Relationships

Table 1 is a summary of the relative toxicity, hydrophobicity and molar volume for each of the 62 chemicals used in these studies. Three chemicals tridecylamine, 4-decylaniline and 4-dodecylaniline did not elicit a toxic response in the *Tetrahymena* system at saturation. Regression analyses of log fish toxicity (log FT) versus log K_{ow} for both the weak acid respiratory uncoupler and amine narcotic mechanism of action are summarized in Table 2. Equations [4] and [5], represent the structure-toxicity models for uncouplers and amine narcotics, respectively. The high r^2 values of each QSAR reflect strong predictability and are an indication of the high quality of the QSARs.

TABLE 1--Relative toxicities, hydrophobicity and molar volume of selected weak acid respiratory uncouplers and amine narcotics.

	Chemical	CAS #[a]	log FT[b]	log CT[c]	log K_{ow}[d]	MV[e]
1	2,6-dinitrophenol	573-56-8	0.666	0.573	1.22	117.0
2	2,4-dinitrophenol	51-28-5-1	1.228	1.096	1.54	118.1
3	2,5-dinitrophenol	329-71-5	1.739	0.929	1.75	117.3
4	2,4-dinitroaniline	97-02-9	1.091	0.716	1.84	121.6
5	2,6-dinitro-4-methylphenol	609-93-8	2.058	1.230	2.47	133.4
6	2,4-dinitro-1-naphthol	605-69-6	1.838	1.585	3.09	156.1
7	4-phenylazophenol	1689-82-3	2.229	1.655	3.18	165.1
8	2,3,5,6-tetrachloroaniline	3481-20-7	2.932	1.762	4.10	134.2
9	2,3,4,5-tetrachlorophenol	4901-51-3	2.752	2.004	4.21	130.3
10	pentachloropyridine	2176-62-7	2.728	1.675	4.34	131.4
11	pentachlorophenol	87-86-5	3.037	2.568	5.12	142.3
12	pentabromophenol	608-71-9	3.720	2.664	5.69	166.4
13	2,6-dinitroaniline	606-22-4	...	0.941	1.37	120.3
14	3,5-dinitroaniline	618-87-1	...	0.941	1.37	121.8
15	4,6-dinitro-2-methylphenol	534-52-1	...	1.329	2.56	132.3
16	4-phenylazoaniline	60-09-3	...	1.421	2.62	168.6
17	2,6-dibromo-4-nitrophenol	99-28-5	...	1.357	3.05	133.8
18	2,4-dichloro-6-nitrophenol	609-89-2	...	1.750	3.21	124.6
19	2,4-dichloro-6-nitroaniline	2683-43-4	...	1.170	3.22	128.1
20	4,5-dichloro-2-nitroaniline	6641-64-1	...	1.714	3.22	128.8
21	2,4-dibromo-6-nitroaniline	827-23-6	...	1.170	3.52	138.0
22	2,6-diiodo-4-nitrophenol	305-85-1	...	1.812	3.76	157.1
23	2,3,5,6-tetrachlorophenol	935-95-5	...	2.219	4.31	131.0
24	2,3,4,5-tetrachloroaniline	634-83-3	...	1.956	4.33	135.5
25	tetrabromo-2-methylphenol	576-55-6	...	2.573	5.70	167.6
26	propylamine	107-10-8	-0.717	-0.851	0.48	71.8
27	(sec)butylamine	33966-50-6	-0.575	-0.803	0.70	87.8
28	aniline	62-53-3	-0.088	0.119	0.90	88.0
29	butylamine	109-73-9	-0.564	-0.704	0.97	88.8
30	benzylamine	100-46-9	0.021	-0.253	1.09	104.1
31	4-toluidine	106-49-0	-0.143	-0.023	1.39	103.6
32	amylamine	110-58-7	-0.308	-0.609	1.49	104.6

TABLE 1--Relative toxicities, hydrophobicity and molar volume of selected weak acid respiratory uncouplers and amine narcotics. (Continued)

	Chemical	CAS #[a]	log FT[b]	log CT[c]	log K_{ow}[d]	MV[e]
33	4-ethylaniline	589-16-2	0.044	0.220	1.96	120.0
34	hexylamine	111-26-2	0.252	-0.336	2.06	122.6
35	heptylamine	111-68-2	0.723	0.101	2.57	137.9
36	1-methylheptylamine	693-16-3	1.403	0.397	2.82	154.2
37	octylamine	111-86-4	1.396	0.505	3.05	155.3
38	4-butylaniline	104-13-2	1.165	1.045	3.15	153.3
39	nonylamine	112-2-9	1.822	1.594	3.57	171.5
40	decylamine	2016-57-1	2.184	1.952	4.10	187.6
41	undecylamine	7307-55-3	2.912	2.261	4.63	203.7
42	4-octylaniline	16245-79-7	3.233	2.337	5.27	218.9
43	tridecylamine	2869-34-3	3.487	NTAS[f]	5.68	235.8
44	4-decylaniline	37529-30-9	3.576	NTAS	6.32	252.4
45	(tert)butylamine	75-64-9	...	-1.009	0.57	88.1
46	1-ethylpropylamine	616-24-0	...	-0.939	1.23	105.2
47	(+/-)1-methylbenzylamine	618-36-0	...	-0.323	1.40	121.4
48	2-phenethylamine	64-04-0	...	0.107	1.43	121.6
49	b-methylphenethylamine	582-22-9	...	-0.312	1.83	137.1
50	3-phenyl-1-propylamine	2038-57-5	...	0.254	1.96	137.4
51	2-(4-tolyl)ethylamine	3261-62-9	...	-0.069	2.08	153.2
52	1-aminonaphthalene	134-32-7	...	0.221	2.09	126.9
53	1-naphthalenemethylamine	118-31-0	...	0.468	2.27	143.8
54	2-isopropylaniline	643-28-7	...	0.013	2.33	136.4
55	4-propylaniline	2696-84-6	...	0.494	2.49	136.0
56	4-phenyl-1-butylamine	2046-18-6	...	0.133	2.49	153.7
57	(+/-)-1-naphthylethylamine	42882-31-5	...	0.414	2.58	159.5
58	2-propylaniline	1821-39-2	...	0.059	2.62	137.3
59	4-pentyaniline	33228-44-3	...	1.678	3.68	169.4
60	4-cyclohexylaniline	6373-50-8	...	1.087	3.69	175.3
61	4-hexylaniline	33228-45-4	...	2.047	4.21	186.2
62	4-dodecylaniline	104-42-7	...	NTAS	7.38	285.2

[a]Chemical Abstract Service registry number.
[b]Log fish toxicity in $(mmol/L)^{-1}$.
[c]Log ciliate toxicity in $(mmol/L)^{-1}$.
[d]Log 1-octanol/water partition coefficient from MEDCHEM CLOGP 3.53.
[e]Molar volume in ml/mol.
[f]Not toxic at saturation.

TABLE 2--Regression analyses of log fish toxicity versus log 1-octanol/water partition coefficient.

Group	Slope	Intercept	r^2	n	Eq.
uncouplers	0.5864	0.2841	0.923	12	4
amine narcotics	0.8083	-1.1774	0.973	17	5

Similarly, log ciliate toxicity (log CT) versus log K_{ow} analyses are summarized in Table 3. Again, the high r^2 values indicate the high quality of each QSAR and show strong predictability. Neither the slopes nor intercepts of the respiratory uncouplers training and validation sets, Eqs. [6] and [7], respectively, were statistically different at $\alpha = 0.05$. The data for Eqs. [6] and [7] were combined and evaluated in Eq. [8]. The QSAR for the amine narcotic training set is presented in Eq. [9]. As previously noted by Schultz et al. (1991a), aniline was an outlier being more toxic than predicted. Removal of this chemical and reevaluation resulted in Eq. [10]. Neither the slopes nor intercepts of Eqs. [9] and [10] are statistically different. However, as expected, the coefficient of determination improved with the latter regression. The QSAR for the amine narcotic validation set is presented in Eq. [11]. Neither the slopes nor intercepts of the amine narcosis training and validation sets, Eqs. [10] and [11], respectively, were statistically different. The data for these equations were combined and evaluated in Eq. [12].

TABLE 3--Regression analyses of log ciliate toxicity versus log 1-octanol/water partition coefficient.

Group	Slope	Intercept	r^2	n	Eq.
uncouplers training set	0.4330	0.1472	0.926	12	6
uncouplers validation set	0.3760	0.3438	0.803	13	7
combined uncouplers	0.4098	0.2279	0.877	25	8
amines training set	0.6958	-1.2364	0.894	17	9
w/o aniline	0.7323	-1.3716	0.927	16	10
amines validation set	0.7925	-1.5600	0.873	17	11
combined amines w/o aniline	0.7453	-1.3729	0.909	33	12

Since both ionization and metabolism can alter bioavailability and, therefore, structure-toxicity relationships, the potential effects of these two points were examined. The addition of ionization measured as pK_a as a second molecular descriptor does not improve the predictability of any of the models reported in Tables 2 and 3. Moreover, in no case was pK_a significant at the 0.5 level. While some of the chemicals examined in these investigations can be readily metabolized, the high r^2 values observed for the structure-toxicity relationships reported in Tables 2 and 3 suggest that for no chemical in either the flow-through fish assay or the static ciliate assay was metabolism significant enough to effect the results of these studies.

Volume Fraction Analyses

The hydrophobicity of the target sites was evaluated by means of the "a" value. The "a" values were analyzed by regression analysis of log $(10^{-6} \cdot C_w \cdot MV \cdot K_{ow})$ versus log K_{ow}. These values along with 95% confidence limits and coefficients of determination for each data set in both test systems are shown in Table 4. In the case of each regression, the r^2 value was high. The MVF was determined for each data set in both test systems. These results, along with 95% confidence intervals are presented in Table 5.

In subsequent analyses, the "a" and MVF values were compared between data sets and test systems using multiple comparisons t-test as described by Jaworska and Schultz (1993). These results are presented in Table 6. The hydrophobicity of the target site is different for each test system and each mechanism of action. The MVF is not significantly different for the two test species but different for the two mechanisms.

TABLE 4--"a" values with 95% confidence intervals.*

Group	Fish "a"	Fish r^2	Ciliates "a"	Ciliates r^2
uncouplers training set	0.438 ± 0.034	0.867	0.592 ± 0.023	0.963
uncouplers validation set	...	...	0.647 ± 0.034	0.922
amines training set	0.233 ± 0.021	0.710	0.366 ± 0.028	0.776
amines validation set	...	...	0.312 ± 0.042	0.509

*$\tilde{X} - ts/\sqrt{n}$ to $\tilde{X} + ts/\sqrt{n}$ where t is determined for n-1 degrees of freedom and $\alpha = 0.975$; n is the number of chemicals; $\tilde{X}$ is the mean volume fraction and s is standard deviation.

TABLE 5--MVF values with 95% confidence intervals.*

Group	Fish		Ciliates	
uncouplers training set	6.8 ± 2.3	e-05	8.6 ± 2.2	e-05
uncouplers validation set	...	...	6.0 ± 2.3	e-05
amines training set	1.8 ± 0.4	e-03	1.8 ± 0.6	e-03
amines validation set	...	...	3.3 ± 1.0	e-03

*$\tilde{X} - ts/\sqrt{n}$ to $\tilde{X} + ts/\sqrt{n}$ where t is determined for n-1 degrees of freedom and $\alpha = 0.975$; n is the number of chemicals; $\tilde{X}$ is the mean volume fraction and s is standard deviation.

TABLE 6--Statistical comparisons at $\alpha = 0.05$ of "a" and MVF values by chemical group and test system.

Group(s)	System(s)	"a"	V_f
training - validation uncouplers	ciliate	same	same
training uncouplers	fish - ciliate	different	same
training - validation amines	ciliate	same	same
training amines	fish - ciliate	same	same

Previously, Jaworska and Schultz (1993) conducted similar analyses on chemicals representing the nonpolar and polar narcosis mechanisms of action. Comparisons of the "a" values for respiratory uncouplers and amine narcotics with those previously reported for nonpolar and polar narcosis for both fish and ciliates, are summarized in Table 7. For fish, the "a" values for uncouplers and polar narcotic were not statistically different. Similarly, for fish the "a" value for amine narcotics and nonpolar narcotics were not statistically different. All other fish comparisons revealed statistical differences. For ciliates, the "a" value for amine narcotics was not statistically distinguishable for either nonpolar or polar narcotics. The "a" value for amine narcotics resided between the values for nonpolar and polar narcotics. All remaining ciliate comparisons showed statistical differences.

TABLE 7--Statistical comparisons at α = 0.05 of "a" values for fish and ciliates by mechanisms of toxic action.

	Fish			
	nonpolar narcotics	polar narcotics	respiratory uncouplers	amine narcotics
nonpolar narcotics	...			
polar narcotics	different	...		
respiratory uncouplers	different	same	...	
amine narcotics	same	different	different	...
	Ciliates			
	nonpolar narcotics	polar narcotics	respiratory uncouplers	amine narcotics
nonpolar narcotics	...			
polar narcotics	different	...		
respiratory uncouplers	different	different	...	
amine narcotics	same	same	different	...

The MVF values for uncouplers and amine narcotics were also compared with the previously reported MVF values for nonpolar and polar narcotics. These results are summarized in Table 8. These results indicate that MVF is specific for a given mechanism of action among all evaluated mechanisms in fish and ciliates. In all cases, the slopes of the V_f versus log K_{ow} regressions were not statistically different from zero.

TABLE 8--Statistical comparisons at $\alpha = 0.05$ of MVF for fish and ciliates by mechanisms of toxic action.

	Fish			
	nonpolar narcotics	polar narcotics	respiratory uncouplers	amine narcotics
nonpolar narcotics	...			
polar narcotics	different	...		
respiratory uncouplers	different	same	...	
amine narcotics	different	different	different	...
	Ciliates			
	nonpolar narcotics	polar narcotics	respiratory uncouplers	amine narcotics
nonpolar narcotics	...			
polar narcotics	different	...		
respiratory uncouplers	different	different	...	
amine narcotics	different	different	different	...

Comparisons of "a" values and MVF between test systems and by mechanism of toxic action are summarized in Table 9. For "a" values nonpolar, polar, and amine narcotics were not statistically different. However, the "a" values for respiratory uncouplers in fish and ciliates were different. Moreover, evaluations of MVF showed no statistical difference between test systems for any of the four mechanisms.

There was a strong correlation between MV and log K_{ow} for the narcotic amines in the training set as indicated by an r^2 value of 0.992. The amines in the validation set were not correlated with log K_{ow}, $r^2 = 0.124$. However, no such correlation was observed for the respiratory uncouplers, $r^2 = 0.352$.

TABLE 9--Statistical comparisons at $\alpha = 0.05$ of "a" values and MVF for mechanisms of toxic action by test system.

	"a"			
Fish \ Ciliate	nonpolar narcotics	polar narcotics	respiratory uncouplers	amine narcotics
nonpolar narcotics	same			

TABLE 9--Statistical comparisons at α = 0.05 of "a" values and MVF for mechanisms of toxic action by test system. (continued)

	"a"			
Fish \ Ciliate	nonpolar narcotics	polar narcotics	respiratory uncouplers	amine narcotics
polar narcotics		same		
respiratory uncouplers			different	
amine narcotics				same

	MVF			
Fish \ Ciliate	nonpolar narcotics	polar narcotics	respiratory uncouplers	amine narcotics
nonpolar narcotics	same			
polar narcotics		same		
respiratory uncouplers			same	
amine narcotics				same

DISCUSSION

The hypothesis that a given toxic effect occurs at a constant V_f for a particular reversible mechanism of action is based on the following assumptions: a) thermodynamic equilibrium was reached for each chemical in each test system and, b) concentration of toxicant in the target phase was such that it may be considered a dilute solution. The first assumption allows toxicity to be related only to partitioning between the phases each toxicant must pass through to reach the site of action.

Despite the general lack of knowledge about the molecular basis for toxic mechanisms, several methods have been developed that are thought to be sufficient to group toxicants by mechanism of action. These include: (1) membership to the same high quality QSAR; (2) strict concentration addition in joint toxic action models, and (3) similar behavioral and cardiovascular-biochemical responses. The latter is the basis for the fish acute toxicity syndrome or FATS (McKim et al. 1987).

The slopes of the log K_{ow}-dependent QSARs for nonpolar narcotics, polar narcotics and respiratory uncouplers have been shown to be different and vary consistently across test systems (Schultz et al. 1986; Cajina-Quezada and Schultz 1990; Schultz et al. 1990a). Broderius and Kahl (1985) have shown that 1-octanol, a classic nonpolar narcotic, and phenol, the model polar narcotic, were not concentration additive in binary mixture. Similarly, the study of Veith and Broderius (1987) stated that strongly acidic anilines and phenols, and oxidative phosphorylase uncouplers, were not concentration additive with either 1-octanol or phenol. In addition, discriminant function analysis of FATS showed that exposure to nonpolar narcotics, polar narcotics and respiratory uncouplers give rise to distinct respiratory-cardiovascular syndromes (McKim et al. 1987; Bradbury et al. 1989). All these approaches suggest that there are at least three mechanisms of reversible, physical toxicity: nonpolar narcosis, polar narcosis and weak acid respiratory uncoupling. The V_f analyses reported here and those of Jaworska and Schultz (1993) also point to nonpolar narcosis, polar narcosis and weak acid respiratory uncoupling being distinct mechanisms of reversible toxicity (see Tables 7 and 8).

The evidence that amine narcosis is a distinct mechanism of toxic action is not as strong. The toxicity of primary amines was recently investigated by Schultz et al. (1991b). They showed that alkyl-substituted primary aromatic amines and saturated aliphatic primary amines modeled well together by a simple log K_{ow} dependent QSAR. The aliphatic amines were more toxic than nonpolar narcotics. Whereas, the 4-position alkyl-substituted anilines were less toxic than other anilines considered to be polar narcotics. As with the other mechanisms of action, there was significant correlation between fish and ciliate toxicity. Similarly, the study of Newsome et al. (1991) showed their QSAR for amine toxicity to fish to be different from that for baseline nonpolar narcotics reported by Schultz et al. (1990b).

The amine narcotics examined in the training set were a congeneric series. The lone structure variation was the hydrocarbon content. In contrast, the amine validation sets and both uncoupler sets were structurally more heterogeneous groups. Although not decisive, the present results suggest amine narcosis is a distinct mechanism of toxic action in fish and in ciliates.

The volume fraction analyses approach is still in its infancy. To date, it has only been used to examine mechanisms of toxic action where penetration to the molecular site of action is the limiting step. Such mechanisms have high quality log K_{ow}-dependent structure-toxicity relationships. It appears unlikely that membrane irritants (McKim et al. 1987) and other direct-acting bioreactive mechanisms of toxicity will be successfully modeled by the approach.

In conclusion, the results of the present study reveals that volume fraction analyses is a potential tool for the determination of the mechanism of toxic action of organic chemicals. Based on this comparison of four mechanisms of action, it appears that target site hydrophobicity quantitated by means of "a" is constant for a mechanism of action, but distinct for a test system. The MVF is constant for a mechanism regardless of the test system.

Acknowledgments

J. S. J. was supported in part by The University of Tennessee's Center of Excellence in Livestock Disease and Human Health. The authors are grateful to S. E. Bryant for her assistance in determining *Tetrahymena* toxicity data for some of the amines. We also wish to thank the National Institutes of Health for the use of the hardware and software used in the computation of the molar volumes.

REFERENCES

Abernethy, S., and Mackay, D., 1987, In QSAR in Environmental Toxicology - II, K. L. E. Kaiser, Ed., D. Reidel Publishing Co., Dordrecht, Holland, 1987, pp. 1-16.

Abernethy, S., MacKay, D., and McCarty, L. S., 1988, Environmental Toxicology and Chemistry, Vol. 7, pp. 469-481.

Anderson, E., Veith, G. D., and Weininger, D., 1987, USEPA Environmental Research Brief EPA/600/M-87 021.

Bradbury, S. P., Henry, T. R., Niemi, G. J., Carlson, R. W., and Snarski, V. M., 1989, Environmental Toxicology and Chemistry, Vol. 8, pp. 247-263.

Broderius, S. J., and Kahl, M., 1985, Aquatic Toxicology, Vol. 6, pp. 307-322.

Cajina-Quezada, M., and Schultz, T. W., 1990, Aquatic Toxicology, Vol. 17, pp. 239-252.

Center for Lake Superior Environmental Studies, University of Wisconsin-Superior, 1984, "Acute Toxicities of Organic Chemicals to Fathead Minnows (*Pimephales promelas*)", Vol. 1, p. 414.

Center for Lake Superior Environmental Studies, University of Wisconsin-Superior, 1985, "Acute Toxicities of Organic Chemicals to Fathead Minnows (*Pimephales promelas*)", Vol. 2, p. 326.

Center for Lake Superior Environmental Studies, University of Wisconsin-Superior, 1986, "Acute Toxicities of Organic Chemicals to Fathead Minnows (*Pimephales promelas*)", Vol. 3, p. 328.

Center for Lake Superior Environmental Studies, University of Wisconsin-Superior, 1988, "Acute Toxicities of Organic Chemicals to Fathead Minnows (*Pimephales promelas*)", Vol. 4, p. 355.

Center for Lake Superior Environmental Studies, University of Wisconsin-Superior, 1990, "Acute Toxicities of Organic Chemicals to Fathead Minnows (*Pimephales promelas*)", Vol. 5, p. 332.

Hunter, R., 1988, In QSAR 88 Proceedings 3rd International Workshop on Quantitative Structure-Activity Relationships (QSAR) in Environmental Toxicology [CONF-880520-9OE 88013180], J. E. Turner, M. W. England, T. W. Schultz and N. J. Kwaak, Eds. NTIS, Springfield, VA, pp. 33-42.

Jaworska, J. S., and Schultz, T. W., 1993, SAR and QSAR in Environmental Research, Vol. 1, pp. 3-19.

Leo, A., and Weininger, D., 1988, MEDCHEM software release 3.53, Pomona Medical Chemistry Project, Pomona College, Claremont, CA.

Lipnick, R.L., 1991, "Studies of Narcosis", C. E. Overton, Chapman & Hall, London, p. 146.

McKim, J. M., Bradbury, S. P., and Niemi, G. J., 1987, Environmental Health Perspective, Vol. 71, pp. 171-186.

Mullins, L. J., 1954, Chemical Review, Vol. 54, pp. 289-323.

Newsome, L. D., Johnson, D. E., Lipnick, R. L., Broderius, S. J., and Russom, C. L., 1991, The Science of the Total Environment, Vol. 109/110, pp. 537-552.

Perrin, D. D., Dempsey, B., and Sergeant, E.P., 1981, pK_a Predictions for Organic Acids and Bases, Chapman and Hall, London, p. 146.

SAS Institute Inc., 1989, SAS/STAT user's guide, version 6, Fourth edition, Vol. 2, Cary, NC, p. 846.

Schultz, T. W., Holcombe, G. W., and Phipps, G. L., 1986, Ecotoxicology and Environmental Safety, Vol. 12, pp. 146-153.

Schultz, T. W., Lin, D. T., and Arnold, L. M., 1991a, The Science of the Total Environment, Vol. 109/110, pp. 569-580.

Schultz, T. W., Lin, D. T., Wilke, T. S., and Arnold, L. M., 1990a, In Practical Applications of Quantitative Structure-Activity Relationships (QSAR) in Environmental Chemistry and Toxicology, W. Karcher and J. Devillers, Eds., Kluwer Academic Publishers, Dordrecht, Holland, pp. 241-262.

Schultz, T. W., Wilke, T. S., Bryant, S. E., and Hosein, L. M., 1991b, The Science of the Total Environment, Vol. 109/110, pp. 581-587.

Schultz, T. W., Wyatt, N. L., and Lin, D. T., 1990b, Bulletin of Environmental Contamination and Toxicology, Vol. 44, pp. 67-72.

Seeman, P., 1972, Pharmacology Review, Vol. 24, pp. 583-655.

Veith, G. D., and Broderius, S. J., 1987, In QSAR in Environmental Toxicology - II, K.L.E. Kaiser, Ed., D. Reidel Publishing Co., Dordrecht, Holland, pp. 385-391.

Sediment Toxicology

David E. Weber[1], Gerald E. Walsh[2], and Matthew A. MacGregor[1]

USE OF VASCULAR AQUATIC PLANTS IN PHYTOTOXICITY STUDIES WITH SEDIMENTS[3]

Reference: Weber, D. E., Walsh, G. E. and MacGregor, M. A., **"Use of Vascular Aquatic Plants in Phytotoxicity Studies with Sediments"**, Environmental Toxicology and Risk Assessment - Third Volume, ASTM STP 1218, Jane S. Hughes, Gregory R. Biddinger, and Eugene Mones, Eds., American Society for Testing and Materials, Philadelphia, 1995.

ABSTRACT: Sediments and rooted aquatic plants are major components of wetland systems. Sediments in these systems act as sinks and reservoirs for organic and inorganic pollutants that are adsorbed to sediment particles or contained in interstitial water that exists between the particle spaces of sediments. Sediments may release toxic materials to aquatic environments through processes that include resuspension, desorption, and bioturbation. In sediment systems, aquatic plants are affected by toxic materials through direct effects on root growth or rhizosphere microorganisms, or by the assimilation and translocation of chemical substances to aerial organs, where they may injure foliage or inhibit growth and seed production. Procedures are being developed to identify the effects of contaminated sediments on aquatic plants through use of laboratory toxicity tests involving natural and artificial sediments, and a group of rooted aquatic species. In these studies, two freshwater species, Echinochloa crusgalli and Sesbania macrocarpa, and a saltmarsh species, Spartina alterniflora, are being evaluated. Artificial substrates proved useful in assessing the effects of contaminants on plant growth and development, and provided techniques for evaluating the role of sediment components on plant response.

KEYWORDS: bioavailability, organic matter, clay minerals, root nodulation, simulated sediments

The increased awareness of environmental problems from contaminated sediments has lead to the need for the development of sediment toxicity tests and sediment quality criteria for use by environmental management programs (Chapman 1989; Shea 1988; Southerland et al. 1992). To address this concern, phytotoxicity tests with rooted aquatic plants in laboratory and greenhouse studies have the potential of providing useful information on the presence and effects of contaminants in sediments.

[1]Research Biologist and Biological Assistant, respectively, U.S. Environmental Protection Agency, 1 Sabine Island Dr, Gulf Breeze, FL 32561.

[2]Research Ecologist, 4401 Wellington Dr., Ft. Collins, CO 80526.

[3]Contribution No. 834 from the Environmental Research Laboratory, Gulf Breeze, FL. Use of trade names in this publication does not constitute endorsement by the U.S. Environmental Protection Agency.

Since these vascular plants grow in direct contact with sediment materials, they are exposed to chemical substances present in the sediment matrix. Within this matrix, chemical nutrients are utilized by both emergent and submersed aquatic plants in normal processes of growth and development. In contaminated sediments, plant growth and development can be adversely affected by toxic chemicals through direct effects on root growth, and by the assimilation and translocation of toxicants to aerial organs, where they may injure foliage and inhibit growth of leaves and stems and production of seed. Only a small number of studies have examined the use of laboratory toxicity tests in evaluating the effects of toxicants on rooted aquatic species growing in contaminated sediments. In evaluations of heavy metals in dredged material, Folsom and Price (1991) used natural sediments in bioassays involving Cyperus esculentus. Knowlton et al.(1983) used pond sediment in studies on the uptake of lead by Potamogeton foliosus. In studies involving a group of submersed aquatic species, Forney and Davis (1981) used a river sediment treated with atrazine in evaluating effects. Washed sand was used in a culture tube system for evaluating the uptake of several xenobiotics by Hydrilla verticillata (Hinman and Klaine 1992).

This article addresses some of the chemical and physical aspects of sediments in relation to their influence on the availability and phytotoxicity of contaminants to vascular aquatic plants. Results are presented from studies involving the use of artificial sediments in toxicity testing; and the use of marsh species in tests to evaluate effects on plant growth, plant development, and root nodulation associated with nitrogen fixation.

Sediment Characteristics

Aquatic sediments can be perceived as consisting of four primary components: inorganic components, organic materials, water, and anthropogenic materials (Power and Chapman 1992).

Inorganic components provide the mineral fabric of sediments. These components include sand and shell fragments, silt, clay, and ionic minerals. The materials are the result of the natural erosion of rocks and soils of terrestrial origin and inorganic substances from atmospheric sources and biological processes. In estuaries, these materials originate from rivers, streams, and coastal areas. The amount of these materials, their size, and their mineralogy are of importance in determining the physical and chemical characteristics of sediments and in understanding the bioavailability of contaminants (Neff 1984; Power and Chapman 1992). Inorganic components are identified by an analysis of the distribution of particle sizes (Mudroch and MacKnight 1991). Through this analysis, sediment components are classified quantitatively into sand, silt, and clay fractions. In the analysis, particles that are greater than 63 μm diameter are identified as sand and other coarse material; particles that are less than 63 μm are classified as fine particles consisting of silt and clay (Förstner 1990), often referred to as "mud" (Folk 1980). The two groups of particles are separated by sieving of a sediment sample through a 63 μm screen; however, some consider 50 μm as the size separation point (Singer and Munns 1991). Silts and clays are identified by measurement of the fine components suspended in water (Burton 1992). The identification of particle classes provides a basis for evaluating process-oriented properties of sediments and properties that are important in regulating phytotoxicity responses.

Sand and silt fractions of sediments consist of crystalline particles that include quartz, feldspar, mica, silica, calcium carbonate, ferromagnesium minerals, and some clay minerals that may be present as large particles. Sand and silt particles are important structurally and their presence affects sediment permeability - the movement of water or chemicals within the spaces of sediment particles (Power and Chapman 1992; Russell 1988).

The clay fraction, usually defined as particles of a diameter smaller than 2 μm, consists of minerals that are the product of weathering processes and include a range of types: vermiculite, smectite (montmorillonite), kaolinite, chlorite, and other types (Russell 1988). In chemical terms, clay minerals are aluminosilicates (crystals consisting of aluminum, silicon, and oxygen). Most clays are in the form of platy sheets of various layers of molecular structure which vary from two- to multiple-layered types (Russell 1988). The multiple layered types have a greater capacity to retain ions and contaminants than clays with fewer surface layers (Means et al. 1979). In most instances, clay minerals of aquatic sediments are coated with aluminum, ferric and manganese oxides, and living and non-living matter (Leenheer 1991). The coatings and clay minerals provide sorption sites for contaminates (Jenne 1977; Förstner 1987). Clay minerals have a larger surface-to-volume ratio than sand and silt components. Singer and Munns (1991) reported surface-to-volume ratios of 20 to 80 m^2/g of clay.

Organic matter constitutes a small volume of sediment and consists of living and non-living materials composed of carbon. This group of materials includes microorganisms (including algae, bacteria, and fungi), invertebrates, non-viable plant and animal material in various stages of decomposition, plant exudates, and animal excretions. Organic matter occurs in sediment systems as particulate matter and dissolved or colloidal substances (humic and fulvic acids). Humic materials are dark-colored and formed by the decomposition of organic matter. Organic colloids are highly charged, have a very large surface area, and an absorptive capacity that is larger than the capacity of clay minerals (Singer and Munns 1991; Wershaw 1991).

Because of a large surface area and the presence of an electrostatic charge, clay and organic particles are important in chemical and biological reactions of sediments (Power and Chapman 1992; Wershaw 1991). The surface charge, which is usually negative, contributes to the overall charge density of sediments, and is measured as the cation exchange capacity (CEC) of sediment. The CEC provides an indication of the capacity of sediment to bind and exchange positively charged substances, including contaminants (Russell 1988; Means et al. 1979, 1980). Within sediment and soil systems, clay and organic matter are considered the major cation exchangers. The chemical adsorbing surfaces of sand and silt particles are of less importance (Russell 1988; Förstner 1987). Values of CEC range from 0 to 7 meq/100g material for sand and silt, 10 to 150 meq/100g for clay, and exceed 200 meq/100g for organic matter (Black 1968).

The sediment matrix also consists of interstitial or pore water that is located in the spaces between sediment particles. Pore water can be considered as the sediment solution, consisting of cations, anions, dissolved organic carbon, and contaminants. The volume or space occupied by interstitial water is characterized as sediment porosity (Power and Chapman 1992; Russell 1988).

The anthropogenic component includes inorganic and organic chemicals from point and non-point sources, including the deposition of particulate matter from soil erosion and dredging. Although contaminated sediment can be considered as a source of pollutants to the water column, the concentration of contaminants is generally larger in sediment than in overlying water (Baudo and Muntau 1990; Neff 1984).

Bioavailability and Phytotoxicity

Bioavailability and the resulting phytotoxicity of contaminants are regulated by a group of factors that include: the movement of contaminants in sediments; the assimilation of contaminants by organisms; and the expression of toxicity responses. The interstitial water of sediments is considered to be the major route of the exposure of organisms, including rooted aquatic plants, to contaminants (Giesy and Hoke 1990; Singer and Munns 1991; Power and Chapman 1992). The processes of dissolution and precipitation, and sorption and desorption, are regarded as important reactions that control the availability of contaminants in sediment systems (Burton 1992; Burgess and Scott 1992; Förstner 1990). Contaminants of interstitial water may become immobilized and unavailable by the processes of sorption and precipitation. Sorption and desorption reactions form the basis for Landrum's model (1989), in which the bioavailable contaminant is conceptualized as existing in a "freely dissolved pool" within interstitial water (Landrum 1989). In this pool, the concentration and bioavailability of contaminants are controlled by sorption and desorption rates, and chemical gradients occurring between interstitial water and sediment particles (primarily clay and organic matter of various forms). Through sorption and desorption processes, a steady-state exists that can result in a continued mobilization of contaminants in interstitial water that may cause toxicity responses. If sorption and desorption rates are very slow, due to the molecular binding of contaminants to sediment particles, the bound contaminants are less available and less toxic. The degree and magnitude of chemical reactions occurring within the sediment solution depend on pH, ionization constants, redox conditions, the concentration of ions in solution, the amounts of clays and organic matter, and thermodynamic interactions. The availability of contaminants is also controlled by microorganisms (Gibson 1984) and uptake by plants and animals.

The characteristics and chemistry of sediments are of considerable importance in growth and development of aquatic plants and in influencing the responses of plants to sediment contaminants. Laboratory studies were designed to examine the use of testing systems with artificial substrates for identifying sediment-associated toxicity responses of several emergent aquatic plants and to evaluate the role of organic matter in regulating toxicity responses.

EXPERIMENTAL METHODS

Emergent freshwater species, two varieties of *Echinochloa crusgalli* (L.) Palisot de Beavois and *Sesbania macrocarpa* Muhl. ex Raf., and a salt marsh plant, *Spartina alterniflora* Loisel were evaluated in toxicological studies involving natural, and artificial sediments. Seeds of freshwater species were obtained from Wildlife Nurseries, Oshkosh, Wisconsin. Seeds of *S. alterniflora* were obtained from Environmental Concern, St. Michaels, Maryland, and maintained in 4 ppt seawater. All seeds were stored at 4°C.

Natural and Artificial Sediments

In initial studies (Walsh et al. 1991a, 1991b), growth of *E. crusgalli* and *S. alterniflora* was compared in natural and artificial sediments. Natural sediments were collected from a freshwater wetland and a saltmarsh, and air dried. Artifical sediments were prepared from commercially available sand, silt, clay and organic matter (peat humus) with particle size ratios and organic contents that were similar to natural sediments (Table 1). Dried sediments were mixed with a range of herbicide concentrations (Walsh et al. 1991a) or complex effluents (Walsh et al. 1991b) in deionized water (freshwater species). Four ppt seawater was used in tests involving the saltmarsh species. Untreated water (deionized) was used for controls. Sediments were mixed, by use of a spatula, at a ratio of 42 mL water:135 g of sediment, which was the amount added to styrofoam pots of a size 7.5 cm diameter x 5.5 cm high. Each treatment and control group consisted of three pots.

Twelve seedlings, grown from seeds in water, were transplanted to each pot containing the sediment formulations. Plants were cultured in a growth chamber under a cycle of 16 h light:8 h darkness at a temperature of 24°C ± 1°C. Plant nutrients were provided by addition of Hoagland's solution. Plants were irrigated with deionized water to maintain a wet sediment environment (Walsh et al. 1991a, 1991b).

At 14 days(*E. crusgalli*)and at 28 days(*S. alterniflora*) after planting, seedlings were removed from sediments, rinsed with deionized water, and counted. Plants from each pot were combined, dried, and weighed. The average weight of individual plants was calculated to provide a measure of plant growth.

TABLE 1--Characteristics of natural and artificial Sediments.[a]

Characteristics	Freshwater Natural	Freshwater Artificial	Saltmarsh Natural	Saltmarsh Artificial
Component Group (Percent by Weight)				
Coarse Sand	0.6	0.6	33.6	28.6
Medium Sand	9.5	8.7	58.8	62.4
Fine Sand	67.4	69.2	4.9	6.3
Silt	10.3	10.2	0.6	1.0
Clay	6.7	6.4	0.7	0.9
Organic matter	4.9	4.9	0.8	0.8
pH/CEC				
pH	5.8	7.5	2.9	7.4
CEC (meq/100g)	16.6	19.0	14.1	19.0

[a]Adapted, in part, from Walsh et al. (1991a).

Organic Matter Comparisons with Artificial Sediments

Four artificial sediments were formulated with different amounts of organic matter (Table 2) to simulate a range of sediment types typical of natural conditions (Walsh et al. 1991c). The procedures for sediment preparation and seedling culture have been described (Walsh et al. 1991c). Sediment components were formulated from materials similar to those presented in Table 3.

TABLE 2--Characteristics of artificial sediments.

Substrate (% Organic Matter)	Percent Composition Sand	Silt	Clay	Cond. (mmho/cm)	pH	CEC (meq/100g)
3	83.4	12.1	4.5	0.17	6.4	5.1
5	81.8	13.2	5.0	0.37	6.8	8.3
7.5	78.4	16.1	5.5	0.83	6.9	18.9
10	76.2	20.0	3.8	1.33	7.2	28.0

The herbicide, hexazinone (3-cyclohexyl-6-(dimethylamino)-1-methyl-1,3,5-triazine-2,4-(1H, 3H)-dione), or a group of complex effluents were mixed with the various sediment formulations. In tests with hexazinone, concentrations ranged from 0 to 0.25 mg/kg of sediment. Complex effluents were collected as single samples from industrial facilities, shipped with ice, and stored at 4°C prior to use in toxicity studies. For each sediment type, ten seedlings of E. crusgalli and three seedlings of S. macrocarpa were transplanted to each of three pots that contained sediment mixed with hexazinone or undiluted effluent, or untreated sediment that served as the control. Washed sand was used as a reference substrate for treated and non-treated conditions. Plants were watered with Hoagland's nutrient solution or undiluted effluent containing nutrients on alternate days of a 5-day week (three times/ week) for the two week duration of each study. Plant growth and survival was measured as described above (Walsh et al. 1991c).

Studies with S. macrocarpa and Rhizobium

An artificial sediment and S. macrocarpa were used in toxicity tests to evaluate the effects of toxic agents on indicators of plant growth and development, from seedling to flower and seed production; and to assess the effects of pollution stress on a symbiotic rhizobium-plant relationship of importance in the fixation of atmospheric nitrogen.

Toxicant Preparation -- An effluent from a metal fabricating facility and the herbicide, norflurazon (4-chloro-5-(methylamino)-2-(a,a,a-trifluoro-m-tolyl)-3(2H)-pyridazinone), were used in toxicity tests.

The effluent was collected, shipped on ice, and stored at 4°C until use. The effluent was light yellow in color with a pH of 8.5. A chemical analysis of the effluent by argon-plasma emission spectrometry (Jarrell-Ash AtomComp 800 Series) revealed the presence of nickel at a concentration of 0.5 mg/L. Prior to the initiation of toxicity studies, the effluent was diluted with deionized water to provide concentrations consisting of 25% and 50% effluent. These mixtures and the undiluted effluent (100%) were used in tests with S. macrocarpa.

Norflurazon, > 98% pure, Sandoz Inc., Homestead, FL, was dissolved in deionized water and prepared to obtain concentrations of 0.2, 0.4, 0.6 and 0.8 mg/kg sediment. Concentrations were measured by extraction of solutions with 40% ethyl acetate/40% hexane (v/v), and analyzed by gas chromatography equipped with an SP-2100 packed column and a nitrogen-phosphorus detector.

Sediment Preparation--Sediments were formulated from components presented in Table 3. Sphagnum and cow manure components were sieved through a 2-mm screen prior to use in sediment preparation. Chemical and physical characteristics of the sediment were evaluated (Table 4). The combustion method described by Jackson (1960) was used in measurement of organic matter. Procedures used in analysis of soil substrates were followed for other measurements (Folk 1980; USDA 1984).

Artificial sediment was mixed with various concentrations of effluent or norflurazon, at a ratio of 38 mL toxicant:100 g of dry sediment. Deionized water was used as the control. Thoroughly mixed samples of sediment (700 g dry weight) were added to plastic vessels that served as pots, 9.5 cm diameter x 15 cm high. Openings were provided on the bottom of each pot. Pots were placed in plastic containers that were used to maintain a constant supply of water to each sediment/plant system. Sediments were prepared 24 h before use.

Toxicity Tests--Five pots per treatment in effluent tests, and eight pots per treatment in tests with norflurazon were planted, individually, with 11-day-old seedlings of S. macrocarpa. During planting, each seedling was inoculated with 100 mg of inoculum of Rhizobium sp. (Nitragin Co.; Milwaukee, WI) that was applied to plant roots in a 5 ml aqueous suspension. An inoculum concentration of 100 mg/pot was also added to the sediment during mixing to ensure that an adequate quantity of inoculum was present in the substrate. Plants were cultured in a growth chamber under a photoperiod of 16 h light/8 h darkness at a day/night temperature of 25°/22° ± 1°C. Light intensity was 225 μmol/m^2/s at the surface of the growth chamber bench.

In effluent tests, plants were watered with 55 mL of the specific effluent concentrations once each week. Undiluted effluent was also applied once every two weeks. Deionized water was applied to all plants between scheduled effluent applications and to untreated controls. In norflurazon tests, plants were watered with 55 mL deionized water three times per week throughout the study.

TABLE 3--Composition of artificial sediment used in toxicity test with *Sesbania macrocarpa*.[a]

Sediment components	Grams per 100 g of dry sediment
Sand	81.1
Silt/clay	14.3
Dolomite	0.5
Cow manure	2.0
Sphagnum moss	2.1
Humic acid	0.01

Sources of components

Sand - Mystic White No. 45
New England Silica, Inc. South Windsor, CT
Silt/clay - ASP-400, Englehard Corp., Edison, NJ
Dolomite - Southern Agri-Mineral Corp., Hartford, AL
Sphagnum moss - Stim-U-Plant, Inc., Columbus, OH
Cow manure - A. H. Hoffman, Inc., Landisville, PA
Humic acid - Aldrich Chemical Co., Milwaukee, WI

[a]Adapted from Walsh et al. (1991c).

TABLE 4-Physical and chemical characteristics of artificial sediment.

Component Classification (% Composition):

Sand (mm)					Fine (μm)		
Very Coarse 1-2 mm	Coarse 0.5-1	Medium 0.25-0.5	Fine 0.125-0.5	Very Fine 0.063-0.125	Silt 2-63	Clay < 2.0	Organic Matter (%)
0.01	13.6	42.7	16.0	4.3	12.7	5.9	4.8

Chemical Characteristics:

CEC (meq/100g)	Extractable Bases (meq/100g)	Extractable Acids (meq/100g)	Base Saturation (%)	pH
6.13	6.11	0.84	87.86	6.9

Plant growth and development, were measured when experiments were concluded at the end of 41 days. The measurements included shoot and root dry weight, plant height, stem diameter, and the number of branches, trifoliate leaves, and root nodules. Root nodules were dried to constant weight and weighed. An estimate of the average weight per nodules was calculated by dividing nodule weight by the number of nodules per plant. The number of flower buds, expanded flowers, and seed pods were determined. Variables are expressed as means for each treatment.

Data Analysis

Means of treatments and controls were calculated and compared by an analysis of variance. Treatment means were compared with the control by multiple range procedures when F values were significant at $P \leq 0.05$ (SAS, 1989).

RESULTS AND DISCUSSION

In the absence of pollutants, plants grown in natural and artificial freshwater sediments appeared normal. Although plant growth tended to be greater in artificial sediments than in natural substrates, this trend was not always statistically significant. In toxicity studies, increasing concentrations of metolachlor and norflurazon inhibited the growth of the two varieties of E. crusgalli in natural and artificial sediments (Walsh et al. 1991a). Inhibitory effects at specific herbicide concentrations were often similar (Table 5). The two effluents also inhibited the growth of the varieties of E. crusgalli in both sediment types (Walsh et al. 1991b). Adverse effects occurred after a single addition of 311 ml effluent/kg sediment (Table 5). In saltmarsh sediments, growth of S. alterniflora was less in natural sediments than in artificial substrates. A growth suppression gradient with increasing concentrations of herbicide was evident in artifical sediments, but was not apparent in natural sediments. Differences in plant response between the two types of sediment were probably caused by the low pH of the natural saltmarsh sediment which resulted from the process of drying and subsequent rehydration during sediment preparation. Due to the adverse influence of pH, artifical sediment provided a more accurate assessment of toxicity responses in tests with S. alterniflora (Table 5).

Both stimulatory and inhibitory responses were observed in studies involving the growth of E. crusgalli and S. macrocarpa in artificial substrates composed of sand and various concentrations of organic matter (Table 6). The absence of effects with increases in the amount of organic matter is illustrative of the probable binding of chemicals to the organic component of sediment. Because of this molecular attraction at organic receptor sites, the availability of chemicals in interstitial water may be limited. As a result, toxicity responses are reduced or not occurring. In instances in which plant growth was affected in sand and at the various organic matter concentrations, the capacity of organic receptor sites to absorb contaminants may have been exceeded. This could have resulted in an increased bioavailability of the chemical agent in the interstitial water of sediment.

In 41-day studies with artificial sediments and S. macrocarpa, trifoliate leaves were injured by the various concentrations of herbicide and effluent. The extent of injury increased with increases in concentration of the toxic substances. In studies with the effluent, injury first developed as a chlorosis of the margins of the apical part of individual leaflets. By the end of 21 days, leaf tissues were necrotic, affecting about one-third of the area of the leaflets of leaves. In this test, nickel was believed to be the toxic agent in the effluent. The metal is known to be toxic and bioavailable in the

TABLE 5--Lowest effect concentrations for growth responses of wetland species exposed to herbicides and effluents from a metal plating and coke plant in natural (Nat.) and artificial (Art.) sediments.[a]

	Lowest Effect Concentration[b]					
Pollutant	Metolachlor		Norflurazon		Effluents	
Plant Species	Nat.	Art.	Nat.	Art.	Nat.	Art.
E. crusgalli						
var *crusgalli*	0.25	0.25	0.25	0.25	311	311
var *zelayensis*	0.1	0.25	0.25	0.25	311	311
S. alterniflora	10	0.5	>2	0.25	...	...

[a] Data adapted from Walsh et al. (1991a, 1991b).
[b] Concentrations expressed as mg herbicide/kg sediment and ml effluent/kg sediment that resulted in a significant inhibition of total dry weight ($P \leq 0.05$) when compared with respective controls.

TABLE 6--Effects of a herbicide and complex effluents on two wetland species in artificial sediments composed of sand or differing amounts of organic matter.[a]

Pollutant	*E. crusgalli*	*S. macrocarpa*
Hexazinone	Toxicity decreased with > organic matter	Not tested
Municipal Wastewater	Stimulation of shoot growth, no effect at 10% organic matter	Inhibition of shoots & roots in sand & organic matter
Pulp Mill Effluent	Increase inhibition of of shoot & root growth with > organic matter	Inhibitory effect in sand, toxicity less with > organic matter
Coke Plant Effluent	Inhibitory effects in sand & at all organic matter concentrations	Inhibition of shoot & root growth, toxicity less with organic matter > 3%
Chemical Plant Effluent	Stimulation effect of shoot growth in sand, no effect in organic matter	Inhibitory effect of shoot growth in sand, slight inhibition in organic matter
Sewage Treatment Effluent	Inhibitory effect only in sand, no effect with organic matter	Inhibition of shoot growth in sand and organic matter

[a]Data adapted from Walsh et al. (1991c, 1991d), and D.E. Weber and G.E. Walsh (unpublished).

aquatic environment (Guilizzoni 1991). Foliar damage of plants exposed to norflurazon began as a chlorosis and bleaching of leaflets. At herbicide concentrations greater than 0.2 mg/kg sediment, some leaves became necrotic and abscised. Plants of the non-exposed controls were green and healthy, and leaves were not injured.

A number of response variables were found to be adversely affected by the toxicants (Table 7 and 8). The growth of shoots and roots, as

TABLE 7--Norflurazon test with Sesbania macrocarpa in artificial sediments.[a]

Response Variable		Mg Norflurazon/Kg Sediment				
	Control	0.2	0.4	0.6	0.8	p>F
Shoot Wt (g)	3.7	1.9*[a]	0.3*	0.05*	0.03*	0.0001
Root Wt (g)	0.7	0.4*	0.1*	0.03*	0.01*	0.0001
Plant Height(cm)	84.6	57.7*	28.6*	19.2*	11.4*	0.0001
No. Branches	3.6	0.6*	0*	0*	0*	0.0015
No. Trifoliates	18.0	15.1*	5.9*	3.9*	3.6*	0.0001
Stem Dia.(mm)	4.9	3.9*	2.5*	1.7*	1.5*	0.0001
No. Nodules	163.4	131.8	25.5*	7.0*	2.4*	0.0001
Nodule Wt(mg)	440.5	235.7*	35.6*	1.3*	1.4*	0.0001
Av. Nodule Wt(mg)	3.2	2.0*	1.2*	0.2*	0.1*	0.0001
No. Flower Buds	15.8	4.6*	1.1*	0*	0*	0.0005
No. Flowers	2.8	1.4	0*	0*	0*	0.0005
No. Seed Pods	2.0	1.9	0*	0*	0*	0.0037

[a] Values are means of 8 samples per treatment. * = significantly different (P ≤ 0.05) from the control by Duncan's multiple range procedure (SAS 1989).

TABLE 8--Effluent test with Sesbania macrocarpa in artificial sediments.[a]

Response Variable	Concentration & Application Frequency					
	Control	Once/Week			Once/ 2 Wks	p>F
	0%	25%	50%	100%	100%	
Shoot Wt (g)	7.0	5.0*[a]	3.7*	1.8*	1.8*	0.0001
Root Wt (g)	1.4	0.7*	0.8*	0.3*	0.3*	0.0001
Plant Ht (cm)	109.6	95.9	73.7*	51.6*	63.9*	0.0039
No. Branches	10.2	7.6	3.0*	0.6*	0.4*	0.0003
No. Trifoliates	21.2	19.6	18.6	14.6*	15.0*	0.0008
Stem Dia.(mm)	5.9	5.1	5.1	3.5*	3.6*	0.0001
No. Nodules	177.4	150.2	170.0	72.8*	75.2*	0.0001
Nodule Wt(mg)	771.9	489.2*	371.9*	186.8*	199.8*	0.0001
Av. Nodule Wt(mg)	4.4	3.3	2.2*	2.5*	2.9*	0.0233
No. Flower Buds	37.4	41.2	13.2	9.2*	9.8*	0.0263
No. Flowers	15.0	8.8	3.8*	1.4*	2.6*	0.0029
No. Seed Pods	6.3	4.3	4.0	2.5*	1.8*	0.0177

[a] Values are means of 5 samples per treatment. * = significantly different (P ≤ 0.05) from the control by Duncan's multiple range procedure (SAS 1989).

determined from dry weights, was suppressed at all norflurazon and effluent concentrations tested. Plants exposed to the pollutants were stunted and produced fewer auxiliary branches than controls. The number of trifoliate leaves and diameter of stems were adversely affected by the pollutants. In effluent tests, the number of leaves and diameter of stems were statistically different from the control only at the concentration of 100%. Nodulation of plant roots and nodule size, as reflected by the average weight of nodules per plant, were less in plants exposed to the contaminants.

The production of floral buds and flowers was inhibited at norflurazon concentrations of 0.2 mg/kg sediment and at effluent concentrations of 50 and 100%. Flowers and seed pods were absent on plants damaged by norflurazon at concentrations of 0.4 mg/kg and greater. The mean number of seed pods per plant was less in toxicant exposures than in the control, but this effect was not always statistically significant. This variation, appeared to be related to an inconsistency in the time required for the production of flowers and pods among individuals of the population. At the end of the 41-day period, one-third of the plants within the control groups failed to produce flowers and pods. These plants required an additional 16-20 days for anthesis; however the data presented in Tables 7 and 8 are reflective of the 41-day experimental period. The delay in anthesis and in the subsequent production of pods and seeds may be genetically controlled.

CONCLUSIONS

The use of emergent aquatic plants and artificial sediments have value in toxicity testing; although, the procedures for these tests should be considered in the initial stages of development. Through a group of studies involving freshwater sediments, artificial substrates have been shown to support plant growth that is similar to growth occurring in natural sediments. In both types of substrates, plants responded to pollutant stress. The use of artificial sediments provided techniques for evaluating the role of organic matter in sediment-plant toxicity studies. In saltmarsh sediments, the use of artificial substrates provided a more accurate indication of pollutant responses than natural sediments, probably due to the low pH of the dried natural sediment when rehydrated.

In tests with S. macrocarpa, artificial substrates proved useful in assessing the effects of contaminants on a group of indicators of vegetative growth and development, and a symbiotic relationship involving the fixation of nitrogen. Results from research with S. macrocarpa provided an example of the potential use of a marsh plant in life-cycle tests within a relatively short time period. Further research, through the selection and development of specific plant cultivars, will be needed to obtain a genetic line that is uniform with respect to the production of flowers and seed pods. Research also is needed to evaluate the influencing effects of different types of clay minerals and the various forms of organic matter, since clay and organic matter are major components in regulating chemical bioavailability and phytotoxicity responses.

Walsh et al. (1992) discuss advantages and limitations associated with the use of artificial substrates. An important advantage of using artificial sediments involves the ability to formulate sediments to achieve specific experimental requirements, such as, the establishment of a non-contaminated control in toxicity tests, or to determine the role of various substrate components on plant responses to contaminates. Another approach for evaluating sediment components could involve the amendment of natural sediments with specific components. This approach was used by Barko and Smart (1986) in nutrient-cycling studies with aquatic plants in which nutrients and organic matter were added to a natural sediment. The procedure may be useful in the assessment of the interactions of sediment components and pollutant responses, and would tend to minimize a concern (Walsh et al. 1992) that artificial substrates may not contain important components present in natural sediments.

REFERENCES

Barko, J. W. and Smart, R.M., 1986, "Sediment-Related Mechanisms of Growth Limitation in Submersed Macrophytes," Ecology, Vol. 67, No. 5, pp. 1328-1340.

Baudo, R. and Muntau, H., 1990, "Lesser Known In-Place Pollutants and Diffuse Source Problems," in Sediments: Chemistry and Toxicity of In-Place Pollutants, R. Baudo, J. P. Giesy, and H. Muntau, Eds., Lewis Publishers, Ann Arbor, MI, pp. 1-14.

Black, C. A., 1968, Soil-Plant Relationships, John Wiley and Sons, New York.

Burgess, R. M. and Scott, K. J., 1992, "The Significance of In-Place Contaminated Marine Sediment on the Water Column: Processes and Effects," in Sediment Toxicity Assessment, G. A. Burton, Ed., Lewis Publishers, Chelsea, MI, pp. 129-165.

Burton, G. A., 1992, "Sediment Collection and Processing: Factors Affecting Realism," in Sediment Toxicity Assessment, G. A. Burton, Ed., Lewis Publishers, Chelsea, MI, pp.37-66.

Chapman , P. M., 1989, "Current Approaches to Developing Sediment Quality Criteria," Environmental Toxicology and Chemistry, Vol. 8, pp. 589-599

Folk, R. I., 1980, Petrology of Sedimentary Rocks, Hemphill Publishing Co., Austin, TX.

Folsom, B.L. and Price, R.A., 1991, "A Plant Bioassay for Assessing Plant Uptake of Contaminants from Freshwater Soils or Dredged Material,"in Plants for Toxicity Assessment: Second Volume, ASTM STP 1115, J. W. Gorsuch, W. R. Lower, W. Wang and M. A. Lewis, Eds., American Society for Testing and Materials, Philadelphia, pp. 172-177.

Forney, D. R. and Davis, D. E., 1981, "Effects of Low Concentrations of Herbicides on Submersed Aquatic Plants," Weed Science, Vol. 29, pp. 677-685.

Förstner, U., 1987, "Sediment-Associated Contaminants -- An Overview of Scientific Bases For Developing Remedial Options," Hydrobiologia, Vol. 149, pp. 221-246.

Förstner, U., 1990, "Inorganic Sediment Chemistry and Elemental Speciation," in Sediments: Chemistry and Toxicity of In-Place Pollutants, R. Baudo, J. P. Giesy, and H. Muntau, Eds., Lewis Publishers, Ann Arbor, MI pp. 61-106.

Gibson, D. T., 1984, Microbial Degradation of Organic Compounds, Microbiology Series, Vol. 13, Marcel Dekker, New York.

Giesy, J. P. and Hoke, R. A., 1990, "Freshwater Sediment Quality Criteria: Toxicity Bioassessment," in Sediments: Chemistry and Toxicity of In-Place Pollutants, R. Baudo, J. P. Giesy, and H. Muntau, Eds., Lewis Publishers, Ann Arbor, MI, pp. 265-348.

Guilizzoni, P., 1991, "The Role of Heavy Metals and Toxic Materials in the Physiological Ecology of Submersed Macrophytes," Aquatic Botany, Vol. 41, pp. 87-109.

Hinman, M. L. and Klaine, S. J., 1992, "Uptake and Translocation of Selected Organic Pesticides by the Rooted Aquatic Plant, Hydrilla verticillata Royle," Environmental Science and Technology, Vol. 26, pp. 609-613.

Jackson, M. L., 1960, Soil Chemical Analyses, Prentice Hall, Englewood Cliffs, NJ.

Jenne, E. A., 1977, "Trace Element Sorption by Sediments and Soils--Sites and Processes," in Symposium on Molybdenum, Vol. 2, Marcel Dekker, New York, pp. 425-553.

Knowlton, M. F., Boyle, T. B., and Jones, J. R., 1983, "Uptake of Lead from Aquatic Sediment by Submersed Macrophytes and Crayfish," Archives of Environmental Contamination and Toxicology, Vol. 12, pp. 535-541.

Landrum, P. F., 1989, "Bioavailability and Toxicokinetics of Polycyclic Aromatic Hydrocarbons Sorbed to Sediments for the Amphipod, Pontoporeia hoyi," Environmental Science and Technology, Vol. 23, pp. 588-595.

Leenheer, J. A., 1991, "Organic Substance Structures That Facilitate Contaminant Transport and Transformations in Aquatic Sediments," in R. A. Baker, Ed., Organic Substances and Sediments in Water--Humics and Soils, Vol. 1, Lewis Publishers, Chelsea, MI, pp. 3-22.

Means, J. C., Hassett, J. J., Wood, S. G., and Banwart, W. L., 1979, "Sorption Properties of Energy-Related Pollutants and Sediments," in P. W. Jones and P. Leber Eds., Polynuclear Aromatic Hydrocarbons, Ann Arbor Science Publishers, Ann Arbor, MI, pp. 327-340.

Means, J. C., Hassett, J. J., Wood, S. G., Banwart, W. L., Ali, S., and Khan, A., 1980, "Sorption Properties of Polynuclear Aromatic Hydrocarbons and Sediments: Heterocyclic and Substituted Compounds," in A. Borseth and A. J. Dennis, Eds., Polynuclear Aromatic Hydrocarbons: Chemistry and Biological Effects, Battelle Press, Columbus, OH, pp. 395-404.

Mudroch, A. and MacKnight, S. D., 1991, CRC Handbook of Techniques for Aquatic Sediments Sampling, CRC Press, Boca Raton, FL.

Neff, J. M., 1984, "Bioaccumulation of Organic Micropollutants from Sediments and Suspended Particulates by Aquatic Animals," Fresenius Z. Analytical Chemistry, Vol. 319, pp. 132-136.

Power, E. A. and Chapman, P. M., 1992, "Assessing Sediment Quality," in Sediment Toxicity Assessment, G. A. Burton, Ed., Lewis Publishers, Chelsea, MI, pp. 1-18.

Russell, E. W., 1988, Russell's Soil Conditions and Plant Growth, 11th edition, John Wiley and Sons, New York.

SAS Institute, Inc., 1989, SAS/STAT Users Guide, Version 6, 4th edition, Vol. 1., SAS Institute, Inc., Cary, NC.

Shea, D., 1988, "Developing National Sediment Quality Criteria," Environmental Science and Technology, Vol. 22, pp. 1256-1261.

Singer, M. J. and Munns, D. N., 1991, Soils -- An Introduction, Second Edition, Macmillan, Inc, New York.

Southerland, E., Kravitz, M. and Wall, T., 1992, "Management Framework for Contaminated Sediments (The U.S. EPA Sediment Management Strategy)," in Sediment Toxicity Assessment, G. A. Burton, Ed., Lewis Publishers, Chelsea, MI, pp. 341-370.

DA/SCS, 1984, "Procedures for Collecting Soil Samples and Methods of Analysis for Soil Survey," U.S. Department of Agriculture, Soil Conservation Service, Soil Survey Investigations Report No. 1, Washington, D.C.

Walsh, G. E., Weber, D. E., Simon, T. L., Brashers, L. K., and Moore, J. C., 1991a, "Use of Marsh Plants for Toxicity Testing of Water and Sediment," in Plants for Toxicity Assessment: Second Volume, ASTM STP 1115, J. W. Gorsuch, W. R. Lower, W. Wang and M. A. Lewis, Eds., American Society for Testing and Materials, Philadelphia, pp. 341-354.

Walsh, G. E., Weber, D. E., Simon, T. L., and Brashers, L. K., 1991b, "Toxicity Tests of Effluents with Marsh Plants in Water and Sediment," Environmental Toxicology and Chemistry, Vol. 10, pp. 517-525.

Walsh, G. E., Weber, D. E., Nguyen, M. T., and Esry, L. K., 1991c, "Responses of Wetland Plants to Effluents in Water and Sediment," Environmental and Experimental Botany, Vol. 31, No. 3, pp. 351-358.

Walsh, G. E., Weber, D. E., Esry, L. K., and Nguyen, M. T., 1991d, "Synthetic Sediments: A Tool for Research", Proceedings, Fifth Federal Interagency Sedimentation Conference, Las Vegas, NV, Vol. 1, Chapter 5, pp.40-47.

Walsh, G. E., Weber, D. E., Esry, L. K., Nguyen, M. T., Noles, J., and Albrecht, B., 1992, "Synthetic Substrata for Propagation and Testing of Soil and Sediment Organisms," Pedobiologia, Vol. 36, pp. 1-10.

Wershaw, R. L., 1991, "The Importance of Humic Substance - Mineral Particle Complexes in the Modeling of Contaminant Transport in Sediment-Water Systems," in R. A. Baker, Ed., Organic Substances and Sediments in Water--Humics and Soils, Vol. 1, Lewis Publishers, Chelsea, MI, pp. 23-33.

Tom M. Dillon[1], D.W. Moore[1], and D.J. Reish[2]

A 28 DAY SEDIMENT BIOASSAY WITH THE MARINE POLYCHAETE, *NEREIS (NEANTHES) ARENACEODENTATA*

REFERENCE: Dillon, T. M., Moore, D. W., and Reish, D. J., **"A 28 Day Sediment Bioassay with the Marine Polychaete, Nereis (Neanthes) Arenaceodentata,"** Environmental Toxicology and Risk Assessment - Third Volume, ASTM STP 1218, Jane S. Hughes, Gregory R. Biddinger, and Eugene Mones, Eds., American Society for Testing and Materials, Philadelphia, 1995.

ABSTRACT: A protocol for conducting a 28 day sediment bioassay with the marine polychaete, *Nereis (Neanthes) arenaceodentata* is described. Primary application is the regulatory evaluation of dredged material. Test endpoints are survival and estimated individual growth rate. Bioassays are initiated by adding juvenile worms to 1L glass beakers (5 worms/beaker) containing aerated seawater (30 ^{o}/oo) and 2-3 cm of sediment. Temperature is 20°C and photoperiod 12h. Worms are fed twice weekly, seawater renewed weekly and water quality monitored throughout. After 28 days, the number of survivors per beaker is recorded. Worms in each replicate are dried as a pool. Estimated individual dry weight is calculated by dividing number of survivors into the pooled dry weight biomass. Growth rate (mg dry weight day^{-1}) is calculated by subtracting initial from final dry weights and dividing by the exposure period (28 d). Performance criteria for positive and negative controls are discussed as well as guidance for interpreting bioassay results. Although designed for the regulatory evaluation of dredged material, this chronic sublethal bioassay can be applied to other assessments of sediment quality.

KEYWORDS: chronic, sublethal, sediment, bioassay, polychaetes, growth, reproduction, population dynamics

Sediment bioassays are used to assess the aggregate toxicity of sediment-associated anthropogenic chemicals. Historically, these bioassays have measured survival in highly sensitive species following acute exposures ($\leq$ 10 days). A new generation of sediment bioassays is being

[1]Research Biologist, USAE Waterways Experiment Station, Environmental Laboratory, CEWES-ES-F, Vicksburg, MS 39180-6199 USA

[2]Emeritus Professor, California State University, Long Beach, Department of Biology, Long Beach, CA 90840 USA

developed in which the subtle, sublethal response of test species is measured following chronic sediment exposures (Dillon 1993). Here, we report a protocol for conducting a chronic sublethal sediment bioassay with juveniles of the marine polychaete, *Nereis (Neanthes) arenaceodentata*.

TARGET APPLICATION FOR THIS SEDIMENT BIOASSAY

This sediment bioassay was developed for the regulatory evaluation of dredged material under §103 of the Marine Protection, Research, and Sanctuaries Act of 1972 (PL 92-532) and §404(b)(1) of the Federal Water Pollution Control Act of 1972 (Public Law 92-500), as amended. It was was designed specifically to assess the toxicity of bedded sediments. Research and test development was targeted for eventual use by the commercial bioassay contracting community. Thus, great emphasis was placed on logistical feasibility, practicality, low capital start-up and run costs. To maximize regulatory utility, interpretive guidance explaining the biological importance of test results was also developed. Although targeted for dredged material toxicity testing, this bioassay can be used in other assessments of sediment quality. For example:

- Bioaccumulation potential - uptake of sediment-associated contaminants
- Suspended sediments - toxicity and bioaccumulation
- Field surveys - spatial distribution of sediment toxicity
- Hazard assessments - strength or magnitude of sediment-associated chemicals (may require spiked sediments)
- Risk assessments - integration of chronic sublethal effects assessments with spatial distributions of sediment toxicity.
- Hypothesis testing - evaluation of specific questions regarding sediment quality (e.g. effects of food on sediment toxicity)

TEST ORGANISM

Taxonomy and Natural History

The test organism for this sediment bioassay is the nereid polychaete, *Nereis (Neanthes) arenaceodentata*. Its taxonomic status is still being debated (for discussion see Dillon et al. 1993). For example, Atlantic and Pacific populations have different karyotypes, are reproductively isolated and are probably different species (Weinberg et al. 1990). Until the taxonomic status of this species is resolved we recommend using the name most familiar to toxicologists (*Neanthes arenaceodentata*) and reporting the original source of worms. *N. arenaceodentata* is widely distributed in shallow marine and estuarine benthic habitats of Europe, North America and throughout the Pacific (Day 1973, Pettibone 1963, Reish 1957, Taylor 1984, Whitlatch 1977). It constructs one or more mucoid tubes in the upper 2 to 3 cm of sediment. This deposit-feeder ingests particles up to 70 μm in diameter with a preference for those around 12 μm (Whitlatch 1980).

Life Cycle

The life cycle of *N. arenaceodentata* is well-documented (Pesch and Hoffman 1983, Reish 1957). As worms approach sexual maturity, males and females establish pairs and occupy a common tube. Eggs are deposited by the female within the tube. The male presumably fertilizes the eggs at this time. The spent female soon exits the tube and dies within 1-2 days or is eaten by the male. The male remains in the tube to incubate and guard the developing embryos. He creates a current of water via rhythmic undulations to remove metabolic wastes and prevent hypoxic conditions. There is no planktonic larval life stage. Development is direct and occurs entirely within the parental tube. Emergent juveniles (EJs) exit the parental tube about 3 weeks after egg deposition. They establish tubes of their own and begin to feed. Juvenile worms grow and eggs become visible in the coelom of females at about 6 weeks post-emergence. The eggs continue to grow in the coelom and deposition occurs 9-13 weeks post-emergence to complete the life cycle. The entire life cycle can be completed in the laboratory in 12 to 16 weeks at 20 to 22°C. The non-planktonic benthic larvae and paternal care are uncommon characteristics among the Nereidae. These features greatly facilitate laboratory culture and experimental investigations of growth and reproductive effects of contaminated sediments.

Laboratory Culture Methods

Laboratory cultures of *N. arenaceodentata* were begun by one of us (D.J.R.) in 1964. In March 1988, approximately 200 juvenile worms were shipped to the USAE Waterways Experiment Station (WES). Continuous worm cultures have been maintained at the WES since that time. Static-renewal culture methods were adapted from the static procedures of Reish (1974) and the flow-through methods of Pesch and Schauer (1988). Worms are maintained at 20°C in 30 °/oo artificial seawater made up with reverse osmosis water (ROW). The photoperiod is 12 h light. EJs are raised to adulthood in 38 L all glass aquaria (100 EJs/aquarium) containing 30 L aerated seawater and a 2-3 cm layer of fine-grain, uncontaminated marine sediment collected near Sequim, WA. Twice weekly finely-ground (≤ 0.50mm) Tetramarin® (100 mg) and alfalfa (50 mg) are added to each aquarium via a seawater slurry. The slurry is prepared and stirred for about 4h prior to feeding. Complete seawater renewal every three weeks is sufficient to maintain good water quality. Initially and at each renewal, approximately 25 cm^3 of frozen green algae (*Enteromorpha sp.*) is provided to each aquarium. The algae is added to diversify the food ration and provide additional tube-building material. After 10 weeks worms are paired using the intrasexual fighting response and the presence/absence of eggs in the coelom (Reish 1974). Unpaired worms are not returned to the culture. Pairs are placed in 600 ml beakers with 500 ml seawater. Each pair is initially fed a slurry containing 4 mg Tetramarin® and 4 mg alfalfa. Gentle aeration is provided via pasteur pipettes and the beakers are covered with watch glasses to reduce evaporation. Seawater is carefully renewed weekly (≃ 80% by volume) in a manner that avoids disturbing worm pairs. Beakers are monitored daily for the presence of eggs and EJs. When discovered, EJs are pooled from different broods and returned to the 38 L aquaria to complete the culture cycle. These culture conditions and feeding rations were used in all experiments described below unless otherwise noted.

Toxicology

N. arenaceodentata is recommended for dredged material toxicity testing by the two Federal agencies having regulatory responsibility; the US Army Corps of Engineers (USACE) and the US Environmental Protection Agency (USEPA) (USEPA/USACE 1991, 1993). It has been used in numerous scientific studies designed to evaluate the chronic sublethal effects of contaminated sediment (Johns et al. 1985, Pastorok and Becker 1990, Pesch et al. 1987). A considerable amount of information has also been reported regarding contaminant-specific toxicity for this species (Moore et al. 1991, Reish 1980, 1985).

STATISTICAL DESIGN

The null hypothesis for this sediment bioassay is that there are no statistically significant (α=0.05) differences between the project or test sediments and the reference sediment. Characteristics and selection of an appropriate reference sediment is discussed in USEPA/USACE (1991, 1993). There are five replicates per treatment and 5 animals per replicate. Treatments should be arranged in a completely randomized block design. The level of variability in the endpoints results in minimum detectable differences (MDD) of 21% for growth and 24% for survival. Johns et al. (1991) report these MDD bracket those observed in sediment bioassays with saltwater amphipods. One liter exposure vessels constitute the experimental replicate.

TEST PROTOCOL

This section describes the protocol for conducting the 28 day chronic sublethal sediment bioassay with *N. arenaceodentata*. General guidance for conducting dredged material toxicity tests can be found in USEPA/USACE (1991, 1993). Supporting information can also be found in Standard Guides produced by the Sediment Toxicology Subcommittee E47.03 of the American Society of Testing and Materials (ASTM 1990, 1993).

Sediment Handling

Sediments are stored cold (4°C) in sealed containers with a minimum of overlying water. One to two days before initiating the bioassay, sediments are removed from cold storage and press-sieved (2 mm screen) without the addition of seawater. This seiving removes macrofauna and large objects which may be present. It also greatly facilitates sediment seiving at test termination to recover surviving worms. After seiving, sediments are thoroughly homogenized and randomly distributed to appropriate exposure vessels. Enough sediment is added to each vessel to create a 2-3 cm layer. Replicate subsamples are removed from the homogenized sediment for grain size analysis, interstitial salinity, pH and ammonia determinations.

Preparation of Exposure Vessels

Exposure vessels are 1L glass beakers. After sediment has been added to pre-labeled beakers, 30 $^{o}/oo$ seawater is slowly added to the 800 ml mark in a manner which minimizes sediment resuspension. Beakers are placed in a temperature- and photoperiod-controlled environment ($20^{o}C$ and 12h light, respectively) physically isolated from other laboratory activities. Trickle-flow aeration is provided via glass pipette after any suspended sediment has settled. Pipettes are secured in such a manner that they will remain several centimeters above the sediment surface without resuspension. Beakers are covered with watch glasses to minimize evaporation and keep out any dust. For logistically reasons, beakers are usually prepared the day before a test is initiated. Blind labeling of exposure vessels is recommended for QA/QC.

Test Initiation

Initial water quality--Highly organic test sediments may release an initial bolus of ammonia and/or hydrogen sulfide when seawater is first added to the beaker (unpublished data). Consequently, overlying water should be carefully renewed prior to test initiation. Following this renewal, but prior to the addition of worms, overlying water quality should be determined in each beaker. At a minimum, temperature, salinity, dissolved oxygen, pH and ammonia should be determined.

Test organisms--Juvenile worms (2-3 weeks old) are used to initiate this sediment bioassay. This age worm is recommended for several reasons. One, they are 10 to 15 mm long and thus, readily visible to the naked eye. Younger worms are much more difficult to see which we find greatly increases the probability of counting errors. Two, very small worms have very low (50%-60%) rates of survival (unpublished data). Three, initiating tests with 2-3 week old worms allows time for a commercial supplier to collect and ship worms to a test facility if they do not maintain laboratory cultures in-house. Finally, if worms older than 2-3 weeks are used to initiate the bioassay, they will be entering active vitellogenesis at test termination. Egg deposition may even occur in some individuals. Since the endpoint for this bioassay is somatic growth (see Measurement of Test Endpoint below), onset of gametic growth should be avoided.

Worms used to initiate the test are selected from a pool containing about twice the number of animals actually needed. Some worms from this pool will not be used; i.e. those physically damaged or exhibiting aberrant behavior, very small or very large worms (see above paragraph). Also, some worms from this common pool will be used to determine initial estimated individual dry weight and in the reference toxicant test (see below). Selected worms are randomly placed in pre-labeled 100 ml holding beakers (5 worms/beaker) containing seawater. Enough holding beakers should be prepared for: 1) the sediment bioassay (5 beakers/treatment), 2) the reference toxicant test (30 beakers) and 3) initial dry weights (5 beakers). For a blind experimental design, the holding beakers may be labeled sequentially then selected at random by someone not involved in worm selection.

The bioassay is initiated when worms are introduced into the 1L exposure beakers containing sediment. Worms are transferred with a No. 3 camel hair brush. They are added one at a time to verify initial census and to visually examine the condition of each worm. Care should be taken to insure worms are not caught in the surface tension when introduced.

Feeding--Once the bioassay is initiated, each beaker is provided a seawater slurry containing finely-ground ($\leq$ 0.50mm) well-hydrated Tetramarin® (5 mg) and alfalfa (2.5 mg). For example, if the bioassay involves 6 treatments (i.e. 30 beakers), a feeding slurry of 350 mls is prepared containing 175 mg of Tetramarin® and 87.5 mg alfalfa. After stirring for about 4 hours, 10 mls of this slurry is added to each beaker via pipette. The food slurry is well mixed each time an aliquot is withdrawn.

Reference toxicant test--A seawater-only 96h reference toxicant test with cadmium chloride is conducted at the same time the sediment bioassay is initiated. We currently use 6 exposure concentrations (0, 3, 6, 12, 24, 48 mg Cd/L), 5 replicate beakers/concentration and 5 worms/beaker. A concentrated stock solution of reagent grade cadmium chloride in cation-exchanged ROW is prepared anew for each test. Using this stock, five liters of each concentration is prepared in 30 $^{o}/oo$ seawater, thoroughly mixed and distributed among the 1L beakers (800 ml solution/beaker). Beakers are placed under trickle flow aeration and covered with watch glasses. Experimental conditions are the same as in sediment bioassays. Worms for the reference toxicant test are drawn from the same pool of animals used to initiate the sediment bioassay. Animals are added to beakers one at a time as described above. Worms are not fed during the test. After 96h the number of survivors in each beaker is recorded. Water quality is determined in each beaker when the test is initiated and at termination. A 30 ml sample is collected from each beaker initially and at test termination to analytically confirm nominal cadmium concentrations. Samples are analyzed for cadmium within 24h. We find in-house analysis of cadmium with an ion-specific electrode to be rapid, accurate and cost-effective.

Initial dry weights--Initial dry weights are determined on a subsample of 25 worms from the pool of animals used to initiate the bioassay. These worms are placed in 5 beakers during selection of test animals (see above). Procedures for dry weight determinations are described below (see Test Termination).

Test Maintenance

Each beaker is visually checked every weekday. Abnormal and/or unanticipated events and observations are recorded in the lab notebook. This includes but is not limited to interruptions in aeration, cloudy water, abnormal appearance/texture/color of the sediment surface, evidence of worm activity or inactivity (e.g. burrow openings, surficial tracks or lack thereof, presence in the water column). Weekly seawater renewals are sufficient to maintain good water quality. At each renewal, approximately 80% of the overlying seawater is removed and refilled to the 800 ml mark. Water quality (dissolved oxygen, salinity, pH, ammonia) should be monitored in each beaker prior to each renewal and at test termination. Temperature should be monitored daily. Worms are fed the Tetramarin®-alfalfa slurry described above twice weekly; after every renewal and 3-4 days later.

Test Termination

The test is terminated after 28 days sediment exposure. A final visual check of each beaker is made and terminal water quality assessed. All surviving worms are removed from each beaker in the following manner. Most of the overlying seawater is carefully poured off retaining any worms that may be in the water column. The beaker is then gently swirled to suspend the surficial sediment. This slurry is gently poured through a stack of nested sieves (2.0, 1.0, 0.5 mm). Experience indicates that all surviving worms will often be recovered in this surficial layer. If survival is 100% (i.e. if 5 worms are recovered) the need to sieve all the sediment in the beaker is eliminated. If < 5 worms are recovered, all remaining sediment must be sieved and checked for survivors. To do this, deposit the sediment from the beaker on top of the nested sieves. Rinse with a gentle stream of seawater. Remove survivors to a beaker with clean seawater. The number of surviving worms/replicate is recorded. They are briefly rinsed in ROW water to remove saltwater and any adhering sediment, pooled and placed on a tared aluminum weighing pan. The ROW rinse has been shown to have no effect on weight determinations compared to a similar rinse in isotonic ammonium formate (Dillon et al. 1993). Tissue samples are oven-dried at 60°C to a constant weight ($\simeq$ 24h), brought to room temperature under desiccation and reweighed. Estimated individual worm weights are calculated by dividing the total dry weight biomass in a replicate by the number of survivors.

DATA ANALYSIS

Data Validation

Data validation procedures generally assume data are valid until they deviate from some performance criteria. Significant deviations in performance criteria can be grounds for rejecting data unless a good explanation can be provided. Standard data validation procedures for sediment bioassays have not formalized. Performance criteria for individual sediment bioassays typically evolve over time in an *ad hoc* fashion rather than by any rigorous numerical analysis. Based on observations in our and other laboratories, we recommend that data validation be carried out using the following assessments.

Performance in the Negative Control Treatment--The negative control for most sediment bioassays are beakers containing sediment in which the animals were either cultured or field-collected. For this bioassay with *N. arenaceodentata*, we recommend performance criteria of $\geq$ 80% survival in any one replicate and $\geq$ 90% mean survival for all replicates containing Sequim Bay, WA sediment.

Performance in the Positive Control--For this bioassay, the survival of *N. arenaceodentata* in the reference toxicant test with cadmium chloride is the positive control. Tests conducted thus far indicate 96h LC_{50s} range between 10 and 15 mg/l. These data will eventually be used to construct a Shewart Control Chart. This chart will be used to identify statistically "out of control" data and thus, invalid sediment bioassays. However, extant guidance (Environment Canada 1990, Shainin and Shainin 1988) suggests 15 to 25 tests are required to construct a legitimate control chart.

Water Quality Data--Mean water quality should meet the following performance criteria: temperature - $20^oC \pm 2^oC$; salinity - 30 $^o/oo \pm 3^o/oo$, dissolved oxygen $\geq$ 6.0 mg/L, pH - 8.0 $\pm$ 1.0, total ammonia - $\leq$ 1.0 mg/L.

Anomalous Events or Deviations from Good Laboratory Practice--Anomalous events or deviations from good laboratory practice can be grounds for rejecting data. However, the impact of those events, if sufficient in magnitude or duration, should be reflected in deviations of the above performance criteria.

Data Reduction

Data reduction and subsequent analysis proceeds only after the data have been validated. For each replicate, survival and juvenile worm growth is calculated. The latter is expressed as a rate function according to the formula

$$G = \frac{DW_t - DW_i}{T}$$

where G = estimated individual growth rate (mg dry weight day^{-1})
DW_t = estimated individual dry weight at termination (mg)
DW_i = mean estimated individual dry weight at initiation (mg)
T = exposure time (days)

DW_i was determined on a subsample from the pool of juvenile worms used to start the bioassay (see Test Initiation above). The advantages of expressing growth as a rate function (mg/d) rather than as an absolute dry weight (mg) is discussed in Dillon et al. (1993).

Statistical Analysis

One-way ANOVA is used to test the null hypothesis that response in the reference sediment is not statistically different from that in the project sediments. This analysis is conducted for both test endpoints; survival and estimated individual growth rate. Homogeneity of variances is evaluated with either Bartlett's test or Levene's test using appropriate transformations as needed. Mean separation may be performed via a Tukey's HSD test, Dunnett's, or other appropriate parametric procedure. All differences are assumed statistically significant at $P<0.05$.

INTERPRETING BIOASSAY TEST RESULTS

We recommend a tiered hierarchy for interpreting bioassay test results.

Tier I: Are the test results valid?

Methods to validate data were discussed above. If the data cannot be validated, and if no reasonable explanation can be provided, the test may be considered invalid. Further analysis would be unwarranted. If the data are acceptable, proceed to Tier II.

Tier II: Are the results statistically significant?

Statistical methods are recommended above. If response in the reference sediment is statistically indistinguishable from that in the project sediments, further data interpretation is unwarranted. If results are significantly different, go to Tier III.

Tier III: Are the results biologically important?

A statistically significant result may or may not be important biologically. For example, if a project sediment causes a statistically significant 5% decrease in survival, is that level of response truly detrimental to the organism? Would a 10% decrease be twice as "bad" or only incrementally injurious? Deciphering the biological importance of sublethal endpoints such as growth is even more problematic. For this bioassay, the technical basis for interpreting test results relies on the relationship between growth and reproductive success. Growth and reproduction are energy antagonists. That is, they represent competing demands on a usually limited energy source. As a result, diminished growth will likely lead to adverse effects on reproduction. Establishing the quantitative nature of this relationship provides the technical basis for interpreting the growth endpoint. Moore and Dillon (1993) examined this relationship quantitatively and observed no significant effects on either survival or reproduction when somatic growth rates were $\geq$ 0.65 mg wet/day. Growth rates $\leq$ 0.45 mg/day resulted in significant reductions in reproduction. Very low growth rates (i.e. 0.05 mg/day) were associated with a nearly complete cessation of reproduction and very poor survival (5%-11%).

Ultimately, the biological importance of ecotoxicology studies should be interpreted in terms of a meaningful population-level response (Barnthouse et al. 1986, Suter 1990). If a contaminant-induced perturbation represents an important environmental hazard, there is a risk that a local population may decline or even become extinct. This risk can be projected quantitatively using demographic population models. Originally developed by actuaries to project trends in human populations (Lotka 1925), demographic models were first used to assess population-level effects of xenobiotics on aquatic animals about 30 years ago Marshall (1962). These models represent a tool for integrating life history observations (i.e. survival, growth, reproduction) into deterministic and risk-based estimates of population viability. WES is currently developing a risk-based demographic model for *N. arenaceodentata*.

QUALITY ASSURANCE (QA)/QUALITY CONTROL (QC)

QA/QC are the administrative and technical steps taken to insure reliable data are produced with specified precision and accuracy. Specific QA/QC measures associated with this chronic sublethal sediment bioassay with *N. arenaceodentata* were discussed above. In a more general sense, QA/QC should include but is not limited to the following subject areas:

- Lab-wide Quality Assurance Management Plan (QAMP)
- Project-specific Quality Assurance Project Plan (QAPP)
- Documented Standard Operating Procedures (SOPs)
- Appropriate staffing and training
- Adherence to Good Laboratory Practices (GLP)
- Performance criteria for negative and positive controls
- Data validation procedures
- Anticipated corrective actions
- Use of control charts

EVALUATE TEST "RUGGEDNESS"

ASTM (1991) defines "ruggedness" as the "insensitivity of a test method to departures from specified test or environmental conditions.". For sediment bioassays, "ruggedness" is evaluated from two perspectives: 1) sensitivity to the physico-chemical properties of sediments and 2) deviations in normal test conditions and protocols. Examples of the former include the effects of grain size, interstitial ammonia, presence of indigenous fauna, organic carbon, etc. These factors are known to bias results of acute lethality sediment bioassays (e.g. DeWitt et al. 1988) and their potential influence will no doubt increase as test duration increases and more sensitive endpoints are examined. The effects of sediment properties and deviations from normal conditions on survival and growth in *N. arenaceodentata* has been reported (Dillon et al. 1993) and are summarized below.

Intraspecific Densities

Survival was high (81%-100%) after 6 weeks in 600 ml beakers containing sediment and up to 12 juvenile worms. Growth after 6 weeks was unaffected at densities $\leq$ 4 worms/beaker but significantly depressed at densities $\geq$ 8 worms/beaker. In the absence of sediment, the adverse effects of intraspecific interactions were magnified.

Grain Size

Juvenile worms can tolerate a wide range of grain sizes. Survival was high (89%-100%) and unaffected after 6 weeks in grain sizes ranging from 5% to 100% sand. Likewise, there was no significant effect on growth. However, there was a consistent trend of reduced worm weight with increasing grain size. This may indicate a possible grain size effect with longer (> 6 weeks) exposures.

Salinity

N. arenaceodentata is cultured in 30 ^{o}/oo seawater at WES. Test sediments may come from areas where the salinity is considerably lower. Survival and growth of *N. arenaceodentata* after 6 weeks was unaffected following acute transfers from 30 ^{o}/oo seawater to salinities $\geq$ 20 ^{o}/oo. However, no juvenile worms survived acute transfers to $\leq$ 15 ^{o}/oo. The effects of gradual acclimation was not examined.

Ammonia Toxicity

Juvenile worms exhibited a sharp threshold response to chronic ammonia concentrations similar to that observed for salinity. Survival and growth were unaffected following a 6 week exposure to total ammonia concentrations $\leq$ 10 mg/L. Survival was 0% at $\geq$ 40 mg/L. At the intermediate test concentration (20 mg/L), both survival and growth were slightly but not significantly diminished.

Hydrogen Sulfide Toxicity

Survival of juvenile worms in short term (96h) exposures was 100% at sulfide concentrations $\leq$ 5.0 mg/L. At 10.0 and 20.0 mg/L, survival was 44% and 0%, respectively.

Resistance to Hypoxia

Survival of juvenile worms in short term (96h) exposures was 100% at $\leq$ 1.5 mg/L. At 1.0 and 0.5 mg/L, survival was 68% and 0%, respectively

FUTURE ACTIVITIES

Although a test protocol can be recommended at this time, we feel additional test development is required. This work falls into the following categories:

- Continue evaluating test "ruggedness"
- Develop a risk-based demographic population model
- Conduct bioassays on a wide range of dredged material
- Evaluate interlaboratory variation
- Compare with other dredged material bioassays

SUMMARY OF BIOASSAY TEST PROTOCOL

A protocol for conducting a 28 day sediment bioassay with the marine polychaete, *Nereis (Neanthes) arenaceodentata* is described. Primary target application is the regulatory evaluation of dredged material. Bioaccumulation potential may also be evaluated under certain conditions. Test endpoints are survival and estimated individual growth rate. The bioassay is conducted at 20°C under a 12h photoperiod in 1L glass beakers containing aerated seawater (30 °/oo) and a 2-3 cm layer of bedded sediment. The test is initiated by randomly adding juvenile worms (2-3 weeks old) to beakers (5 worms/beaker and 5 beakers/treatment). Worms are quantitatively fed twice weekly a seawater slurry containing finely-ground Tetramarin® and alfalfa. Seawater is renewed weekly (ca. 80% volume replacement). Water quality is monitored at least weekly prior to each renewal and at termination. After 28 days, worms are removed via seiving and the number of survivors in each beaker is recorded. Survivors from each treatment are pooled, placed on a tared weighing pan, dried to a constant weight (24h at 60°C) and weighed to the nearest 0.01 mg. Estimated individual worm weight is determined for each replicate by dividing total dry weight biomass by the number of survivors. Growth is expressed as a rate (mg dry weight day^{-1}) for each replicate by subtracting initial dry weight from final values and dividing by the exposure period (28 d). Quality control performance criteria for positive and negative controls are reported. Interpretive guidance for this bioassay is based on the relationship between growth and subsequent reproductive success. Although designed for the regulatory evaluation of dredged material this bioassay can be applied to other assessments of sediment quality.

ACKNOWLEDGMENTS

Insightful reviews were provided by Dr. Todd Bridges and Ms. Alfreda Gibson of the USAE Waterways Experiment Station, Dr. Jack Word, Battelle Northwest Marine Laboratory, as well as anonymous reviewers. Funding for this work was provided by the USAE District, San Francisco, as well as the U.S. Army Corps of Engineers (USACE) Long-Term Effects of Dredging Operations (LEDO) Program, Work Unit 32468. The LEDO Program is sponsored by the Headquarters, USACE. Permission was granted by the Chief of Engineers to publish this information.

REFERENCES

ASTM, 1990, "Standard Guide for Collection, Storage, Characterization, and Manipulation of Sediment for Toxicological Testing," ASTM Standard No. E 1391-90, (American Society for Testing and Materials, Philadelphia, PA).

ASTM, 1991, "Standard Terminology Relating to Quality and Statistics," ASTM Standard No. E 456-91a, (American Society for Testing and Materials, Philadelphia, PA).

ASTM, 1993, "Standard Guide for Designing Biological Tests with Sediment," " ASTM Standard No. E 1525-93, (American Society for Testing and Materials, Philadelphia, PA).

Barnthouse, L.W., O'Neill, R.V., Bartell, S.M., and Suter, G.W. II, 1986, "Population and Ecosystem Theory in Ecological Risk Assessment", *Aquatic Toxicology and Environmental Fate: Ninth Volume*, Poston, R.M. and Prudy, R., eds., ASTM STP 921, American Society for Testing and Materials, Philadelphia, PA, pp. 82-96.

Day, J., 1973, "New Polychaeta from Beaufort with a key to all species recorded from North Carolina," NOAA Tech. Report 375. National Oceanic and Atmospheric Adminstration, National Marine Fisheries Service, Washington, DC.

DeWitt, T.H., Ditsworth, G.R., and Swartz, R.C., 1988, "Effects of natural sediment features on survival of the phoxocephalid amphipod *Rhepoxynius abronius*," Mar. Environ. Res., Vol. 25, pp. 99-124.

Dillon, T.M., 1993, "Developing Chronic Sublethal Sediment Bioassays: A Challenge to the Scientific Community," *Environmental Toxicology and Risk Assessment: 2nd Volume*, Gorsuch, J.W., Dwyer, F.J., Ingersoll, C.G. and La Point, T.W., eds., ASTM STP 1173, American Society for Testing Materials, PA, (*in press*).

Dillon, T.M., Moore, D.M., and Gibson, A.B., 1993, "Development of a chronic sublethal sediment bioassay with the marine polychaete worm, *Nereis (Neanthes) arenaceodentata*," Environ. Toxicol. Chem., Vol. 12, pp. 589-605.

Environment Canada, 1990, "Guidance document on control of toxicity test precision using reference toxicants," Report EPS 1/RM/12, Ottawa, Ontario.

Johns, D.M., Gutjahr-Gobell, R., and Schauer, P., 1985, "Use of Bioenergetics to Investigate the Impact of Dredged Material on Benthic Species: A Laboratory Study with Polychaetes and Black Rock Harbor Material," Technical Report D-85-7, U. S. Army Waterways Experiment Station, Vicksburg, MS.

Johns, D.M., Pastorok, R.A., and Ginn, T.C., 1991, "A sublethal toxicity test using juvenile *Neanthes* sp. (Polychaeta: Nereidae)," *Aquatic Toxicology and Risk Assessment: 14th Volume*, Mayes, M.A. and Barron, M.G., eds., ASTM STP 1124, American Society for Testing and Materials, Philadelphia, PA, pp. 280-293.

Lotka, A.J., 1925, Elements of Physical Biology, Williams and Wilkins Co., Baltimore.

Marshall, J.S., 1962, "The effects of continuous gamma radiation on the intrinsic rate of natural increase of *Daphnia pulex*," Ecology, Vol. 43, pp. 598-607.

Moore, D.W., Dillon, T.M., and Suedel, B.S., 1991, "Chronic toxicity of tributyltin on the marine polychaete worm, *Neanthes arenaceodentata*," Aquatic Toxicol., Vol. 21, pp. 181-198.

Moore, D.W. and Dillon, T.M., 1993, "The relationship between growth and reproduction in marine polychaete *Nereis (Neanthes) arenaceodentata* (Moore): Implications for chronic sublethal sediment bioassays," J. exp. Mar. Biol. Ecol. (*in press*).

Pastorok, R.A. and Becker, D.S., 1990, "Comparative sensitivity of sediment toxicity bioassays at three Superfund sites in Puget Sound," *Aquatic Toxicology and Hazard Assessment*, Landis, W.G. and van der Schalie, W.H., eds., ASTM STP 1096, American Society for Testing and Materials, Philadelphia, PA, pp. 123-139.

Pesch, C.E. and Hoffman, G.A., 1983, "Interlaboratory comparison of a 28-day toxicity test with the polychaete *Neanthes arenaceodentata*," *Aquatic Toxicology and Hazard Assessment*, Bishop, W.E., Cardwell, R.D., and Heidolph, B.B., eds., ASTM STP 802, American Society for Testing and Materials, Philadelphia, PA, pp. 482-493.

Pesch, G., Mueller, C., and Pesch, C.E., 1987, "Sister Chromatid Exchange in Marine Polychaetes Exposed to Black Rock Harbor Sediment," Technical Report D-87-5, U. S. Army Engineer Waterways Experiment Station, Vicksburg, MS.

Pesch, C.E. and Schauer, P.S., 1988, "Flow-through culture techniques for *Neanthes arenaceodentata* (annelida: polychaeta), including influence of diet on growth and survival," Environ. Toxicol. Chem., Vol.7, pp. 961-968.

Pettibone, M.H., 1963, "Marine polychaete worms of the New England region. 1. Aphroditidae through Trochochaetidae," Smithsonian Institution Museum of Natural History, Washington, D.C., 356 pp.

Reish, D.J., 1957, "The life history of the polychaetous annelid *Neanthes caudata* (delle Chiaje), including a summary of development in the family Nereidae," Pacific Sci., Vol. 11, pp. 216-228.

Reish, D.J., 1974, "The establishment of laboratory colonies of polychaetous annelids," Thalassia Jugoslavica, Vol. 10, pp. 181-195.

Reish, J.D., 1980, "Use of polychaetous annelids as test organisms for marine bioassay experiments," *Aquatic Invertebrate Bioassays*, Buikema, A.L., Jr. and Cairns, J., Jr., eds., ASTM STP 715, American Society for Testing and Material, Philadelphia, PA, pp. 140-154.

Reish, D.J., 1985, "The use of the polychaetous annelid *Neanthes arenaceodentata* as a laboratory experimental animal," Tethys, Vol. 11, pp. 335-341.

Shainin, D. and Shainin, P.D., 1988, "Statistical Process Control," *Juran's Quality Control Handbook*, fourth edition, Juran, J.M. and Gryna, F.M., eds., McGraw-Hill, Inc., New York, NY, pp. 23.1-23.121.

Suter, G.W. II, 1990, "Endpoints for regional ecological risk assessments," Environ. Manag., Vol. 14, pp. 9-23.

Taylor, J.L., 1984, "Family Nereidae Johnston, 1845, "Taxonomic guide to the Polychaetes of the Northern Gulf of Mexico," Uebelacker, J.M. and Johnson, P.G., eds., U.S. Department of the Interior, Minerals Management Service, Metairie, LA, pp. 14-15.

U.S. Environmental Protection Agency/U.S. Army Corps of Engineers, 1991, "Evaluation of dredged material proposed for ocean disposal (testing manual). Implementation Manual for §103 of Public Law 92-532 (Marine Protection, Research, and Sanctuaries Act of 1972," U.S. Army Engineer Waterways Experiment Station, Vicksburg, MS.

U.S. Environmental Protection Agency/U.S. Army Corps of Engineers, 1993, "Evaluation of dredged material proposed for inland and near-shore disposal. Draft Testing Manual for §404(b)(1) of Public Law 92-500 (Federal Water Pollution Control Act of 1972, as amended" U.S. Army Engineer Waterways Experiment Station, Vicksburg, MS.

Weinberg, J.R., Starczak, V.R., Meuller, C. Pesch, G.C., and Lindsay, S.M., 1990, "Divergence between populations of a monogamous polychaete with male parental care: premating isolation and chromosome variation," Mar. Biol., Vol. 107, pp. 205-213.

Whitlatch, R.B., 1977, "Seasonal changes in the community structure of the macrobenthos inhabiting the intertidal sand and mud flats of Barnstable Harbor, Massachusetts," Biol. Bull., Vol. 152, pp.275-294.

Whitlatch, R.B., 1980, "Patterns of resource utilization and coexistence in marine intertidal deposit-feeding communities," J. Mar. Res., Vol. 38, pp. 743-765.

Michael H. Salazar[1] and Sandra M. Salazar[2]

IN-SITU BIOASSAYS USING TRANSPLANTED MUSSELS: I. ESTIMATING CHEMICAL EXPOSURE AND BIOEFFECTS WITH BIOACCUMULATION AND GROWTH

REFERENCE: Salazar, M. H., and Salazar, S. M., **"In-Situ Bioassays Using Transplanted Mussels: I. Estimating Chemical Exposure and Bioeffects with Bioaccumulation and Growth,"** Environmental Toxicology and Risk Assessment - Third Volume, ASTM STP 1218, Jane S. Hughes, Gregory R. Boddinger and Eugene Mones, Eds., American Society for Testing and Materials, Philadelphia, 1995.

ABSTRACT: Using transplanted mussels as an *in-situ* bioassay to assess marine environmental quality has provided important information on bioavailability of contaminants and associated bioeffects that would not have been available with traditional chemical monitoring, biomonitoring, or laboratory bioassays. It is one of the most promising field bioassay systems because of the relative ease in making synoptic measurements of bioaccumulation and growth to estimate chemical exposure and bioeffects, respectively. *In-situ* field studies that utilize transplanted animals combine the advantages of environmental realism associated with field monitoring and experimental control associated with laboratory testing. Because they are sedentary and concentrate contaminants, resident mussels have been used extensively to estimate exposure by measuring contaminants in their tissues. The use of resident mussels as a response indicator has been very limited because of the difficulties associated with measuring biological processes and defining the exposure period in natural populations. Transplanting caged mussels facilitates measurements of bioeffects and clearly defines the exposure period. Data from a series of mussel (*Mytilus galloprovincialis*) transplants in San Diego Bay, California, demonstrate how this methodology can be used to assess the extent of contamination and associated biological effects. Although more than 18 sites were studied in nine separate transplants between 1987 and 1990, emphasis will be placed on two sites in the Shelter Island Yacht Basin separated by only 3 meters vertical distance. The mussel field bioassay was used to identify the following: (1) site-specific differences, (2) temporal and spatial variability, (3) short-term and long-term trends, (4) potential sources of contamination, and (5) dose-response relationships.

KEYWORDS: mussel transplants, sediments, bioaccumulation, growth, contamination, *in-situ* bioassay, standard protocols

Biological monitoring systems are needed to identify the presence of potentially toxic chemicals, quantify their presence in animal tissues, and provide meaningful measurements of biological effects (Mearns 1985; U.S. Environmental Protection Agency 1988). Although there has been extensive use of filter-feeding bivalves to measure bioaccumulation in both laboratory and field studies, synoptic field measurements of exposure and bioeffects have been extremely limited.

[1]NOAA Bioeffects Branch, 7600 Sand Point Way NE, Seattle, WA, 98115
[2]EVS Consultants, 200 West Mercer Street, Suite 403, Seattle, WA 98119

Transplanted mussels are an effective tool to obtain information about exposure and bioeffects associated with chemical contamination that is not provided by traditional chemical monitoring of water, sediment, and tissue or from laboratory bioassays (Phillips 1980; Martin 1985; Nelson 1990; Widdows and Donkin 1992; Phillips and Rainbow 1993; Salazar and Salazar 1994). Traditional approaches do not adequately measure bioavailability or the potential effects of contaminants. The exposure period is always uncertain in chemical monitoring of resident mussels, there is little experimental control, and bioeffects are difficult to measure. In laboratory bioassays, bioeffects are easily measured but the experimental control may introduce unwanted artifacts and the environmental significance is always questionable. Even the most comprehensive approaches that combine chemical measurements of seawater or sediment with laboratory bioassays and community assemblages (Long and Chapman 1985) should be augmented with field bioassays that include more direct measurements of actual exposure and associated biological effects.

Currently, there are no ASTM protocols for *in-situ* bioassays to estimate exposure or bioeffects. There is a need to standardize protocols for the use of transplanted mussels as indicators of exposure and effects because the few protocols that have been developed differ significantly (Martin 1985; Foe and Knight 1987; Weber 1988; Phillips 1988; Clark 1989; Nelson 1990; Salazar and Salazar 1991). Standardization would help ensure consistent and comparable data and interpretation of the results. *In-situ* bioassays should undergo the same level of scrutiny for standardization as any laboratory bioassay, and biological effects monitoring should be emphasized as much as chemical monitoring.

Because of the relative ease in chemical monitoring of mussel tissues, extensive protocols have been developed for collection, tissue extraction, and subsequent chemical analysis. Since only live animals are collected, maintenance during the exposure period has not been an issue and animal health at the time of collection has generally been ignored. The robust nature of mussels and the emphasis on using mussel tissues for estimates of exposure to contaminants has probably led to the lack of appropriate care by inexperienced investigators using caged mussels as an *in-situ* bioassay.

Established in 1977, the State of California has the longest running Mussel Watch program, but the emphasis has been on measuring bioaccumulation in resident populations and mussel transplants to estimate "hot spots" of contamination (Martin and Severeid 1984; Martin 1985). The National Oceanic and Atmospheric Administration (NOAA) National Mussel Watch Program measures bioaccumulation in mussels and oysters throughout the United States (National Oceanic and Atmospheric Administration 1989). As evidenced by these two major monitoring programs, biological processes are seldom measured in the field, and they are clearly not part of routine monitoring (Roesijadi et al. 1984; Foe and Knight 1987). Few studies have been conducted to validate laboratory bioassay results in the field. Although the methods for conducting *in-situ* exposure and bioeffects studies with mussels are relatively simple, few studies with synoptic measurements have been conducted. Furthermore, problems associated with experimental design and handling have commonly led to spurious data and inappropriate data interpretation (White 1984; Salazar 1992). In advocating the use of biological indicators for environmental monitoring, Phillips (1980) has stressed the potential power of bioindicators, but has also cautioned against the potential pitfalls in data interpretation. There are a number of unexplained inconsistencies in survival, bio-accumulation, and growth of mussels in response to contaminant exposure in the laboratory and the field (Kiorboe et al. 1981; Chapman 1983; Cossa 1989; Salazar 1989; Lobel et al. 1990, 1991, 1992; Salazar 1992).

We have successfully transplanted mussels in San Diego Bay and Puget Sound to assess the extent of contamination and associated bioeffects. In all of our studies, both exposure and bioeffects were measured in the same test animals. Data from mussel transplants in San Diego Bay, California, will be used as a case study to demonstrate how this methodology can be used in an environmental assessment. Although more than 18 sites were studied in nine separate transplants between 1987 and 1990, emphasis will be placed on two sites in the Shelter Island Yacht Basin (the most contaminated area) separated by only 3 meters vertical distance. The Puget Sound data are discussed elsewhere (Salazar et al. this volume) and are used to demonstrate how the protocols presented here can be varied to address different issues, such as sediment effects. This "protocol" paper has three primary objectives: (1) Describe the advantages of using transplanted mussels as *in-situ* indicators of chemical exposure and bioeffects; (2) Present the basic protocols that we found successful; and (3) Present data supporting the utility of the approach.

ADVANTAGES OF *IN-SITU* MUSSEL BIOASSAYS

Advantages of Transplants

Transplanted mussels can be used as an *in-situ* bioassay to obtain information on marine environmental quality that would not be available through routine chemical monitoring, biological monitoring, or laboratory bioassays. The transplant approach combines the experimental control of laboratory testing and the environmental realism of field testing (Green et al. 1985; Salazar and Salazar 1994). There is control of integrated sampling over space and time (Martin 1985) with a clearly defined exposure period. As shown in Fig. 1, caged mussels can be strategically deployed along physical and chemical gradients and at sites in the assessment area where resident mussels would not normally be found; subtidally in the water column and away from the shoreline. Caged mussels can be transplanted near suspected sources of contamination, such as sediment or outfalls, to confirm the relative bioaccumulation and bioeffects associated with those sources. Caged animals can be used to sample an infinite matrix over space and time. Transplants also help avoid some of the factors that add to the variability associated with sampling natural populations that have been detailed by Lobel et al. (1990, 1991, 1992). For example, different populations may be at different tidal heights, have a different size/age structure, and may even be composed of different species.

Transplant studies conducted with caged animals also permit repetitive, non-destructive measurements of individuals to increase the statistical power of the test and the ability to identify site-specific differences. Repetitive measurements during a given bioassay and successive transplant studies in a given area allow estimates of temporal and spatial variability. Caging facilitates tracking individuals and making measurements of bioeffects over time to identify short- and long-term trends. Lastly, serial, sequential studies permit quantification of dose-response relationships over a variety of environmentally realistic test conditions. This can be used as a first-order-approximation to predict environmental risk.

Several investigators have used differences in accumulation of contaminants in transplanted mussels for source identification. Sediments were shown to be the source of dichloro diphenyl trichloroethane (DDT) and polychlorinated biphenyls (PCB) contamination by measuring tissues of mussels transplanted at various depths from the surface to the bottom. The concentration of contaminants in tissues decreased with distance from the bottom (Young et al. 1976). Tissues from mussels nearest the bottom had concentrations 10 times higher than

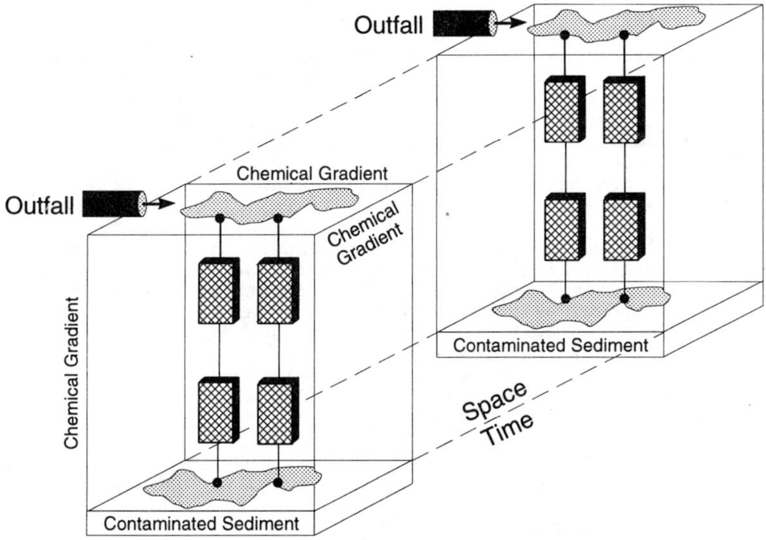

FIG. 1--Diagram of environmental sampling over space and time using *in-situ* transplants of caged mussels along gradients of chemical contamination. Two suspected sources (outfall and sediment), two sites, two depths, and two sampling intervals are shown.

those nearest the surface. In a related study, it was shown that resident mussel populations in the area also reflected temporal and spatial changes in the ambient concentrations of DDT and PCB. There was no correlation with depth for mercury in tissues of mussels transplanted at various depths in the same assessment area (Eganhouse and Young 1978). These data suggest that, in contrast to DDT and PCBs, mercury associated with sediments was not leaching to the water column and becoming bioavailable. As part of the environmental assessment for the *Exxon Valdez* oil spill, transplanted mussels were used to show that particulate oil in subsurface waters was bioavailable and bioavailability decreased with water depth (Short and Rounds 1993). In a related *Exxon Valdez* study, Shigenaka and Henry (1993) showed that the concentration of oil in tissues from transplanted mussels was 100 times greater than sediment concentrations and two times higher than oil accumulated by lipid bags. These results suggest that although the semi-permeable membrane devices may be more convenient and provide more experimental control, they are not a perfect surrogate for live mussel bioaccumulation and they cannot predict bioeffects. In comprehensive reciprocal transplant experiments, Roesijadi et al. (1984) and Widdows et al. (1990) were able to identify sources of contamination and show rates of accumulation and depuration for several different contaminants.

Advantages of Mussels

Mussels are particularly well-suited to the transplant methodology because they are sedentary; their hard shells make them easy to collect, handle, cage, and measure. They survive well under most environmental conditions. Mussels are probably the most common *in-situ* bioindicator for marine environments because they are ubiquitous, sedentary, and responsive to their environment at both the micro- and macrogeographical scales and at all levels of biological organization (Green et al. 1985). They integrate bioavailable contaminants at concentrations that can be orders of magnitude above those found in other environmental compartments (water or sediment). There is a tremendous amount of background material available based on bioaccumulation in the field (State of California 1988; National Oceanic and Atmospheric Administration 1989) and in the laboratory (Bayne et al. 1985; Widdows and Donkin 1992). Other advantages of using mussels as *in-situ* bioindicators have been documented elsewhere (Goldberg et al. 1978; Phillips 1980; Farrington et al. 1987; Phillips and Rainbow 1993).

Although the use of mussels as a bioindicator is sometimes criticized for relative insensitivity to contaminants, their ability to survive under sub-optimal conditions is a strength of the approach (Phillips and Rainbow 1993). We have refined measurement protocols for a sublethal response (growth) to increase the sensitivity and the discriminating power of the bioassay. Transplants could be used as an exposure system to facilitate measuring any clinical biomarker of environmental effects (McCarty 1991). This includes the most sensitive biomarkers that are being developed to assess effects at the cellular and the molecular level of organization. Almost any hypothesis regarding bioaccumulation and bioeffects relationships over space and time is testable using the transplant approach with mussels.

Advantages of Bioaccumulation

Mussels have been used extensively as indicators of exposure for several reasons: (1) they are capable of concentrating contaminants in their tissues at concentrations that are frequently orders of magnitude above those found in seawater or sediment, (2) they provide integrated information about environmental conditions and the bioavailability of contaminants that cannot be defined with chemical measurements of discrete water or sediment samples, and (3) they can provide a more direct link between exposure and bioeffects. This is why bioaccumulation is used to estimate exposure. Tissue concentrations of contaminants better represent *actual* exposure whereas concentrations of contaminants in environmental media (e.g., water and sediments) only represent *apparent exposure*. Actual exposure can lead to biological effects. Even if contaminants were detectable and bioavailability could be estimated by chemical analysis of water samples, the number of samples that would be necessary to adequately describe the ephemeral nature of contaminants in the water column would be cost-prohibitive. In a recent study where tributyltin (TBT) could not be detected in sediment at many locations in the assessment area, TBT was measured in all natural populations of oysters (Espourteille et al. 1993). Similarly, PCBs and polycyclic aromatic hydrocarbons (PAHs) were measured in tissues of transplanted mussels when concentrations were below the limits of detection in seawater (Green et al. 1986; Short and Rounds 1993).

Advantages of Growth

Growth, a commonly used indicator of biological effects, is a sensitive and environmentally realistic biological response because it is a sublethal effect that shows a quantifiable dose-response relationship. It is a biological response that represents the integration of all internal biological processes and has been identified as a significant effect to be measured in environmental assessments (Bayne et al. 1985; Widdows and Donkin 1992). It also integrates total environmental exposure and can be related to adverse effects at the population level (Bayne et al. 1985). Reductions in growth are easily quantified and correlated with adverse environmental effects. However, since both natural and pollution-related stresses have been shown to reduce mussel growth rates, cause-and-effect is not easily proven

(Widdows and Donkin 1992). Repetitive measurements and the experimental control associated with the transplant methodology facilitate isolating the variables in question and providing essential information to help establish causality; particularly when used in combination with laboratory bioassays and field measurements of factors affecting growth.

There is an increasing trend toward measuring sublethal responses like growth in laboratory and field studies; instead of, or in addition to measuring mortality. Reduced mussel growth has been associated with a variety of contaminants in both laboratory and field bioassays (Stromgren 1982, 1986; Stephenson et al. 1986; Salazar and Salazar 1987, 1988, 1991, 1994; Stromgren and Bongard 1987; Widdows et al. 1990; Valkirs et al. 1991; Widdows and Donkin 1992). Juvenile mussel growth was the most sensitive sublethal indicator of TBT measured in San Diego Bay microcosm experiments (Salazar and Salazar 1987; Salazar et al. 1987).

Advantages of Synoptic Measurements

The *in-situ* mussel bioassay assesses environmental quality with direct, synoptic measurements of tissue accumulation and mussel growth in field exposures. It is important to make the distinction between the use of biological indicators as detectors of environmental contamination by monitoring tissue accumulation versus their use as indicators of environmental effects by measuring biological responses like growth. Bioaccumulation is an exposure measurement and is used to determine the relative bioavailability of contaminants; growth is a bioeffect measurement and is used to identify adverse effects associated with that exposure. Both must be used to address the question of whether elevated concentrations of contaminants in the environment (water, sediment, or tissues) and reduced growth constitute an environmental problem. The *in-situ* mussel bioassay facilitates the synoptic measurements of bioaccumulation and growth to help answer that question. It should also be recognized that bioaccumulation can be regarded as both a chemical and a biological process and that bioaccumulation in itself, should not be considered an adverse biological effect. Synoptic measurements have other applications in the risk assessment process. Widdows has pioneered using synoptic measurements of bioaccumulation and physiological responses (scope for growth) to predict tissue concentrations where adverse effects are expected in mussels (Widdows and Donkin 1992). This approach is gaining importance because of the applications to ecological risk assessment and several investigators have advocated moving toward criteria based on tissue burdens; in addition to, or instead of the concentration of contaminants in water or sediment (McKim and Schmieder 1991; Calabrese and Baldwin 1993). Although these predictions can be based on chemical models, the best method is to establish the dose-response curves from direct, synoptic measurements of the dose and the associated response.

METHOD SUMMARY AND RECOMMENDED PROTOCOLS

Most of the protocols presented here were developed between 1987 and 1990 as part of a long-term research program during which nine transplant studies with juvenile mussels were conducted in San Diego Bay, California, (Salazar and Salazar 1994). In summary, the exposure period was 12 weeks, 18 caged juvenile mussels were deployed at each site, and growth was measured with whole-animal wet-weights weekly or on alternate weeks. These were water column studies to evaluate the distribution and effects of TBT antifouling coatings associated with vessels. At most sites, mussels were transplanted 1 meter below the surface, but some sites like the Shelter Island Yacht Basin (the most contaminated) also had mussels 1 meter above the bottom. The emphasis was on juvenile mussels 10 to 12 mm in length. A single 12-week study was conducted in Elliott Bay, Washington, during the winter of 1990 to

1991 (Salazar et al. 1994). In summary, the exposure period was 12 weeks, and 18 to 54 juvenile mussels and 200 to 300 adult mussels were caged at each site. Juvenile mussel growth measurements were made at the beginning and end of the test. Individual adult mussels were only measured at the end of the test; adults were sized (not measured individually) for the 50 to 60 mm range at the beginning of the test. Juvenile mussels from 24 to 30 mm were also used. Bioaccumulation was measured at the end of the tests in San Diego Bay and Elliott Bay.

Based on the San Diego Bay and Elliott Bay results, and subsequent studies, we recommend that mussel transplant studies be conducted with both juvenile (≤30 mm) and adult (≥50 mm) animals. The size range should be minimized in each group and synoptic measurements should include bioaccumulation and growth. It is also important to make multiple measurements on individual mussels to estimate growth. This increases the statistical power of the test and maximizes the ability to discriminate differences among sites. We recommend measuring whole-animal wet-weights and lengths as a non-destructive method to achieve those multiple measurements on individuals. We also recommend cages or bags with individual cells to facilitate the measurements. The collection site is largely dependent on the question to be answered and the availability of test animals. Regardless, animals should be collected with extreme care to avoid injury and other experimentally-induced stressors that might affect bioaccumulation and growth. An exposure period of approximately 90 days is recommended. It should be remembered that the purpose of the *in-situ* mussel bioassay is to estimate both exposure and bioeffects in a minimum period of time and to use those data to detect differences among sites in assessing relative environmental quality.

Experimental Design

Size--We recommend minimizing the size range for juvenile and adult mussels to reduce variability in bioaccumulation and growth attributable to size. A target range of 2 to 5 mm is suggested. Since size and reproduction are two of the most important factors influencing mussel bioindicator results (Bayne et al. 1981; Lobel et al. 1990, 1991, 1992; Widdows and Donkin 1992; Phillips and Rainbow 1993), these effects can be minimized by restricting the size range as we have done. The absolute size is less important than the range of test animals. We have successfully completed juvenile mussel transplant studies using animals 10 to 12 mm, 24 to 30 mm, and 26 to 30 mm. The majority of our work was conducted with juvenile mussels in the smallest size group (10 to 12 mm). We used small juveniles almost exclusively in the San Diego Bay studies for the following reasons: (1) to avoid the effects of gametogenesis on bioaccumulation and growth; (2) to maximize growth potential throughout the test and allow for greater separation among sites; and (3) to utilize what we believed was greater sensitivity to contaminants in juvenile mussels. We used adult mussels less frequently, but animals 50 to 60 mm and 59 to 65 mm were successfully used in San Diego Bay and Elliott Bay. Although the target size range of 2 mm is realistic, it is not always practicable and adjustments should be made to minimize the range to the extent possible. It is more difficult to use a broad size range to estimate bioaccumulation or growth because of the differences in bioaccumulation and growth attributable to size and associated physiological differences.

By limiting the overall size range (2 to 5 mm in length), the discriminating power of the bioassay improves dramatically. Statistically significant differences among sites based on growth can be identified even if growth rates differ by only 25 mg/wk (≈ 25%) (Salazar et al. this volume). Similarly, sites can be differentiated by the concentration of contaminants in tissues even if tissue residues differ by a factor of two or less (≤100%). We believe these statistical differences are also environmentally significant and could not be as easily identified with a wider size range of animals. The Mussel Watch Program initially set a goal of identifying "hot spots" of contamination with differences exceeding a factor of 10, or greater than 1,000% (Goldberg et al. 1978), but the recommended size ranges in adult mussels vary from 10 to 30 mm (Stephenson et al. 1980; Weber 1988; National Oceanic and Atmospheric Administration 1989).

Based on results from our studies, we recommend using juvenile mussels between 10 and 30 mm with a minimum range. The smallest recommended size is 10 mm, for several reasons. First, it is the minimum practicable size to collect, cage, and measure. Secondly, more somatic tissue is added in animals between 10 and 40 mm than in any other size range. To take advantage of the potential for rapid tissue gain, it is better to start with the smallest practicable animals. The maximum recommended size for the juvenile component of the *in-situ* mussel bioassay at the beginning of the test is 30 mm. At 30 mm, animals are still growing rapidly and they will usually not exceed 50 mm during the test. At a length of approximately 50 mm, gamete production begins to exceed somatic production (Rodhouse et al. 1986). Most monitoring programs use mussels >50 mm but the recommended range is 10 to 30 mm (Stephenson et al. 1980; Weber, 1988; National Oceanic and Atmospheric Administration 1989).

Juveniles may be more representative of short-term changes than adults because of their more rapid growth rates and corresponding addition of tissue and contaminants (Fischer 1983, 1988). In the San Diego Bay study, animals that began the test in the range 10 to 12 mm provided sufficient tissue for chemical analysis at the end of the test since the contaminants of concern were limited to TBT, selected metals, and a few organic compounds. In the Elliott Bay study, we used larger juveniles (24 to 30 mm) to increase the amount of tissue available for chemical analysis. Even so, it was not enough for the complete priority pollutant list of analytes using regional EPA protocols. Low winter temperatures and high concentrations of contaminants reduced growth rates and the amount of tissue available for chemical analysis. Therefore, juvenile mussel tissues were only analyzed for metals and TBT. Since analytical laboratories differ in the amount of tissue required to achieve a particular level of detection, this criterion should be used to determine the amount of tissue (and the number of mussels) required for chemical analysis. Survival and growth rates both affect available tissue and should be taken into account.

For adults, we recommend using animals ≥50 mm within the 2 to 5 mm range. Adult mussels provide substantially more biomass for chemical analysis and they provide important information on exposure and bioeffects that is significantly different from that provided by measuring bioaccumulation and growth in juveniles alone. We have previously used growth in juveniles to assess effects and bioaccumulation in adults to assess exposure, but results based on this partial characterization could be misleading. Although their growth rates are much slower than juvenile mussels, adults may be more sensitive to contaminants during gametogenesis, as well as during temperature and nutritive stress (Bayne et al. 1985). It is generally believed that juveniles, and larvae in particular, are the most sensitive life stage. However, Widdows and Donkin (1992) suggest that adult mussels are more sensitive to contaminants than both juvenile and larval mussels. This elevated sensitivity may be attributable to a reduction in the efficiency of the immune response system of the older, larger individuals (Hole et al. 1992). Adult mussels could also be more sensitive to particular contaminants. Based on our most recent San Diego Bay transplant study (1993), adult growth rates, as estimated by whole-animal wet-weights, may be more sensitive to PAHs than juvenile growth rates.

Number of Test Animals/Frequency of Measurement--For both juvenile and adult mussels, we recommend using 50 to 100 test animals per site to achieve the resolution that is necessary to detect statistical differences in growth, to provide sufficient tissue for chemical analysis, and to provide a reasonable estimate of population exposure and response. Based on our previous studies with juveniles, 100 data points are usually necessary to detect statistically significant differences. In San Diego Bay, this was accomplished by transplanting 18 animals/site and measuring them weekly or biweekly. Using a 12-week exposure period, this provided 234 and 126 data points per site, respectively (including measurements at the beginning of the test). In Elliott Bay, a similar level of replication was achieved by transplanting 54 animals per site and making growth measurements only at the beginning and end of the test (54 x 2 = 108), and we found statistically significant differences. No statistically significant differences in adult growth were found among any of the Elliott Bay sites by measuring individuals only at the end of the test (100 measurements). This was probably attributable to the 10 mm size range and associated variability in growth, and the uncertainty regarding differences in size among cages at the beginning of the test.

We recommend a minimum of 50 juveniles per site to provide enough tissue for chemical analysis. More animals might be required depending on analytical requirements, growth rates, and mortality. For example, 50 juveniles (24 to 30 mm at the start of the test) did not provide enough tissue for analyzing all the priority pollutants in the Elliott Bay studies, whereas tissues from 100 adult animals did. In the San Diego Bay experiments, 18 juvenile mussels provided sufficient tissue for chemical analysis of TBT and some metals. The use of more animals than the minimum for tissue analysis better represents the population and reduces the overall variability in the chemical measurements attributable to differences among individuals. Gordon et al. (1980) recommend a sample size of 16 to 30 individuals in order to detect a statistically significant difference in tissue concentrations when the means differ by 20 to 40%. However, analyses were conducted on individual mussels and only for selected contaminants.

Collection Site-- The source of test animals is largely dependent on three factors: (1) the question to be answered; (2) the availability of test animals; (3) logistics involved in collection, initial measurements and sorting, and transport to the test site. Animals should be collected from a site where environmental conditions have been documented, contaminant concentrations are low, and the animals are in good health. Options include collection from a natural site or purchase from commercial culturing facilities that utilize field or laboratory grow-out. For repetitive studies, population effects can be eliminated by always collecting animals from the same population as we did in the 3-year San Diego Bay study. A similar approach has been used by the State of California Mussel Watch program for over 17 years (Martin and Severeid 1984). Population effects can also be eliminated by using hatchery-raised animals. The transplant methodology facilitates studying population effects and site effects by reciprocal transplants of animals from different populations (Dickie et al. 1984; Roesijadi et al. 1984; Mallet et al. 1987).

We have used animals from a variety of sources and obtained useful information with each. In the San Diego Bay studies, mussels (*Mytilus galloprovincialis*) were collected from a site near the mouth of the bay where contaminant concentrations were lower than those further inside the bay. These intertidal animals were alternately submerged and exposed to air during normal tidal cycles. In the Elliott Bay study, mussels (*Mytilus trossulus*) were collected from a mussel farm situated in relatively pristine waters near Whidbey Island. These animals were attached to floating platforms and were continuously submerged. (The effects of submergence could also be studied with reciprocal transplants.) We have also used oysters (*Crassostrea virginica*) from a laboratory culture facility for field transplant studies in Tampa Bay, Florida, and microcosm tests in San Diego, California. These three different approaches demonstrate the versatility of stock choice for optimizing transplant methodologies.

Exposure Period-- We recommend an exposure period of approximately 90 days if the major priority pollutants are being assessed. This should provide sufficient time for mussel tissues to reach equilibrium with contaminants in the environment, maximize the period where growth is most rapid, and still avoid most of the effects of gametogenesis on bioaccumulation and growth. We used a 12-week exposure period in all the San Diego Bay and Puget Sound studies to accomplish this. Preliminary San Diego Bay experiments on the rate of TBT uptake in transplanted adult mussels and in microcosm exposures suggested that approximately 60 days was required to reach equilibrium (Fig. 2). A subsequent reciprocal transplant with juveniles and adults suggested that TBT equilibrium was reached in 21 days or less (Fig. 3) but the apparent exposure concentration was significantly lower (72 vs 500 ng TBT/L). Depuration was also quite rapid in this experiment. With all other conditions in the microcosm experiment relatively equal, there was a good correlation between seawater concentration and tissue concentration. Another bioaccumulation experiment in southern California with transplanted mussels has shown that DDT equilibrium was reached in approximately 90 days (Young et al. 1976). The California State Mussel Watch routinely uses 4 to 6 months exposure for bioaccumulation studies of all contaminants (Martin and Severeid 1984; Martin 1985) but has used 3 to 4 month deployment periods for growth studies (Stephenson et al. 1986). Alternatively, for some petroleum hydrocarbons, equilibrium is approached with mussel tissues within days or weeks (Widdows and Donkin 1992). Widdows et al. (1990) transplanted tropical mussels for only 11 to 12 days and achieved elevated concentrations of PAHs, TBT, PCBs, and lead. Although we have found statistically significant differences in growth after only one week when comparing the most contaminated site (Shelter Island Yacht Basin - surface) with other sites, this exposure period may not be long enough to detect more subtle differences and chronic effects.

Cages

We recommend cages that maximize water flow, confine yet maintain adequate space among individuals, and facilitate monitoring growth of individual mussels. Measuring individual mussels for growth improves the statistical power of the test because there are multiple measurements of the same individuals, even if measurements are only made at the beginning and end of the test. This is facilitated by using compartmentalized cages (i.e., trays or mesh bags with one mussel per cell). Compartmentalized cages are preferred because each animal is provided similar holding conditions and animals are not permitted to clump. Clumping could limit exposure to water and contaminants for animals in the center of the clump. With clumped mussels, the bags themselves can also restrict valve opening that, in turn, could affect bioaccumulation and growth. In all our work, plastic mesh cages with individual compartments were used for the juvenile mussels and mesh bags were used for the adult mussels. We have never used marking methods for the following reasons: (1) marks can be obscured by fouling or rubbed off; (2) marking increases the time out of water; (3) some methods could affect the results, and (4) marking increases preparation time at a time-critical portion of the study.

Rigid plastic cutlery trays (Hutzler Manufacturing, Canaan, Connecticut) were subdivided with semi-rigid plastic mesh to create 18 individual cells per cage. Overall dimensions of the cage were 30 x 16

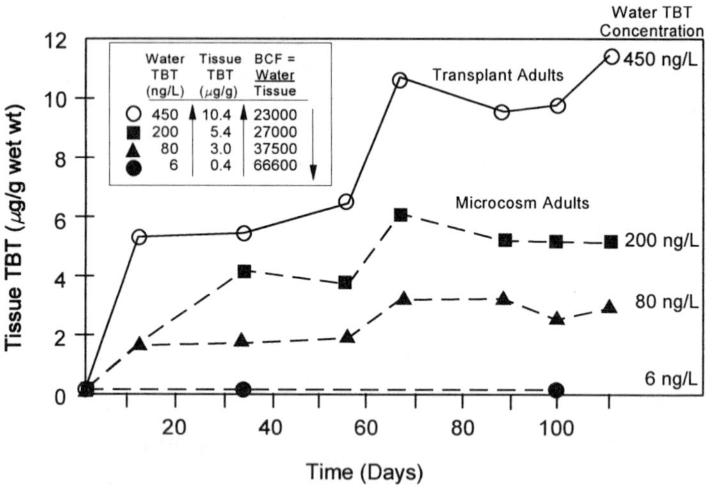

FIG. 2--Tissue concentrations of TBT in adult mussels over time in a field transplant (Shelter Island Yacht Basin) and a flow-through microcosm tank experiment. Results suggest equilibrium is reached in approximately 60 days. The inverse relationship between BCF and TBT concentration is also shown with arrows.

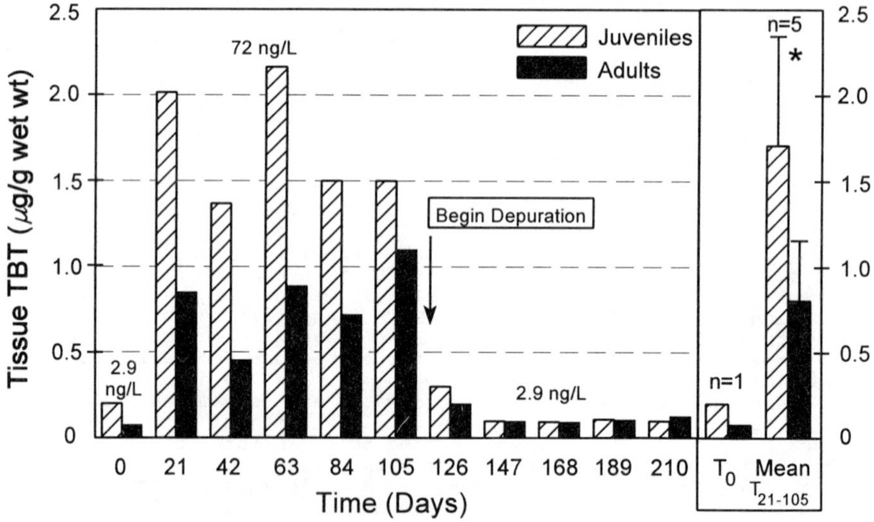

FIG. 3--Tissue concentrations of TBT in juvenile and adult mussels over time in a reciprocal transplant experiment (Shelter Island and a reference site). Results suggest TBT equilibrium is reached in approximately 21 days and concentrations are higher in juveniles than adults. Means from days 21 - 105 (± 2 Standard Errors) are also shown. * = statistically significant difference (α =0.05).

x 3.5 cm with a mesh size of approximately 3 mm. Individual cells were approximately 5 x 5 x 1.6 cm. Flexible plastic mesh (3 to 6 mm mesh size) was used as a top. Increasing mesh size maximized water flow through the cages with larger mesh tops used as the animals grew. The cages and protocols used for the adult mussels in the Elliott Bay study were similar to those developed by the California State Mussel Watch (Stephenson et al. 1980). Oyster culch netting, a plastic mesh tube with a mesh size of approximately 15 mm (Norplex Enterprises, Auburn, Washington), was used to hold the adults. Previous work has shown that clumps of 10 or more mussels can reduce bioaccumulation and growth (Stephenson et al. 1980; Okamura 1986) so we adopted the protocol of 10 adult mussels per clump. Each clump was separated by plastic cable ties. Each deployment consisted of 10 clumps (i.e., 100 mussels).

We now believe that bioaccumulation and growth should be measured in juvenile and adult mussels and that flexible mesh bags are more versatile than rigid trays. The mesh bag approach is being modified to include monitoring individual juvnile and adult mussels. Bags will be compartmentalized to include one animal per clump. A commercially available netting (Norplex Industries, Auburn, Washington) will reduce set-up as well as cleanup time and allow unlimited flexibility in the number of animals deployed at each site. There are no limits to bag length, number of bags that can be prepared for deployment, and the number of individuals per bag. The bags are also disposable. Rigid trays may still be preferable for field tests with a large number of repetitive measurements due to time savings in placing the animals back in the trays. Using beginning and end-of-test measurements only, the mesh bag approach seems best.

Collection and Sorting

We recommend that all animals be carefully collected and sorted by hand. The primary concerns during collection and sorting are animal health and chemical contamination. The collection and processing procedures for chemical monitoring have been carefully developed over many years to avoid cross contamination. Bioresponse protocols are poorly developed because mussels have been traditionally used to estimate only exposure, and animal health has largely been ignored. As is the case with laboratory bioassays, care must be taken in all stages of a field bioassay to prevent stress attributable to experimental protocols. Improper handling techniques can have marked adverse effects on mussel survival and growth (Salazar 1992). Even when we thought our protocols were conservative in terms of experimentally-induced stress, we discovered that weekly measurements had an adverse effect on juvenile mussel growth. During collection, sorting, and measurement, byssal threads should be cut with scissors or gently broken at the point of attachment to avoid injury. Mechanical sorting or ripping mussels apart can remove or tear the byssal gland and lead to death. Mussels can be exposed to air during collection and sorting, but they should be kept cool and moist. Mussel clumps with attached organisms and debris should not be kept in seawater during sorting because the water quickly becomes fouled.

To achieve the minimum recommended size range (2 to 5 mm in length), animals are first "rough sorted" into the approximate size range desired and then "fine sorted" into 0.1 mm groupings for distribution. For both the juvenile and adult mussels, a "rough sort" is done by eye or coarse measuring device to verify that there are enough animals in the appropriate size range to begin the test. The "rough sorted" mussels should be placed in containers filled with clean seawater. They are held in seawater from this point on because initial weights are significantly influenced by air in the mantle cavity. Submergence provides mussels an opportunity to open their valves and release captured air bubbles (burping). For the "fine sort," length measurements to the nearest 0.1 mm are made with plastic vernier calipers and animals are divided into groups of 0.1 mm increments. Prior to placement in the cage, whole-animal wet weights are measured with an electronic balance (nearest 0.01 g) and the length remeasured. Animals that are floating on the surface of the water prior to measurement are generally not used to begin the test because floating indicates the presence of air within the mantle cavity. If animals float prior to weighing at the end of the test, they are given additional time to purge the trapped air and reduce measurement error.

After the fine sort, the size range for both juvenile and adult mussels should be selected based on the minimum range with the most animals. To assure an even distribution of test animals among sites, all animals in a particular 0.1 mm grouping are distributed among the cages. This process is repeated for the remaining size groups until the cages are filled; each cage then has approximately the same number of individuals from each size group. To ensure statistical similarity among cages, an Analysis of Variance (ANOVA) is run on both length and whole-animal wet-weight data. If the means are statistically different, test animals are redistributed to bring the means closer together. Using this method, we have never found a statistically significant difference among cages in weights or lengths after the fine sort. Even if the distributions are not statistically different, any differences in mean weights or lengths can be minimized by replacing or switching individual mussels. If a size range of 5 mm cannot be achieved, the range should still be minimized and animals evenly distributed (not randomly) to the extent practicable. Using size ranges above 5 mm may necessitate larger groupings for the "fine sort;" eg., 1 mm intervals.

<u>Measurements</u>

The *in-situ* mussel bioassay is based on measurements of growth and bioaccumulation, but survival is recorded during the process and could add significant information to the study. In combination with growth, survival can be used to determine if the test was successful. Poor survival at the control/reference site (<50%) is a good indication that the test animals have been mishandled and that test results should be rejected (Salazar 1992). The number of surviving individuals should be recorded at each measurement interval. Since the methods for chemical analysis are well developed, they will not be addressed here. We have already discussed the importance of measuring individual mussels at the beginning of the test to minimize variability. The primary growth metrics are whole-animal wet-weight and shell length. Length measurements should be made to the nearest 0.1 mm and weight to the nearest 0.01 gram. Lengths can also be used to estimate weights and compare test results with other studies since length is a commonly measured parameter in mussels and is also used in the mariculture industry.

Weight measurements are more accurate than length measurements because of variability in shell shape. Weight is also closer to a constantly increasing function than length, which levels off as the maximum length is approached. Whole-animal wet-weights can also provide a good estimate of wet and dry tissue weights (Dauble et al. 1985) although dry weights are more accurate than wet weights due to variability in water (Widdows and Donkin 1992). Shell weights and tissue weights can also increase at different rates (Widdows and Donkin 1992). Nevertheless, measuring whole-animal wet-weights using the transplant methodology provides the opportunity for multiple, non-destructive measurements on individuals. Although we have never made dry weight measurements because of the time and effort involved, research should be conducted to confirm the differences in the discriminating power of the two methods. We have always measured tissue and shell weights at the end of each test because we feel they provide useful data and the measurements are easily made as the tissues are being removed for chemical analysis. We recommend making these measurements in both juvenile and adult mussels.

Due to the economy of scale, it is probably most efficient to measure growth at the beginning and end of the test. To understand physiological and toxicological processes, however, it would be better to measure animals more frequently, but not more than once every two weeks. Although we attempted to maximize replication with weekly measurements, this frequency reduced mussel growth rates and caused additional stress to the test animals (Salazar and Salazar 1994). The effects of handling were minimized by measuring animals on alternate weeks in subsequent tests. Similar growth rates were obtained when mussels were measured on alternate weeks or only at the beginning and end of tests.

Data Analysis and Interpretation

The bioaccumulation and growth data can be statistically analyzed to determine if there are differences among sites. The recommended statistical procedures are an ANOVA followed by Duncan's New Multiple Range Test. For analysis of the growth data, the individual mussels in each cage are treated as replicates to increase the statistical power of the test. Only data for surviving individuals are used in the final analyses to reduce data biases due to mortalities (Dauble et al. 1985). To evaluate the data from two sites in the Shelter Island Yacht Basin, we compared the weighted mean growth slopes for each site by test and across tests with a t-test (Zar, 1974). Although the discriminating power in determining the short-term changes and variability in bioaccumulation and growth is reduced with only beginning and end of test measurements, the statistical power is enhanced by using more animals at the start of the test (i.e., 50 to 100). A similar procedure was followed for the seawater data. In order to conduct statistical analyses on bioaccumulation data, it is necessary to have replicated deployments. We pooled the bioaccumulation data by site across tests and made a single comparison using a t-test.

Short- and long-term trends can be analyzed to determine if there is a significant regression over time. Then the regressions for different sites are compared for statistically significant differences. Temporal and spatial variability can be assessed by measuring that variability over time and then comparing the variability among sites and across tests. Bioaccumulation can be calibrated for specific contaminants by comparing bioaccumulation versus growth to estimate these correlations and comparing them statistically. Dose-response can be evaluated by calculating the regression for bioeffects vs exposure (growth vs bioaccumulation) to determine if the regression is significant. The next procedure is to determine the inflection point and estimate where the critical concentrations occur. This information can be used in an ecological risk assessment to predict the concentrations where effects are expected, where they are not expected, and where effects are uncertain.

SAN DIEGO BAY CASE STUDY

We successfully used the mussel transplant bioassay to identify site-specific differences in bioaccumulation and growth at sites in San Diego Bay (Salazar and Salazar 1991) and Elliott Bay (Salazar et al. this volume). We also used seawater TBT concentrations in San Diego Bay and sediment contaminant concentrations in Elliott Bay to distinguish differences among sites and correlated contamination in environmental media with bioaccumulation and growth in mussels. The discriminating power of the mussel transplant approach will be illustrated primarily with data obtained for two sites in the Shelter Island Yacht Basin: a surface and bottom site separated by only 3 meters vertical distance. The surface site had the highest concentrations of contaminants and the lowest growth rates of all San Diego Bay sites. Since these two sites were so close together, they were expected to be more similar than most other sites. If the *in-situ* bioassay method can detect differences between these sites, it seems reasonable to assume that it could also detect differences among other sites. Fig. 4 shows seawater TBT, tissue TBT, and juvenile mussel growth rates for the surface and bottom sites: by test and by means for all tests. Since bioaccumulation was only measured at the end of the test there was only one measurement per test and there are no error bars on a per-test basis. This figure and those that follow show the utility of the mussel field bioassay in conjunction with chemical monitoring to identify short-term and long-term trends, temporal and spatial variability, site-specific differences, source identification, and dose-response. Since the Elliott Bay study was a single experiment at one point in time, the data do not address trends, variability or dose-response. Serial transplants at the test sites could address those issues, as we have shown with the San Diego Bay data. However, the Elliott Bay data were used to identify site-specific differences and potential contamination sources (Salazar et al. this volume).

Short-term and Long-term Trends

Short-term trends can be estimated by comparing measurements made during one test period with those made during another. Long-term trends can be estimated by serial transplants over time and comparing several tests over a longer time period. The short- and long-term trends in seawater TBT concentration, tissue TBT concentration, and growth for the Shelter Island sites are illustrated in Fig. 4. The seawater concentration of TBT decreased significantly at both sites between 1987-1990, although the decrease at the surface site was much more dramatic. The concentration of TBT in mussel tissues also decreased concomitantly over the first four tests at the surface site, but then showed a dramatic increase before declining again. Since we have shown that weekly measurements reduced mussel growth rates, and a correlation between growth rate and bioaccumulation, we believe that this increase in tissue TBT may be attributable to higher growth rates associated with the switch to measurements on alternate weeks in Test 5. Growth rates increased steadily at both sites through Test 7 and we attribute the decrease in Test 8 to the extremely low winter temperatures. We did not have enough replication over seasons, or enough synoptic measurements of temperature and chlorophyll-*a* to extract seasonal effects, or the effects of other natural factors. Other comparisons could be made between seawater TBT and natural factors to assess covariance. By making multiple measurements of seawater TBT during each test, it is possible to estimate variability and calculate a regression for the rate of change and determine if the change is statistically significant.

Temporal and Spatial Variability

Compared to seawater TBT concentrations and growth rates, it appears that tissue TBT concentrations for these two Shelter Island sites were the most variable over space and time (Fig. 4). The relationship between seawater TBT and growth is better than the relationship between tissue TBT and growth (Salazar and Salazar 1994). By comparing scales however, the tissue concentrations only varied by a factor of two or three. Seawater TBT concentrations and individual growth measurements varied by more than a factor of six (twice as much) on a weekly basis during the same tests (Salazar and Salazar 1988; Salazar and Chadwick 1991). This variability is one of the reasons for measuring tissue concentrations; to normalize exposure concentrations. The variability in tissue measurements may be attributable, at least in

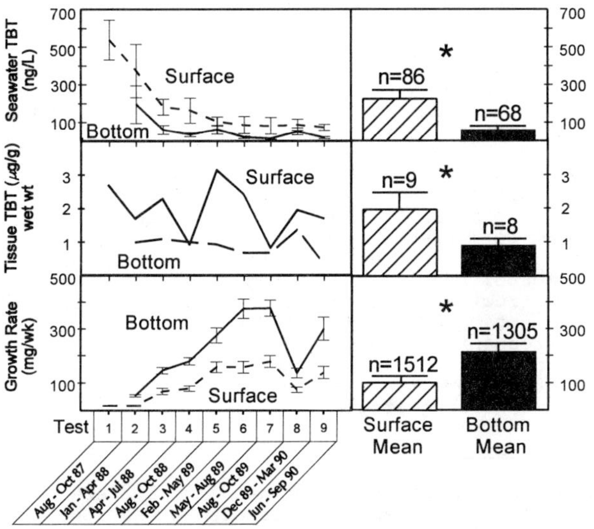

FIG. 4--Temporal and spatial variability and differences in seawater TBT concentrations, tissue TBT concentrations and mussel growth rates at two mussel transplant sites (Shelter Island). Data points for seawater and growth represent 12 week means (±2 Standard Errors). Tissue TBT data points represent end-of-test measurements only. * = statistically significant difference (α = 0.05).

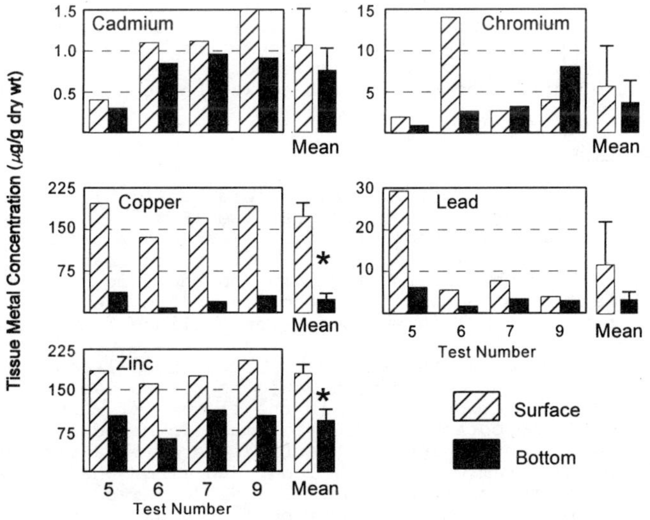

FIG. 5--Concentrations of five metals in juvenile mussel tissues from the surface and bottom site shown in Fig. 3, during the same tests (5, 6, 7, 9) and mussels from the same cages. Means across tests ± 2 Standard Errors are also shown. * = statistically significant difference (α = 0.05).

part, to the lack of replication in tissue measurements. Although the variability in mussel growth appears low, variability in growth rate among individual mussels and between seasons is high. We were able to normalize some of this variability by making many individual growth measurements for each individual mussel. Similar replication is accomplished by increasing the number of test animals and only measuring at the beginning and end of the test as we did in Elliott Bay. It should also be remembered that variability in seawater TBT concentrations decreased at both sites over time as the absolute concentrations decreased. Variability in mussel growth rates increased at both sites over time as the absolute growth rates increased. Although the long-term trends shown here are very similar to those shown for TBT in a monitoring program for water, sediment, and tissues of resident adult mussel populations in San Diego Bay (Valkirs et al. 1991), the fine structure of temporal and spatial variability that we have shown would not have been detected using only resident mussels and measuring less frequently. Mussels are not found at the bottom site in the Shelter Island Yacht Basin, quarterly monitoring did not capture the weekly variability we observed, and bioeffects were not measured in the resident mussel monitoring program.

Site-specific Differences

Even with the variability associated in all three measurements, we found statistically significant differences between the two Shelter Island sites in seawater TBT, tissue TBT, and mussel growth rates across tests ($\alpha = 0.05$). Even though these sites were separated by only 3 meters, they were very different. Growth was significantly different in every test; seawater TBT concentrations were significantly different in all tests but two. Fig. 5 shows the differences in cadmium, chromium, copper, lead, and zinc for the Shelter Island surface and bottom sites. In almost every comparison, the tissue concentrations are higher at the surface site. For copper and zinc, these differences are statistically significant ($\alpha = 0.05$). We also found significant differences in temperature and chlorophyll-*a* between the sites (Salazar and Salazar, 1994). Copper, zinc, and temperature were higher at the surface and chlorophyll-*a* was higher at the bottom. Because the differences in temperature and chlorophyll-*a* were small, we do not believe they were the primary cause of differences in mussel growth between the Shelter Island sites.

Source Identification

Since the concentrations of TBT were significantly higher in both seawater and mussel tissues from the surface site (Fig. 4), it appears that the primary source of TBT contamination is associated with the surface water and not the bottom sediment. This is reasonable since the primary source of TBT is the antifouling paint on the ship hulls moored in the Shelter Island Yacht Basin. With the ban on the use of TBT in 1988, the concentration of TBT in surface water declined dramatically and mussel growth rates increased significantly. This would seem to confirm that the source was at the surface. It was speculated that high concentrations of TBT in bottom sediment would be bioavailable, but we did not find high concentrations of TBT in the tissues of mussels suspended 1 meter off the bottom. Similarly, mussels caged at the surface site had consistently higher concentrations of five different metals (i.e., cadmium, chromium, copper, lead, and zinc) when compared to mussels from the bottom site (Fig. 5). The differences were statistically significant for copper and zinc ($\alpha = 0.05$). Similar differences were found for other metals as well. Collectively, the TBT and metals data all suggest that the source of this contamination was in the surface water and not the bottom sediment.

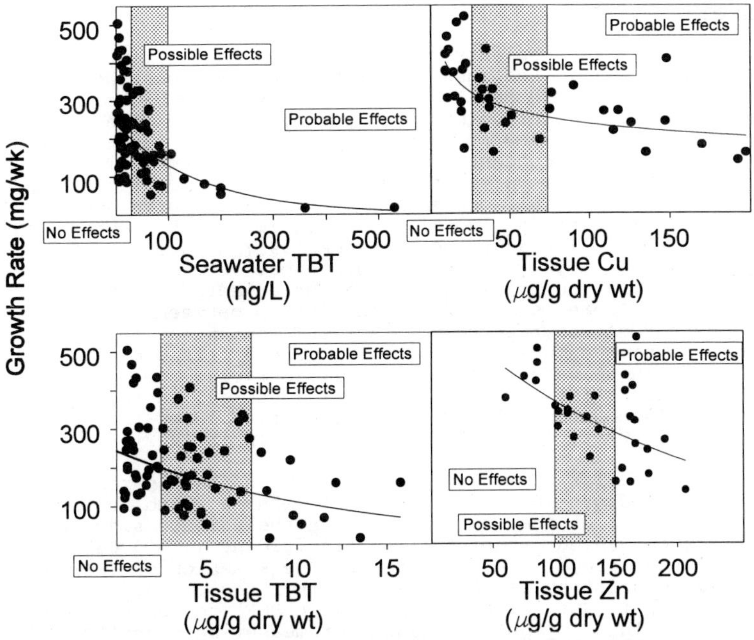

FIG. 6--Statistically significant relationships between juvenile mussel growth rates and seawater concentrations of TBT, and tissue concentrations of three different contaminants: TBT, copper, and zinc. Also shown are first order approximations of effects zones.

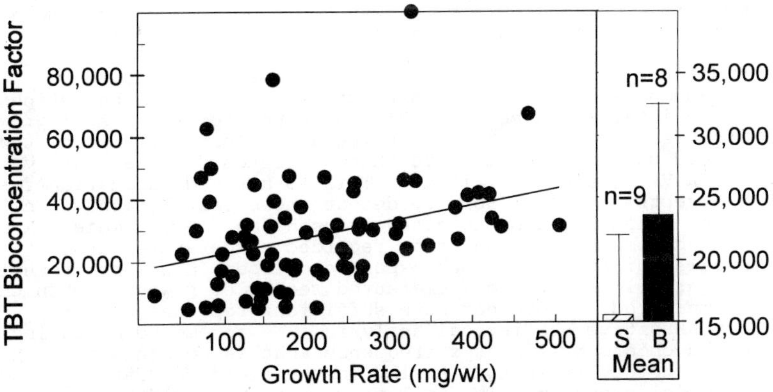

FIG. 7--The relationship between growth rate and apparent bioconcentration factor for TBT is statistically significant (α = 0.05). The mean BCFs from the bottom (B) site in Fig. 3 are much higher than the surface (S) site, but the difference is not statistically significant. Error bars represent ± 2 Standard Errors.

Dose-response

By using serial transplants with repetitive measurements of seawater TBT, tissue TBT, and mussel growth rates, we constructed dose-response curves using field data. Although these field bioassays are more variable than laboratory bioassays, the results are more environmentally realistic and it is possible to achieve first-order approximations for water concentration and tissue concentration effects. Fig. 6 shows dose-response curves for seawater TBT concentrations and concentrations of tissue TBT, copper, and zinc. Each curve is statistically significant ($\alpha = 0.05$). The details of the regressions are provided elsewhere (Salazar and Chadwick 1991; Salazar and Salazar 1994). By using the inflection points in the curves, it is possible to predict first-order approximations of apparent-effects-thresholds and no-effect levels. There is a better relationship between seawater TBT concentrations and growth rate than tissue TBT concentrations and growth rate because the bioaccumulation process is more affected by natural factors than TBT in seawater. Interestingly, our predicted threshold tissue concentrations for effects are almost identical to those predicted for TBT and copper in mussel tissues from scope-for-growth measurements (Widdows et al. 1990; Widdows and Donkin 1992).

Although there was tremendous variability in the apparent bioconcentration factors (BCF) associated with surface and bottom sites, BCFs were much higher at the bottom site than the surface site (Fig. 7), but the difference was not statistically significant ($\alpha = 0.05$). Similar differences are often attributed to the kinetics of TBT, but we attribute them to differences in mussel growth rates. There is a statistically significant relationship between BCF and mussel growth rate ($\alpha = 0.05$). This is another reason for measuring mussel growth rate — to calibrate bioaccumulation. Just as there are criteria for animal survival in bioassays to confirm animal health, mussel growth could be used to confirm animal health in the field bioassay. Clearly, if animals are close to death, they will accumulate lower concentrations of contaminants. If growth rates are extremely low, it could be a signal to evaluate the results of bioaccumulation with more caution than is customary. Just as laboratory bioassays have a standardized survival requirement for acceptance, the *in-situ* bioassay could have a similar survival requirement. Additionally, since survival is not a very sensitive measure of animal health, growth could be used to provide a finer assessment of animal health and associated bioaccumulation.

Using data from synoptic measurements of seawater TBT, temperature, and growth rates, we constructed three-dimensional graphs to evaluate the interaction between TBT and temperature on mussel growth (Fig. 8). Interestingly, the optimum temperature for growth predicted from these field data is identical to that predicted from laboratory studies (Almada-Villela et al., 1982). This is a field validation for temperature effects. We were able to detect these correlations with temperature and differences among sites by using an *in-situ* meter (Ryan Instruments, Redmond, Washington) that recorded temperatures at 30-minute intervals during the 12-week exposure period. Since chlorophyll-*a* was highly variable and was only measured weekly or biweekly when the animals were measured, we did not have sufficient replication for appropriately sensitive statistical analysis. We recommend measuring temperature and chlorophyll-*a* at a frequency that is commensurate with variability in the environment to assist in the field validation using the *in-situ* mussel bioassay. The following approach could be used in a field validation process: quantifying exposure-response in the field; quantifying exposure-response in the lab; quantifying the effects of other variables. Laboratory experiments could be used to isolate particular variables and field manipulations could be used to achieve various combinations of test conditions with more *in-situ* measurements of natural factors affecting growth.

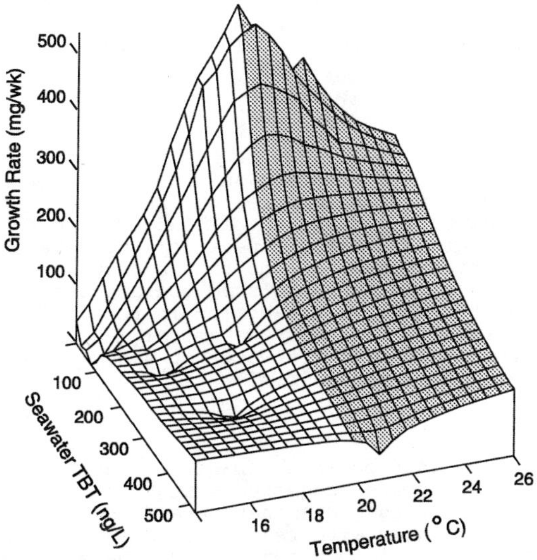

FIG 8.--Effects of seawater TBT concentrations and temperature on growth predicted from 3-dimensional surface plots using weighted means. Shaded area represents growth rate reductions at temperatures above 20°C. Reduced growth at low temperatures and high concentrations of TBT in seawater (>100 ng/L) are also apparent.

SUMMARY AND CONCLUSIONS

The most unique feature of our approach is the combined use of the following: (1) synoptic measurements of bioaccumulation and growth using both juvenile and adult mussels; (2) mussel growth as an indicator of bioeffects; (3) individual measurements to minimize the initial size range and maximize statistical power by multiple measurements of individuals; and (4) compartmentalized cages to facilitate individual, repetitive measurements.

Advantages

The mussel transplant approach combines the advantages of experimental control and environmental realism. Control is gained by manipulating the exposure time and the exposure site. These parameters cannot be controlled if natural populations of mussels are used to estimate exposure and bioeffects. Environmental realism, which is often lacking in laboratory tests, is achieved because the animals are deployed *in-situ*. Other advantages of this approach include the ability to make repetitive, synoptic measurements on individual animals, the ability of test animals to integrate bioavailable contaminants, and the effects of natural factors that provide a meaningful dose and a natural response. The technique is relatively simple, does not require specific expertise or sophisticated equipment, and is relatively inexpensive. There is also a vast mussel literature that can be used to help provide mechanistic explanations for observed responses as well as help direct the coordination of laboratory and field studies that can be used to establish the dose-response relationships used in ecological risk assessments. Almost all clinical measurements are possible, and the *in-situ* mussel bioassay, in essence, could be viewed as simply an exposure system.

Disadvantages

The *in-situ* mussel bioassay also has a number of disadvantages and potential pitfalls. Bioaccumulation and growth are both affected by natural factors that cannot be controlled, such as external abiotic factors and internal biotic factors. It should also be mentioned that growth effects are not contaminant-specific. Mussels are not equally sensitive to all contaminants, nor do they accumulate them equally. Mussels can actually close to avoid some contaminants, and since multiple contaminant exposures are common in the field, this makes discrimination difficult. Extensive chemical measurements are required to document apparent exposures (in water or sediment), and a true field control site is virtually impossible.

Prospectus

Even with these shortcomings, *in-situ* bioassays are powerful assessment tools. Many have suggested using laboratory bioassays in conjunction with monitoring contamination and community assemblages, and this approach has been used with reasonable effectiveness in many monitoring programs. We suggest that field bioassays using more direct measurements of bioaccumulation and growth to estimate chemical exposure and bioeffects should be included as part of a comprehensive program for sediment or water quality monitoring. An integration of laboratory and field bioassays could provide very useful information. Although we used mussels in refining this *in-situ* bioassay, the generic approach is applicable to many bivalve species indigenous to freshwater, estuarine, or marine environments. We have outlined the utility of mussel transplants as a field bioassay, demonstrated the need to standardize protocols for this approach, and presented basic protocols that could be used as a framework for standardization.

REFERENCES

Almada-Villela, P. C., Davenport, J., and Gruffydd, L. D., 1982, "The Effects of Temperature on the Shell Growth of Young *Mytilus edulis* L.," Journal Experimental Marine Biology and Ecology, Vol. 59, pp. 275-288.

Bayne, B. L., Brown, D. A., Burns, K., Dixon, D. R., Ivanovici, A., Livingstone, D. R., Lowe, D. M., Moore, N. M., Stebbing, A. R. D., and Widdows, J., 1985, The Effects of Stress and Pollution on Marine Animals, Praeger Special Studies, Praeger Scientific, New York.

Bayne, B. L., Clarke, K. R., and Moore, M. N., 1981, "Some Practical Considerations in the Measurement of Pollution Effects on Bivalve Molluscs, and Some Possible Ecological Consequences," Aquatic Toxicology, Vol. 1, pp. 159-174.

Calabrese, E. J. and Baldwin, L. A., 1993, Performing Ecological Risk Assessments, Lewis Publishers, Boca Raton.

Chapman, G. A., 1983, "Do Organisms in Laboratory Toxicity Tests Respond Like Organisms in Nature?," Aquatic Toxicology and Hazard Assessment: Sixth Symposium, ASTM STP 802, W. E. Bishop, R. D. Cardwell, and B. B. Heidolph, Eds., American Society for Testing and Materials, Philadelphia, pp. 315-327.

Clark, J. R., 1989, "Field Studies in Estuarine Ecosystems: A Review of Approaches for Assessing Contaminant Effects," Aquatic Toxicology and Hazard Assessment: Twelfth Volume, ASTM STP 1027, U. M. Cowgill and L. R. Williams, Eds., American Society for Testing and Materials, Philadelphia, pp. 120-133.

Cossa, D., 1989, "A Review of the Use of *Mytilus* sp. as Quantitative indicators of Cadmium and Mercury Contamination in Coastal Waters," Oceanologica Acta, Vol. 12, No. 4, pp. 417-432.

Dauble, D. D., Daly, D. S., and Abernethy, C. S., 1985, "Factors Affecting Growth and Survival of the Asiatic Clam, *Corbicula* sp., under Controlled Laboratory Conditions," Aquatic Toxicology and Hazard Assessment: Seventh Symposium, ASTM STP 854, American Society for Testing and Materials, Philadelphia. pp. 134-144.

Dickie, L. M., Boudreau, P. R., and Freeman, K. R., 1984, "Influences of Stock and Site on Growth and Mortality in the Blue Mussel (*Mytilus edulis*)." Canadian Journal of Fisheries and Aquatic Sciences, Vol. 41, pp. 134-140.

Eganhouse, R. P. and Young, D. R., 1978, "*In situ* Uptake of Mercury by the Intertidal Mussel, *Mytilus californianus*," Marine Pollution Bulletin, Vol. 9, pp. 214-217.

Espourteille, F. A., Greaves, J., and Huggett, R. J., 1993, "Measurement of Tributyltin Contamination of Sediments and *Crassostrea virginica* in the Southern Chesapeake Bay," Environmental Toxicology and Chemistry, Vol. 12, pp. 305-314.

Farrington, J. W., Davis, A. C., Tripp, W. P., Phelps, D. K., and Galloway, W. B., 1987, "Mussel Watch -- Measurements of Chemical Pollutants in Bivalves as One Indicator of Coastal Environmental Quality," New Approaches to Monitoring Aquatic Ecosystems, ASTM STP 940, T. P. Boyle, Ed., American Society for Testing and Materials, Philadelphia, pp. 125-139.

Fischer, H., 1983, "Shell Weight as an Independent Variable in Relation to Cadmium Content of Molluscs." Marine Ecological Progress Series, Vol. 12, pp. 59-75.

Fischer, H., 1988, "*Mytilus edulis* as a Quantitative Indicator of Dissolved Cadmium. Final Study and Synthesis," Marine Ecological Progress Series, Vol. 48, No. 2, pp. 163-174.

Foe, C. and Knight, A., 1987, "Assessment of the Biological Impact of Point Source Discharges Employing Asiatic Clams," Archives of Environmental Contamination and Toxicology, Vol. 16, No. 1, pp. 39-52.

Goldberg, E. D., Bowen, V. T., Farrington, J. W., Harvey, G., Martin, J. H., Parker, P. L., Risebrough, R. W., Robertson, W., Schneider, E., Gamble. E., 1978, "The Mussel Watch," Environmental Conservation, Vol. 5, No. 2, pp. 101-125.

Gordon, M., Knauer, G. A., and Martin, J. H., 1980, "*Mytilus californianus* as a Bioindicator of Trace Metal Pollution: Variability and Statistical Considerations," Marine Pollution Bulletin, Vol. 11, pp. 195-198.

Green, R. H., Singh, S. M. and Bailey, R. C., 1985, "Bivalve Mollusks as Response Systems for Modeling Spatial and Temporal Environmental Patterns," Science of the Total Environment, Vol. 46, pp. 147-170.

Green, D. R., Stull, J. K., and Heesen, T. C., 1986, "Determination of Chlorinated Hydrocarbons in Coastal Waters using a Moored *In situ* Sampler and Transplanted Live Mussels," Marine Pollution Bulletin, Vol. 17, pp. 324-329.

Hole, L. M., Moore, M. N., and Bellamy, D., 1992, "Age-Related Differences in the Recovery of Lysosomes from Stress-Induced Pathological Reactions in Marine Mussels," Marine Environmental Research, Vol. 34, pp. 75-80.

Kiorboe, T., Mohlenberg, F. and Nohr, O., 1981, "Effect of Suspended Bottom Material on Growth and Energetics in *Mytilus edulis*," Marine Biology, Vol. 61, pp. 283-288.

Lobel, P. B., Belkhode, S. E., Jackson, S. E., and Longerich, H. P., 1990, "Recent Taxonomic Discoveries Concerning the Mussel *Mytilus*: Implications for Biomonitoring," Archives of Environmental Contamination and Toxicology, Vol. 19, pp. 508-512.

Lobel, P. B., Belkhode, S. P., Bajdik, C., Jackson, S. E., and Longerich, H. P., 1991, "Improved Protocol for Collecting Mussel Watch Specimens Taking Into Account Sex, Size, Condition, Shell Shape, and Chronological Age," Archives of Environmental Contamination and Toxicology, Vol. 21, pp. 409-414.

Lobel, P. B., Bajdik, C., Belkhode, S. P., Jackson, S. E., and Longerich, H. P, 1992, "General Characteristics of the Frequency Distributions of Element Concentrations and of Interelemental Correlations in Aquatic Organisms," Marine Environmental Research, Vol. 33, pp. 111-126.

Long, E. R., and Chapman, P. M., 1985, "A Sediment Quality Triad: Measures of Sediment Contamination, Toxicity and Infaunal Community Composition in Puget Sound," Marine Pollution Bulletin, Vol. 16, No. 10, pp. 405-415.

Mallet, A. L., Carver, C. E., Coffen, S. S., and Freeman, K. R., 1987, "Winter Growth of the Blue Mussel *Mytilus edulis* L.,: Importance of Stock and Site," Journal Experimental Marine Biology and Ecology, Vol. 108, pp. 217-228.

Martin, M., 1985, "State Mussel Watch: Toxics Surveillance in California," Marine Pollution Bulletin, Vol. 16, No. 4, pp. 140-146.

Martin, M. and Severeid, R., 1984, "Mussel Watch Monitoring for the Assessment of Trace Toxic Constituents in California Marine Waters," Concepts in Marine Pollution Measurements. H. H. White, Ed., Maryland Sea Grant Publication, University of Maryland, College Park, pp. 291-323.

McCarty, L. S., 1991, "Toxicant Body Residues: Implications for Aquatic Bioassays with Some Organic Chemicals," Aquatic Toxicology and Risk Assessment: Fourteenth Volume, ASTM STP 1124, M.A. Mayes and M. G. Barron, Eds., American Society for Testing and Materials, Philadelphia, pp. 183-192.

McKim, J. M. and Schmieder, P. K., 1991, "Bioaccumulation: Does It Reflect Toxicity?," Bioaccumulation in Aquatic Systems: Contributions to the Assessment, R. Nagel and R. Loskill, Eds., Proceedings, International Workshop, Berlin, 1990. VCG Publishers, New York, pp. 161-188.

Mearns, A. J., 1985, "Biological Implications of the Management of Waste Materials: The Importance of Integrating Measures of Exposure, Uptake, and Effects," Aquatic Toxicology and Hazard Assessment: Seventh Symposium, ASTM STP 854, R. D. Cardwell, R. Purdy, and R. C. Bahner, Eds., American Society for Testing and Materials, Philadelphia, pp. 335-343.

National Oceanic and Atmospheric Administration, 1989, National Status and Trends Program for Marine Environmental Quality, Progress Report: A Summary of Data on Tissue Contamination from the First Three Years (1986-1988) of the Mussel Watch Project, NOAA Technical Memorandum NOA OMA 49.

Nelson, W. G., 1990, "Use of the Blue Mussel, *Mytilus edulis*, in Water Quality Toxicity Testing and *In situ* Marine Biological Monitoring," Aquatic Toxicology and Risk Assessment: Thirteenth Volume, ASTM STP 1096, W. G. Landis and W. H. van der Schalie, Eds., American Society for Testing and Materials, Philadelphia, pp. 167-175.

Okamura, B., 1986, "Group Living and the Effects of Spatial Position in Aggregations of *Mytilus edulis*," Oecologia, Vol. 69, pp. 341-347.

Phillips, D. J. H., 1980, Quantitative Aquatic Biological Indicators, Applied Science Publishers, Ltd., London.

Phillips, D. J. H., 1988, "Monitoring of Toxic Contaminants in the San Francisco Bay-Delta: A Critical Review, Emphasizing Spatial and Temporal Trend Monitoring," San Francisco Bay-Delta Aquatic Habitat Institute.

Phillips, D. J. H., and Rainbow, P. S., 1993, Biomonitoring of Trace Aquatic Contaminants, Elsevier Applied Science, London.

Rodhouse, P. G, McDonald, J. H., Newell, R. I. E., and Koehn, R. K., 1986, "Gamete Production, Somatic Growth and Multiple-locus Enzyme Heterozygosity in *Mytilus edulis*," Marine Biology, Vol. 90, pp. 209-214.

Roesijadi, G., Young, J. S., Drum, A. S., and Gurtisen, J. M., 1984, "Behavior of Trace Metals in *Mytilus edulis* During a Reciprocal Transplant Field Experiment," Marine Ecological Progress Series, Vol. 18, pp. 155-170.

Salazar, M. H., 1989, "Mortality, Growth and Bioaccumulation in Mussels Exposed to TBT: Differences Between the Laboratory and the Field," Proceedings, Oceans 1989 Conference, 18-21 September 1989, Seattle, Washington, Organotin Symposium, Vol. 4, pp. 1188-1197.

Salazar, M. H., 1992, "Use and Misuse of Mussels in Natural Resource Damage Assessment," Proceedings, MTS 92, Washington, D.C, October 19-21, 1992, Vol. 1, Global Ocean Resources, pp. 257-264, Marine Technology Society.

Salazar, M. H. and Chadwick, D. B., 1991 "Using Real-Time Physical/Chemical Sensors and *In-situ* Biological Indicators to Monitor Water Pollution," Water Pollution: Modelling, Measuring and Prediction, L. C. Wrobel and C. A. Brebbia, Eds., First International Conference on Water Pollution Modelling, Measuring and Prediction, 1991. Elsevier Applied Science, London, pp. 463-480.

Salazar, M. H., Duncan, P. B., Salazar, S. M., and Rose., K. A., 1994, "Bioaccumulation of Contaminants and Reduced Growth in Transplanted Mussels as a Function of Location and Sediment Concentration Around a Superfund Site," Third Symposium on Environmental Toxicology and Risk Assessment, ASTM STP 1218, J. Hughes, G. Biddinger, and E. Mones, Eds., American Society for Testing and Materials, Philadelphia.

Salazar, M. H. and Salazar, S. M., 1987, "TBT Effects on Juvenile Mussel Growth," Proceedings, Oceans 1987 Conference, Halifax, Nova Scotia, Canada, 28 Sept. - 1 Oct. 1987, Organotin Symposium. Vol. 4, pp. 1504-1510.

Salazar, M. H. and Salazar, S. M., 1988, "Tributyltin and Mussel Growth in San Diego Bay," Proceedings, Oceans 1988 Conference, Baltimore, Maryland, 31 Oct. - 2 Nov. 1988, Organotin Symposium. Vol. 4, pp. 1188-1195.

Salazar, M. H. and Salazar, S. M., 1991, "Assessing Site-Specific Effects of TBT Contamination with Mussel Growth Rates," Marine Environmental Research, Vol. 32, pp. 131-150.

Salazar, M. H. and Salazar, S. M., 1994, "Mussels as Bioindicators: Effects of TBT on Survival, Bioaccumulation and Growth under Natural Conditions," Tributyltin: Environmental Fate and Effects. M. A. Champ and P. F. Seligman, Eds., Elsevier. In press.

Salazar, S. M., Davidson, B. M., Salazar, M. H., Stang, P. M., and Meyer-Schulte, K., 1987, "Field Assessment of a New Site-Specific Bioassay System," Proceedings, Oceans 1987 Conference, Halifax, Nova Scotia, Canada, 28 Sept. - 1 Oct. 1987, Organotin Symposium, Vol. 4, pp. 1461-1470.

Shigenaka, G. and Henry, C. B., 1993, "Use of Mussels and Semipermeable Membrane Devices to Assess Bioavailability of Residual Polynuclear Aromatic Hydrocarbons Three Years After the Exxon Valdez Oil Spill," Exxon Valdez Oil Spill: Fate and Effects in Alaskan Waters, ASTM STP 1219. P. G. Wells, J. N. Butler, and J. S. Hughes, Eds. American Society for Testing and Materials, Philadelphia.

Short, J. W. and Rounds, P., 1993, "Determination of Petroleum-derived Hydrocarbons in Seawater Following the Exxon Valdez Oil Spill II," Exxon Valdez Oil Spill Symposium, Program and Abstracts, pp.186-187; Alaska Sea Grant.

State of California, Water Resources Control Board, 1988, "California State Mussel Watch: Ten Year Data Summary 1977-1987," Water Quality Monitoring Report No. 87-3, Division of Water Quality.

Stephenson, M. D., Martin, M., and Martin, J. H., 1980, State Mussel Watch - Volume IV: Trace Metal Concentrations in Mussels from Bays of California, California Department of Fish and Game.

Stephenson, M. D., Smith, D. R., Goetzl, J., Ichikawa, G., and Martin, M., 1986, "Growth Abnormalities in Mussels and Oysters from Areas with High Levels of Tributyltin in San Diego Bay," Proceedings, Oceans 1986 Conference, Washington D. C., 23-25 Sept. 1986, Organotin Symposium, Vol. 4, pp. 1246-1251.

Stromgren, T., 1982, "Effects of Heavy Metals (Zn, Hg, Cu, Cd, Pb, Ni) on the Length Growth of *Mytilus edulis*," Marine Biology, Vol. 72, pp. 69-72.

Stromgren, T, 1986, "The Combined Effect of Copper and Hydrocarbons on the Length Growth of *Mytilus edulis*," Marine Environmental Research, Vol. 19, pp. 251-258.

Stromgren, T. and Bongard, T., 1987, "The effect of tributyltin oxide on growth of *Mytilus edulis*," Marine Pollution Bulletin, Vol. 18, No. 1, pp. 30-31.

U.S. Environmental Protection Agency, 1988, "Report to Congress on Administration of the Marine Protection, Research, and Sanctuaries Act of 1972, as Amended, No. P.L. 92-532. 1984-1986," U. S. Environmental Protection Agency. Office of Marine and Estuarine Protection, EPA-503/8-88/002.

Valkirs, A. O., Davidson, B., Kear, L. L., and Fransham, R. L, 1991, "Long-term Monitoring of Tributyltin in San Diego Bay California," Marine Environmental Research, Vol. 32, pp. 151-167.

Weber, C. I., 1988, Methods for Use of Caged Molluscs for *In-situ* Biomonitoring of Marine Discharges, Report Developed Jointly by the Office of Research and Development, Office of Acid Deposition, Environmental Monitoring, and Quality Assurance, US EPA, Cincinnati, OH, and the Office of Water, US EPA, Washington, DC, March 1988.

White, H. H., 1984, "Mussel Madness: Use and Misuse of Biological Monitors of Marine Pollution," Concepts in Marine Pollution Measurements, H. H. White, Ed., Maryland Sea Grant Publication, University of Maryland, College Park, pp. 325-337.

Widdows, J., Burns, K. A., Menon, N. R., Page, D. S., and Soria, S., 1990, "Measurement of Physiological Energetics (Scope of Growth) and Chemical Contaminants in Mussels (*Arca zebra*) Transplanted Along a Contamination Gradient in Bermuda," Journal of Experimental Marine Biology and Ecology, Vol. 138, pp. 99-117.

Widdows, J., and Donkin, P., 1992, "Mussels and Environmental Contaminants: Bioaccumulation and Physiological Aspects," Chapter 8, The Mussel *Mytilus*: Ecology, Physiology, Genetics and Culture, Developments in Aquaculture and Fisheries Science, E. Gosling, Ed., Elsevier, Amsterdam, pp. 383-424.

Young, D.R., Heesen, T. C., and McDermott, D. J., 1976, "An Offshore Biomonitoring System for Chlorinated Hydrocarbons," Marine Pollution Bulletin, Vol. 7, No. 8, pp. 156-159.

Zar, J. H., 1974, Biostatistical Analysis. Prentice-Hall, Englewood Cliffs.

Michael H. Salazar[1], P. Bruce Duncan[2], Sandra M. Salazar[3], and Keith A. Rose[2]

IN-SITU BIOASSAYS USING TRANSPLANTED MUSSELS: II. ASSESSING CONTAMINATED SEDIMENT AT A SUPERFUND SITE IN PUGET SOUND

REFERENCE: Salazar, M. H., Duncan P. B., and Salazar, S. M., and Rose, K. A., **"In-Situ Bioassay Using Transplanted Mussels: II. Assessing Contaminated Sediment at a Superfund Site in Puget Sound,"** Environmental Toxicology and Risk Assessment, - Third Volume, ASTM STP 1218, Jane S. Hughes, Gregory R. Biddinger, and Eugene Mones, Eds., American Society for Testing and Naterials, Philadelphia, 1995.

ABSTRACT: In a pilot study for the U.S. EPA, bioaccumulation and growth in mussels (*Mytilus trossulus)* were used to assess the bioavailability of contaminants and potentially adverse bioeffects in water overlying contaminated sediments. Caged juvenile and adult mussels were transplanted to 12 locations around a Superfund Site (Harbor Island), and a reference site (Carr Inlet) in Puget Sound, Washington. The exposure period was 82 days and animals were held 1 meter from the bottom. Accumulation of contaminants in adult mussel tissues was used to help identify the extent and magnitude of contamination in the overlying water. Reduced growth in juvenile mussels was used as an indicator of adverse bioeffects. Sites were ranked for these potentially adverse biological impacts. Juvenile mussel growth rates combined with toxicity-normalized sediment chemistry and toxicity-normalized tissue chemistry, provided a first-order approximation of potential biological effects associated with chemicals of concern in sediment and mussel tissues. Mussels from Harbor Island accumulated higher concentrations of contaminants and had significantly lower growth rates than the reference site mussels. Some differences were detected among the Harbor Island sites. Mussels from one site were much more contaminated than the others and, based on extremely low growth rates, exhibited the greatest potential for adverse biological effects. TBT and copper were the contaminants of greatest concern in both tissues and sediments; lead and zinc were an additional concern in sediments. A statistically significant inverse relationship was found between growth rate, toxicity-normalized tissue accumulation, and toxicity-normalized sediment contamination. Based on our results, we recommend the following integrated approach for evaluating contaminated sediments: (1) conduct *in-situ* bioassays, (2) estimate bioaccumulation in addition to bioeffects, and (3) evaluate water overlying the sediments.

KEYWORDS: mussel transplants, sediments, bioaccumulation, growth, Superfund, contamination, *in-situ* bioassay

[1]NOAA Bioeffects Branch, 7600 Sand Point Way NE, Seattle, WA, 98115
[2]U.S. EPA, Region 10, 1200 - 6th Ave, Seattle, WA, 98101
[3]EVS Consultants, 200 West Mercer St., Suite 403, Seattle, WA, 98119

INTRODUCTION

Harbor Island is a 400-acre industrial island which was added to the Superfund National Priority List in 1983. It is located at the mouth of the Duwamish River and adjacent to Elliott Bay, in Seattle, Washington (Fig. 1). The Island was constructed with dredged sediments from the Duwamish River at the turn of the century. In 1982, the U.S. Environmental Protection Agency (EPA) completed a preliminary assessment to identify sources of industrial contaminants and the potential for human exposure. Potential sources of industrial contaminants included a secondary lead smelter, shipyards, metal recycling operations, foundries, a metal plating facility, ship and railroad cargo operations, and petroleum bulk fuel storage and transfer operations (Weston 1993).

Many studies have shown high concentrations of contaminants in both sediments and biota from the Harbor Island area, as well as associated adverse biological effects. Long and Chapman (1985) report that, among urban waterways in Puget Sound, the concentrations of metals and organic compounds were among the highest in the Duwamish Waterway. Adverse effects in sediment bioassays have been reported for amphipods, worms, and fish (Chapman et al. 1985). The Elliott Bay Action Program (EBAP) used sediment chemistry, laboratory bioassays, effects on benthic infauna, bioaccumulation potential, and persistence in the environment to assess contaminated sediment. This EBAP study identified PAHs, PCBs, and trace elements as the contaminants of concern (PTI and Tetra Tech 1988). There is strong evidence that contaminants in sediment are accumulated by, and are affecting fish in this area. For example, relative to other contaminated Puget Sound sites, the concentrations of PCBs in English sole and chlorinated hydrocarbons in juvenile Chinook salmon, have been among the highest in the vicinity of the Duwamish Waterway (Malins et al. 1987; McCain et al. 1990; Varanasi et al. 1993). Tissue accumulations at similar sediment concentrations have been associated with reduced immunocompetence and reproduction (Varanasi et al. 1993). The highest incidences of fin erosion and liver lesions have been repeatedly found in bottom-dwelling fish collected from the Duwamish River (Malins et al. 1987; Stein et al. 1992; Varanasi et al. 1992).

In 1992, EPA completed a Phase II Remedial Investigation (RI) for Harbor Island which included sampling sediments at 119 locations and analyzing them for priority pollutants. The objective of that study was to define the areas of sediment contamination which exceed the State of Washington sediment management standards (SMS) (Washington State Department of Ecology 1991) and identify those areas that require remediation. The SMS are based on the Apparent Effects Threshold (AET) concept that identifies sediment contaminant concentrations above which statistically significant biological effects are expected to occur in marine organisms (Barrick et al. 1989). This approach was developed using Puget Sound data. As in the EBAP study, the Phase II investigation concluded that sediments in a large number of areas around Harbor Island contained elevated concentrations of several contaminants. In contract to the EBAP data, cadmium concentrations frequently exceeded the state management standard. Tributyltin (TBT) contamination was widespread and usually exceeded reference area concentrations (Weston 1993), but TBT was not measured as part of EBAP.

As part of the Phase II Remedial Investigation, caged mussels were transplanted around Harbor Island to assess the potential for bioaccumulation and adverse biological effects. The value of biological testing in assessing contamination is well known and bioaccumulation studies using transplanted bivalves can demonstrate the extent to which chemicals have migrated into food webs (Lee et al. 1993). Laboratory bioassays have been used to identify toxic sediments at Superfund sites in Puget Sound (Chapman and Long 1983; Pastorok and Becker 1990). The importance of laboratory bioassays and integrated approaches have been emphasized in the Sediment Quality Triad, which includes sediment chemistry, laboratory bioassays, and benthic community assemblages (Long and Chapman 1985). The use of *in-situ* bioassays is gaining wider acceptance as a potentially powerful tool because it combines the control of laboratory studies with the realism of field evaluations (Salazar and Salazar this volume), and the evaluation of sediments must ultimately be based on an ability to predict or measure biological effects at specific sites (Long and Chapman 1985; U.S. EPA 1992).

Our primary objective was to evaluate the utility of transplanted mussels in augmenting standard approaches to ranking contaminated sediments for regulatory purposes. In this paper we propose holistic assessments by combining mussel growth rates with estimates of potential sediment and tissue toxicity; thereby expanding sediment evaluations to include the overlying water. We also answer the following: 1) Did mussels accumulate the contaminants of concern associated with the sediments?; 2) Did the stations differ with respect to bioaccumulation and growth in mussels?, 3) Was there a relationship between sediment contamination, bioaccumulation, and mussel growth?, and 4) Which sites and which contaminants are of most concern?

EXPERIMENTAL METHODS

Mussel Deployment & Retrieval

Juvenile and adult mussels (*Mytilus trossulus*) were collected from the Penn Cove Mussel Farm, Coupeville, Washington (Fig. 1). Mussels were separated from the grow-out lines by carefully cutting the byssal threads. Since previous studies have shown that excessive handling can reduce mussel survival and growth rate, extreme care was taken to avoid injury that could stress the test animals (Salazar and Salazar this volume). Adult mussels in the 50 to 60 mm length size range were selected with sizing bars (i.e., a sorting device with two sets of fixed bars, the interval between representing the lower and upper acceptable size limits). This approach does not provide individual measurements. One hundred (100) adult mussels were selected at random and then placed into each of 33 bags of flexible vexar mesh tubing (Norplex Industries, Auburn, WA) approximately 1.5 m long. To control crowding and allow equal exposure of all individuals, each bag was subdivided into 10 clumps of 10 mussels each by constricting the mesh with plastic cable ties. Ample slack was provided within each clump to allow sufficient space for valve opening and growth during the test.

Juvenile mussels (24 to 30 mm length) were also selected by length, but individuals were measured with vernier calipers to the nearest 0.1 mm. In addition to recording length data, whole-animal wet-weight measurements (nearest 0.01 gm) were made for each juvenile mussel. Eighteen (18) juvenile mussels were placed into each of 24 cages. Cages were made of rigid plastic mesh cutlery trays (20 x 30 x 4.5 cm; Hutzler Manufacturing, Canaan, CT) modified to provide 18 separate compartments. We placed one individual per compartment to facilitate tracking survival and growth of individuals during the study. To ensure an equivalent distribution of juveniles among cages, the T_0 weight and length data were subjected to statistical analyses before deployment. No significant differences were found ($\alpha = 0.05$). On a per-cage basis, mean whole-animal wet weights ranged from 1.46 to 1.61 g (overall range of individuals: 1.05 to 2.28 g), and mean length from 26.3 to 26.7 mm (overall range 23.9 to 29.7 mm).

After distribution to their respective cages, all adults and juveniles were tied to a pier and suspended in Penn Cove overnight. After this 12-hour holding period, animals were put into ice chests without seawater and transported to the 13 test sites: 12 sites around Harbor Island (E05, E18, K01, K09, N02, N06, N07, W06, W21, W31, W38,

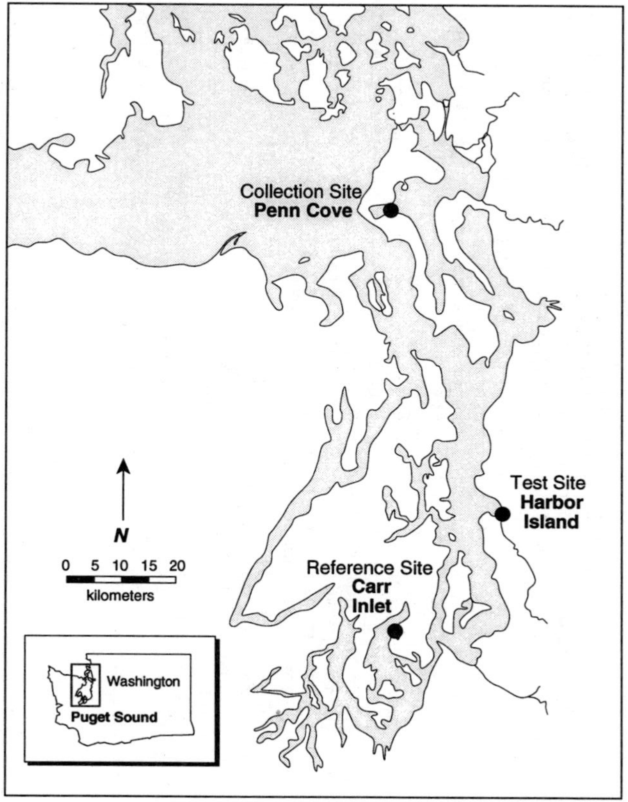

Fig. 1--The Puget Sound study area showing the Penn Cove collection site, the Carr Inlet reference site, and the Harbor Island Superfund site.

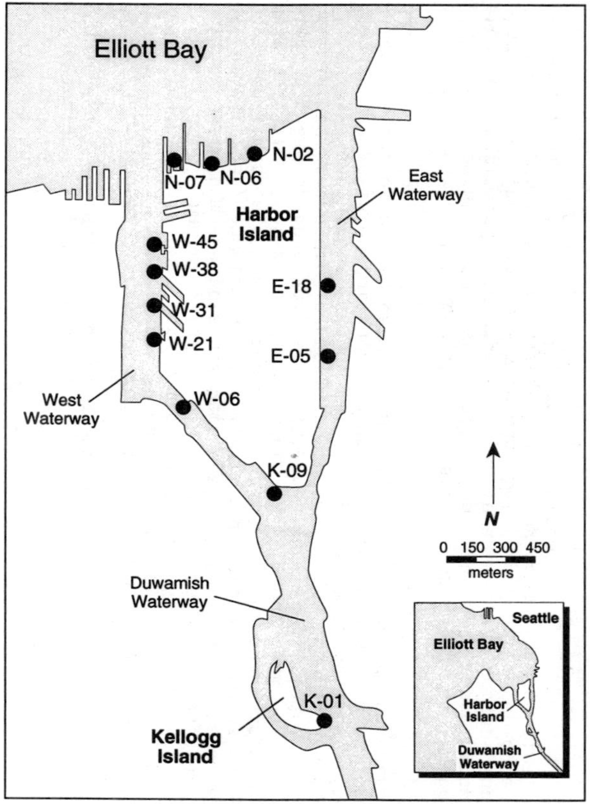

Fig. 2--The Harbor Island Superfund site showing the transplant sites, the Duwamish Waterway and Elliott Bay.

and W45) and the Carr Inlet (CAR) reference site (Fig. 2). Deployment site selections were based on the areal extent of elevated sediment contamination, as described in the RI, and the location of known contamination sources on Harbor Island. Using the convention of the RI, areas around the Island are designated as West (W) or East (E)Waterways, and North (N), or Kellogg Island (K). CAR was used as a reference site because this area is commonly used as a sediment reference site for other investigations in Puget Sound (Washington State Department of Ecology 1991). Test animals were out of seawater between three to six hours during deployment by divers. Around Harbor Island, mussels were deployed by divers approximately 1 m above the bottom in the vicinity of storm water outfalls, shipyards, and other industrial activities. The exposure period was 82 days (16 October 1991 to 7 January 1992). Two bags of 100 adult mussels (200 total) and one cage of juvenile mussels (18 total) were placed at most sites. Replication was used at the CAR reference site as well as K01 and K09 (the Harbor Island sites with the lowest concentrations of contaminants in sediments as measured in previous studies), and N07 (the Harbor Island site suspected of being the most contaminated). Three bags of 100 adult mussels (300 total) and three cages of 18 juvenile mussels (54 total) were transplanted at these sites. A total of 3000 adult mussels and 378 juvenile mussels were transplanted during this study.

Cages were either attached to nylon lines secured between adjacent pilings or to buoyed weights. At the end of the exposure period, mussels were retrieved by divers. While underwater and near the bottom, mussels were placed in plastic bags to isolate test animals from contamination in surface water as they were brought to the surface. Aboard the boat, mesh bags with adult mussels were opened and the mussels were sorted. Dead animals were discarded, and the number of survivors was recorded. Survivors, contained in plastic zip-lock bags with ≤ 100 animals per bag, were then placed in a large plastic trash can for transport. Cages with juvenile mussels were removed from the large plastic transfer bags and placed directly into the plastic trash can without any field processing. All adult and juvenile mussels were transported to the laboratory within 6 hours of collection. They were held overnight at the laboratory in a constant temperature room (4°C) without seawater, until processing the next day.

Adult mussel processing consisted of removing and homogenizing tissues according to the Puget Sound Estuary Protocols (Tetra Tech 1989). Each sample used for chemical analysis was a composite of tissues from 100 individuals. Tissue homogenates were frozen until analyzed. Adult mussel tissues were analyzed for trace metals, PAHs, pesticides, PCBs, and tributyltin (TBT). Analytical methods and detection limits are summarized in the sampling and analysis plan (Weston 1991). Contaminants of concern used in our ranking process were selected based on three criteria: (1) they were identified as contaminants of concern in previous studies of the Duwamish Waterway, Elliott Bay, and Harbor Island, (2) an ambient water quality criterion or equivalent existed for each contaminant of concern, and (3) there was at least a factor of two between the highest and lowest concentration in adult mussel tissues.

Juvenile mussel processing consisted of whole-animal length and weight measurements, and tissue collection. Juvenile mussel growth rates were estimated from changes in whole-animal wet weights and lengths. These measurements were made before and after deployment. Differences in growth were also estimated by comparing the final weights and lengths among sites at the end of the test.

RI & EBAP Sediment Data

To provide the best estimate of sediment contamination at each mussel deployment site, we calculated the mean concentration of contaminants using data for sampling stations located within a 150-m radius of each mussel deployment site. Both RI and EBAP (PTI and Tetra Tech 1988) sediment chemistry data were used in these calculations. We selected the same suite of contaminants that met our selection criteria for tissue contaminants of concern. Three to ten sediment sampling stations from either the EBAP or RI data sets fell within the 150-m radius for each mussel station. These means were used in normalization, ranking, and statistical analyses. Details regarding sediment sampling, handling, and analytical techniques are provided in Weston (1991, 1993).

Potential problems have recently been identified for the RI sediment data including: changes in detection limits among samples, low recovery of chemicals in some spiked samples, and the presence of high contaminant concentrations in the blanks. The cadmium and TBT data presented in the RI were inexplicably higher than previously reported values. This is particularly important because in many areas around Harbor Island the cleanup rankings are being driven by both cadmium and TBT. Although the concentration of cadmium in sediment was reported as an order of magnitude higher relative to previous studies, the tissue cadmium concentrations did not vary enough to meet our selection criteria, so we did not use cadmium in the rankings. We used TBT in the rankings because concentrations were elevated in both sediment and tissue.

Toxicity Normalization & Statistical Analysis

Growth in juvenile mussels (mg/wk/mussel) and bioaccumulation in adult mussel tissues (from the present study) were combined with previously collected sediment chemistry data and used in a preponderance-of-evidence approach to rank contaminated sites. Juvenile mussel growth rates, as estimated by increases in weight (mg/wk) were ranked from 1 (low) to 13 (high). We used growth rate based on weight rather than growth rate based on length, final weights, or final lengths because weight-growth measurements have been more informative in previous studies (Salazar and Salazar this volume). For replicated stations, significant differences in growth among stations were determined with an Analysis of Variance (ANOVA) and Duncan's New Multiple Range Test (Zar 1974; STATISTICA, StatSoft Inc., Tulsa, OK, 1991).

The tissue chemistry data from adult mussels were toxicity-normalized and ranked. To normalize the data, the concentrations of contaminants in tissues were divided by their respective Chronic Ambient Water Quality Criteria (AWQC) (U.S. EPA, 1986) to estimate relative potential toxicity. We chose these criteria because: (1) there are no tissue-based toxicity criteria, (2) concentrations of contaminants in mussel tissues have been related to water concentrations (Salazar and Salazar this volume), (3) there is a relationship between tissue concentrations and bioeffects in mussels (Salazar and Salazar this volume), and (4) there is some support for this procedure (Cook et al. 1992). In the tissue residue approach, maximum allowable tissue concentrations (MATCs) are estimated by multiplying chronic water quality criteria by bioconcentration factors (Cook et al. 1992), recognizing these MATCs may underestimate or overestimate measured tissue concentrations that elicit adverse effects (McKim and Schmieder, 1991; McCarty, 1991). Since there is no AWQC for TBT, we used the proposed State of California criterion (Water Resources Control Board 1991). Ensuing quotients for metals (arsenic, copper, lead, silver, and zinc), total PAHs (TPAHs = sum of Acenaphthylene, Ancenaphthene, Anthracene, Benzo(a)anthracene, Benzo(a)pyrene, Benzo(b)fluoranthene, Benzo(g,h,i)perylene, Benzo(k)fluoranthene, Chrysene, Fluoranthene,

Fluorene, Ideno(1,2,3-cd)pyrene, Phenanthrene, and Pyrene), PCBs (sum of six congeners), and TBT were summed for each station. Stations were then ranked from lowest (1) to highest (13) using the summed quotients of these tissue contamination units. A tissue contamination unit >1 suggests potential adverse effects.

Relative sediment toxicity was estimated by dividing the mean contaminant concentrations at each station by their respective Effects Range - Median (ERM) concentration (Long and Morgan 1991; Long and MacDonald 1992). These ERM guidelines were developed using three basic methods to evaluate data gathered in a variety of geographic areas: equilibrium partitioning, sediment bioassays, and synoptic chemical and biological data from field surveys. The ERM is the concentration approximately midway in the range of reported values associated with biological effects. Since there was no published ERM for TBT, we used the Puget Sound Dredged Disposal Analysis (PSDDA 1989) screening guideline which is similar to that suggested by MacDonald (personal communication). We normalized the data because contamination is not a bioeffect and rankings based on absolute concentrations do not account for potential sediment toxicity. A potential sediment toxicity contamination unit > 1 indicates possible adverse effects. Potential sediment toxicity units for metals (arsenic, chromium, copper, lead, mercury, and zinc), total PAHs, total PCBs, and TBT were summed for each station and ranked from lowest (1) to highest (13).

Overall comparisons among stations based on sediment chemistry, tissue chemistry, and growth were made using ranks, scatterplots, and regression analyses. An overall rank was calculated for each station by summing the individual ranks for sediment chemistry, tissue chemistry, and growth. The relationship between growth, sediment toxicity, and tissue toxicity was examined using a three-dimensional scatterplot. The sediment data were log-transformed to spread out the data points along that axis. Various models of growth, as a function of potential sediment and tissue toxicity, were evaluated to determine which transformations would provide (1) improved normality and linearity, (2) the highest r^2 (greatest overall significance), and (3) significant independent contributions by toxicity-normalized sediment and tissue data. A multiple linear regression was performed and residuals were tested for normality and outliers. The correlation coefficient relating normalized tissue and sediment data was calculated (STATISTICA, StatSoft Inc., Tulsa, OK, 1991).

RESULTS

Sediment Chemistry

The concentrations of almost all contaminants were significantly higher in sediments around Harbor Island than in sediments from the Carr Inlet reference site (Table 1). The biggest differences occurred with TBT and lead where the most contaminated sites had concentrations that were factors of 920 and 230 above reference. Several of the least-contaminated Harbor Island sites were similar to CAR with respect to sediment contamination. The potential for toxicity associated with these contaminated sediments is shown in Table 2, where Station N07 has the highest ranking using ERM-normalized data. Station N07 had the greatest exceedances of the ERM for more contaminants than any other station and exhibited the greatest separation between both the other Harbor Island sites and the reference site. The ranking process was driven primarily by TBT. Other contaminants also contributed to potential sediment toxicity. PCBs, for example, were highest in the East Waterway stations (E05 and E18).

Table 1--Contaminant concentrations (mg/kg) in sediments from Harbor Island and the Reference Site in Carr Inlet (CAR). Also shown are highest and lowest Harbor Island values relative to CAR and the ERM used to create normalized concentrations in Table 2.

	As	Cr	Cu	Pb	Hg	Zn	TPAH	PCBs	TBT
CAR	2.4	40	18	1.3	0.035	42	3.9	0.033	0.02
E05	12	56	127	77	0.844	159	16	0.655	1.42
E18	12	76	119	96	0.442	187	9	0.638	1.16
K01	8	44	142	22	0.134	107	8	0.178	0.18
K09	10	81	85	34	0.128	117	11	0.296	0.21
N02	11	51	66	31	0.213	127	50	0.177	0.40
N06	23	92	275	88	0.679	280	28	0.094	5.21
N07	57	55	965	297	1.950	592	37	0.503	18.41
W06	9	47	90	60	0.331	121	8	0.148	0.62
W21	16	84	166	86	0.538	222	19	0.168	2.01
W31	22	84	276	261	0.582	362	20	0.209	3.37
W38	23	93	221	221	0.739	299	15	0.292	0.38
W45	24	89	228	194	0.888	281	15	0.280	1.07
High CAR	24	2	53	230	56	14	13	20	920
Low CAR	3	1	4	17	4	3	2	3	9
ERM	85	145	390	110	1.3	270	35	0.4	0.03

Table 2--ERM-normalized contaminant concentrations in sediments from Harbor Island and the Reference Site in Carr Inlet (CAR). TPAH and PCBs as in Table 1. R = overall rank; ∑NC = sum of normalized concentrations.

	As	Cr	Cu	Pb	Hg	Zn	TPAH	PCBs	TBT	∑NC	R
CAR	0.03	0.28	0.05	0.01	0.03	0.16	0.11	0.08	0.67	1	1
K01	0.10	0.30	0.36	0.20	0.10	0.40	0.23	0.45	6	8	2
K09	0.12	0.56	0.22	0.31	0.10	0.43	0.32	0.74	7	10	3
N02	0.13	0.35	0.17	0.28	0.16	0.47	1.42	0.44	13	17	4
W38	0.27	0.64	0.57	2.01	0.57	1.11	0.43	0.73	13	19	5
W06	0.10	0.32	0.23	0.54	0.25	0.45	0.23	0.37	21	23	6
W45	0.29	0.61	0.59	1.76	0.68	1.04	0.43	0.70	36	42	7
E18	0.15	0.52	0.30	0.87	0.34	0.69	0.26	1.60	39	43	8
E05	0.14	0.39	0.32	0.70	0.65	0.59	0.45	1.64	47	52	9
W21	0.19	0.58	0.42	1.35	0.41	0.82	0.53	0.42	67	72	10
W31	0.26	0.58	0.71	2.37	0.45	1.34	0.57	0.52	112	119	11
N06	0.26	0.63	0.70	0.80	0.52	1.04	0.80	0.24	174	179	12
N07	0.67	0.38	2.48	2.70	1.50	2.19	1.05	1.26	614	626	13

Tissue Chemistry

The differences in tissue concentrations of contaminants among sites (Table 3) were not nearly as great as those for sediment, even following normalization (Table 4). The small differences observed were largely due to copper and TBT, but PCBs were also a factor. In general, mussels at the most contaminated sites accumulated more contaminants than the reference animals (note that arsenic and zinc were higher in reference mussels than those deployed at the least contaminated sites). As with sediment, station N07 had the highest concentrations of most contaminants as well as the highest ranking with AWQC-normalized data. Tissue concentrations of TBT and copper (both before and after normalization) were highest at N07. Adult mussels at the most contaminated sites had the greatest elevations above reference for PCBs (18 times higher) and TPAHs (17 times higher), but these contaminants were only considered to have a low toxicity potential based on our normalizations (Table 4). Normalized TPAHs were orders of magnitude below predicted toxicity thresholds. PCBs were highest in mussel tissues at E05, E18, and N07, but normalization suggested these concentrations were not potentially toxic. It was surprising that tissue concentrations of TBT in mussels transplanted to Harbor Island were only up to three times higher than reference mussels (Table 3), because sediment concentrations of TBT were up to three orders of magnitude higher than reference sediment concentrations (Table 1). After normalization (Table 4), tissues accumulated TBT at potentially toxic concentrations at all stations, even the reference site. The toxicity-normalized data suggest that mercury was a problem as well, but measurements were all at or below the limits of detection.

Mussel Growth

For mussels deployed at CAR, final whole-animal wet weights, growth rates expressed as mg/wk, final lengths, and growth rates expressed as mm/wk were significantly higher ($\alpha = 0.05$) when compared with mussels deployed at the Harbor Island sites. Mean growth rates (mg/wk/mussel) for juvenile mussels at CAR were approximately 3 to 5 times higher than for mussels transplanted to any of the Harbor Island sites (Table 5). Mussels at N07 had the lowest growth rates. However, the Multiple Range Test did not detect significant differences in growth among any of the cages deployed around the Harbor Island sites when all sites were compared. Because the growth rates were not different among replicate cages, data were pooled for the four stations where replicate cages were deployed.

Analysis of pooled data for the four sites showed the same significant differences among sites in all four mussel metrics; i.e., final weights, final lengths, growth rate based on length, and growth rate based on weight ($n = 190$, $p < 0.001$). Duncan's New Multiple Range Test (Zar, 1974; STATISTICA, StatSoft Inc., Tulsa, OK, 1991) separated growth rates for these sites into the following three groups:

CAR > K01 = K09 > N07

Survival

Compared to most standard laboratory bioassays which run from four to 21 days, this 82-day exposure was a relatively long-term field experiment. Even so, survival was high and within standards commonly accepted for laboratory bioassays. Adult survival by station ranged from 72 to 88% with a mean of approximately 80%. Juvenile survival by station ranged from 78 to 100% with a mean of approximately 90%. This difference in survival between juvenile and adult mussels is statistically significant ($\alpha = 0.05$). Since survival is not a sensitive measure of bioeffects, it was not surprising that there were no

Table 3--Contaminant concentrations (mg/kg) in tissues from Harbor Island and the Reference Site in Carr Inlet (CAR). Also shown are the highest and lowest Harbor Island values relative to CAR and the chronic ambient water quality criteria. TBT value is from the State of California proposed water quality criterion.

	As	Cr	Cu	Pb	Hg	Zn	TPAH	PCBs	TBT
CAR	1.71	0.15	0.92	0.072	0.04	17.2	0.036	0.0012	0.017
E05	0.54	0.27	0.93	0.232	0.04	16.9	0.134	0.0081	0.042
E18	0.98	0.22	0.97	0.112	0.04	14.7	0.121	0.0048	0.047
K01	1.67	0.17	1.07	0.177	0.04	17.4	0.165	0.0024	0.034
K09	1.11	0.16	1.01	0.172	0.04	16.0	0.118	0.0019	0.023
N02	1.34	0.18	1.09	0.132	0.04	18.0	0.227	0.0222	0.019
N06	1.20	0.23	1.18	0.155	0.04	17.8	0.169	0.0021	0.025
N07	1.52	0.23	3.01	0.186	0.04	22.1	0.21	0.0017	0.046
W06	1.75	0.20	1.17	0.252	0.04	16.4	0.289	0.0026	0.021
W21	1.69	0.23	1.46	0.269	0.04	18.5	0.597	0.0016	0.026
W31	0.67	0.26	1.31	0.298	0.04	20.0	0.279	0.0021	0.029
W38	1.47	0.25	1.35	0.521	0.04	20.6	0.196	0.0017	0.032
W45	1.25	0.20	1.11	0.329	0.04	20.0	0.379	0.0027	0.032
High / CAR	1.0	1.9	3.3	7.2	1.0	1.3	16.6	18.0	2.8
Low / CAR	0.3	1.1	1.0	1.6	1.0	0.9	3.3	1.3	1.1
AWQC	36	50	1.5	8.5	0.025	86	150	0.03	0.01

Table 4--AWQC-normalized contaminant concentrations in tissues from Harbor Island and the Reference Site in Carr Inlet (CAR). R = overall rank; ∑NC = sum of normalized concentrations.

	As	Cr	Cu	Pb	Hg	Zn	TPAH	PCBs	TBT	∑NC	R
CAR	0.048	0.003	0.612	0.008	2	0.200	0.000	0.041	1.7	4.21	1
W06	0.049	0.004	0.780	0.030	2	0.191	0.002	0.088	2.1	4.84	2
K09	0.031	0.003	0.670	0.020	2	0.186	0.001	0.062	2.3	4.87	3
N06	0.033	0.005	0.787	0.018	2	0.207	0.001	0.071	2.5	5.22	4
N02	0.037	0.004	0.727	0.016	2	0.209	0.002	0.740	1.9	5.23	5
W21	0.047	0.005	0.973	0.032	2	0.215	0.004	0.054	2.6	5.53	6
W31	0.019	0.005	0.873	0.035	2	0.233	0.002	0.068	2.9	5.73	7
W45	0.035	0.004	0.740	0.039	2	0.233	0.003	0.091	3.2	5.94	8
K01	0.046	0.003	0.715	0.021	2	0.202	0.001	0.080	3.4	6.07	9
W38	0.041	0.005	0.900	0.061	2	0.240	0.001	0.057	3.2	6.10	10
E05	0.015	0.005	0.618	0.027	2	0.197	0.001	0.271	4.2	6.93	11
E18	0.027	0.004	0.647	0.013	2	0.171	0.001	0.159	4.7	7.32	12
N07	0.042	0.005	2.003	0.022	2	0.256	0.001	0.058	4.6	8.59	13

Table 5--Juvenile mussel growth data. Also shown are the highest and lowest Harbor Island values relative to the Reference Site in Carr Inlet (CAR). Initial n = 432; survival ranged from 78 to 100% ($\bar{x}$ = 90%).

Site	n	$\bar{x}$ % Survival	T_0 Whole Animal Weight (g)	T_F Whole Animal Weight (g)	Growth Rate (mg/wk)	T_0 Length (mm)	T_F Length (mm)	Growth Rate (mm/wk)	Rank
CAR	54	83	1.49	4.74	276	26.5	39.2	1.09	1
W45	18	89	1.53	2.54	89	26.6	31.6	0.44	2
N02	18	94	1.50	2.51	84	26.6	32.0	0.45	3
K01	54	92	1.53	2.47	82	26.6	31.3	0.41	4
K09	54	94	1.52	2.47	82	26.5	31.3	0.42	5
W38	18	94	1.48	2.38	77	26.6	31.3	0.40	6
N06	18	94	1.51	2.39	76	26.6	30.9	0.36	7
W31	18	89	1.57	2.44	74	26.6	30.7	0.35	8
W06	18	94	1.49	2.34	71	26.4	30.6	0.37	9
E05	18	100	1.61	2.37	64	26.6	30.4	0.32	10
E18	18	94	1.53	2.30	64	26.5	30.1	0.30	11
W21	18	78	1.51	2.21	62	26.3	30.0	0.33	12
N07	54	81	1.50	2.19	59	26.5	29.6	0.26	13
CAR High				1.87	3.10		1.2	2.42	
CAR Low				2.16	4.68		1.3	4.19	

statistically significant differences in survival among sites. Unlike growth, where the highest growth rates were associated with low sediment and tissue contamination, no associations with contaminant concentrations in either tissue or sediment could be made for survival. Survival was actually lowest at the CAR reference site.

Overall Relationship between Bioaccumulation, Growth and Sediment

Based on the combined rankings for growth, normalized sediment toxicity, and normalized tissue toxicity (Table 6), the biggest difference was found between the CAR reference site and N07. CAR ranked first in terms of lowest normalized sediment and tissue contamination, and first in terms of highest growth rates. By contrast, N07 had the highest potential sediment and tissue toxicity, and lowest growth rate. There are two orders of magnitude difference in potential sediment toxicity (Table 2), a factor of two difference in potential tissue toxicity (Table 4), and a factor of five difference in juvenile mussel

Table 6--Overall ranks by station computed from sum of ranks for normalized sediment toxicity, normalized tissue toxicity, and growth rate (mg/wk/mussel).

Site	Sediment Rank	Tissue Rank	Growth Rank	∑ Rank	Overall Rank
CAR	1	1	1	3	1
K09	3	3	5	11	2
N02	4	5	3	12	3
K01	2	9	4	15	4
W06	6	2	9	17	5
W45	7	8	2	17	6
W38	5	10	6	21	7
N06	12	4	7	23	8
W31	11	7	8	26	9
W21	10	6	12	28	10
E05	9	11	10	30	11
E18	8	12	11	31	12
N07	13	13	13	39	13

growth rate (Table 5). CAR and N07 are also separated from the other Harbor Island sites. It is difficult to separate the remaining Harbor Island sites based on the overall rankings. K09 and N02 appear to be two of the least potentially toxic sites, while E05, E18, and N07 are the most potentially toxic. Growth, normalized sediment toxicity, and normalized tissue toxicity are plotted in Figs. 3 and 4 to provide a graphical representation of separation among sites. Both figures show the largest differences attributable to normalized sediment contamination and the least difference attributable to normalized tissue contamination. Some stations with higher sediment contamination were lower in overall ranking due to a combination of higher growth rate and lower tissue contamination (Table 6).

The scatterplot of growth, normalized sediment, and tissue toxicity (Fig. 4) helps visualize the separation of stations into three major groups: CAR, N07, and the rest of the Harbor Island sites. As shown in all the previous data, the biggest difference among test sites by far, using any data set, normalized or non-normalized, is between CAR and N07. These sites also appeared different than the other Harbor Island sites. Sites E05 and E18 are potentially less toxic than N07, but more toxic than the remaining sites. This is based primarily on tissue and growth rankings with the sediment ranking having less impact. Mussels at E05 and E18 accumulated relatively high concentrations of PCBs.

Regression Analysis

The regression of potential sediment toxicity (inverse transformation, S^{-1}) and potential tissue toxicity (T) on juvenile mussel growth (inverse transformation, G^{-1}) is highly significant ($r^2 = 0.89$, $n = 13$, overall model $p < 0.0001$). This indicates that

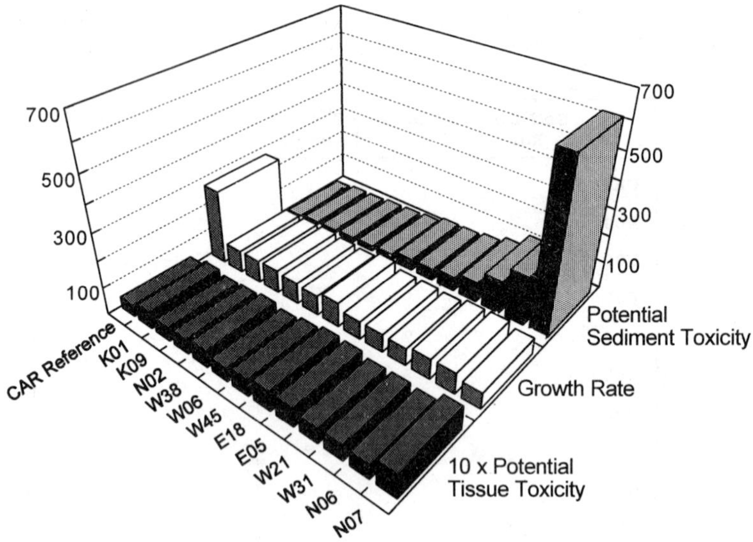

Fig. 3--Bar graph showing potential sediment and tissue toxicity and juvenile mussel growth rates (mg/wk/mussel). Stations are arranged in ascending order of potential sediment toxicity.

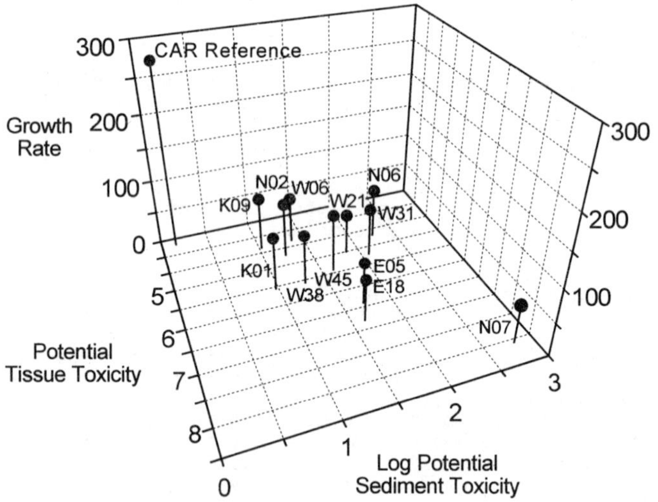

Fig. 4--Three dimensional scatterplot showing growth rate, potential tissue toxicity, and log potential sediment toxicity.

almost 90% of the observed variability in growth across stations could be accounted for by our estimates of potential sediment and tissue toxicity. The resulting equation is:

$$G^{-1} = 0.009 - 0.012(S^{-1}) + 0.00087(T) \quad (1)$$

The independent contributions of S^{-1} and T are also both significant ($p < 0.001$ and $p < 0.05$, respectively). The squared semipartial correlations, which indicate the proportion of total variability in G^{-1}, explained by these two parameters are 40% and 8%, respectively. These results suggest that potential sediment toxicity is more closely associated with growth than potential tissue toxicity. Potential tissue and sediment toxicity were significantly, but moderately correlated ($r^2 = 0.46$, $n = 13$, $p < 0.05$). A plot of residuals versus deleted residuals showed that the regression was influenced by CAR data, but not by N07 data. Without the CAR data, the overall regression analysis model was still significant ($r^2 = 0.53$, $n = 12$, $p < 0.05$) and the regression equation was very similar. However, the ability to account for variability in growth decreases to 53% and the independent contributions of S^{-1} and T are not significant ($p = 0.14$, $p = 0.08$). In addition, the proportion of total variability in G^{-1} explained by S^{-1} and T changed to 13% and 21%, respectively.

DISCUSSION

In this pilot study for EPA, we developed a first-order estimation of potential biological harm from contaminated sediments and tissues using direct measurements of animals exposed *in-situ*. We evaluated the utility of transplanted mussels to augment standard approaches to evaluate contaminated sediments. Mussels accumulated contaminants of concern associated with sediments, stations differed with respect to bioaccumulation and growth, there was a statistically significant relationship between sediment chemistry, tissue chemistry, and growth, and we identified the sites and contaminants of most concern. Based on these results, we recommend that standard approaches to evaluating contaminated sediments be augmented to include: (1) *in-situ* bioassays, (2) bioaccumulation in addition to bioeffects measurements, and (3) evaluations of water overlying the sediments. We used transplanted mussels to accomplish this, but any similar approach could be used.

Bioaccumulation

The tissue chemistry data demonstrate that there is a connection between contaminants in the sediments and contaminants in the water column around Harbor Island. Our results show that the biota in the water column are exposed to and can accumulate these contaminants. Similar results have been reported by others (Young et al. 1976; Widdows et al. 1990; Widdows and Donkin 1992). Even though we have not proven that the contaminants in the mussel tissues came from the sediment (the experiment was not designed to show this) nor investigated the relative contribution of dissolved versus particulate-associated contaminants, we have shown a significant correlation between contaminants in the sediments and contaminants in the tissues. Although it is unclear if bottom sediments or land-based activities were the primary source of contaminants measured in mussel tissues, the accumulation was from one of these sources. Source control has greatly reduced or eliminated contamination from storm drains and many other land-based activities on Harbor Island. This circumstantial evidence combined with the strong statistical relationships suggests that contaminated sediments were the source of the contaminants measured in mussel tissues.

It is well established that suspended particulates adsorb a number of contaminants and that this process reduces the bioavailability of those contaminants to organisms that do not utilize those particles as food. Mussels have been used to estimate potentially bioavailable contaminants because of their ability to filter seawater for dissolved, phytoplankton-associated, and sediment-sorbed contamination (Hermsen et al. 1994; Ekelund et al. 1987; Widdows and Donkin 1992; Salazar 1986). One of the reasons that many of these sediment-sorbed contaminants are available to mussels is that mussels are able to utilize the organic coatings on these particles as food (Kiorboe et al. 1981). The presence of suspended sediments in laboratory bioassays has been shown to enhance the bioaccumulation of TBT (Waldock and Thain 1983; Laughlin et al. 1986) and other chemicals (Hermsen et al. 1994; Ekelund et al. 1987).

Because the mussels in our study were not depurated after field exposure and retrieval, bioaccumulation may have been overestimated. Previous investigators have shown that the mussel gut can contain significant amounts of sediment-sorbed contaminants (Lobel et al. 1991; Metcalfe-Smith et al. 1992; Robinson et al. 1993). It is not clear to what extent this may have biased our results, but the limited data available suggests that this may not be a problem for all of the contaminants measured in our study. Furthermore, even if the contaminants were not bioavailable and had not been incorporated into mussel tissues, the transplanted animals served as effective accumulators of contaminated, suspended sediment. Unless the contaminants were adsorbed on particles to be rejected as pseudofeces, these accumulated contaminants could be available. Nevertheless, the significant correlation between growth and tissue accumulation suggests that the contaminants were available to mussels and that this measurement may be more appropriate for predicting bioeffects than measuring contaminants in sediment.

Growth

We used juvenile mussel growth as an indicator of water column effects associated with contaminated sediments. As in previous studies, our results (Table 5) show that growth is a more sensitive indicator of biological effects than survival and that growth based on increase in weight is more discriminating than growth based on increase in length (Salazar and Salazar this volume). For the replicated sites, juvenile mussel growth could discriminate bioeffects between the control site and some contaminated sites around Harbor Island (Table 2). This suggests that increased replication could help discriminate differences among other Harbor Island sites.

It is possible that growth rates around Harbor Island could be significantly lower than those in Carr Inlet because of differences in the natural physical and chemical factors that affect mussel growth rates such as temperature, salinity, current speed, etc. Similarly, factors such as sediment grain size, diet, and pre-exposure conditions can affect the results of laboratory bioassays. However, despite the influence of other factors that could affect growth, we are convinced that contaminants played a major role in affecting growth since the highest growth rates were associated with the lowest toxicity-normalized sediment and tissue contamination, and vice versa. In addition, after controlling for sediment toxicity, higher growth rates were significantly ($p < 0.05$) associated with lower concentrations of contaminants (Equation 1).

Since mussel growth is such an important component of this assessment procedure and there are so many natural factors affecting growth, these factors should be more thoroughly evaluated in future studies. To evaluate site-specific effects, *in situ* measurements of appropriate natural factors should be included. To help explain the effects of these factors on growth, laboratory bioassays controlling these factors should also be included.

Normalizing and Combining Sediment and Tissue Concentrations

There are inherent problems in any scheme used to estimate the combined potential toxicity attributable to a suite of contaminants. Despite this limitation, we have demonstrated the utility of producing a single estimate of potential tissue or sediment toxicity for comparison with mussel growth rates. The extent to which this approach may have biased the results is unknown, because the toxicity of our selected contaminants may not be additive. We attempted to weight contaminants on the basis of available and biologically relevant factors. Because the ERMs include sediment chemistry, community effects, laboratory bioassays, and equilibrium partitioning, they are one of the most integrative guidelines that can be used to normalize sediment concentrations. Further, the ERM is only the 50th percentile (median) effects level and as such provides a midpoint estimate of the potential for toxicity. We did not feel it was reasonable to use elevations above reference to rank tissue chemistry data (as previously reported in the remedial investigation [Weston 1993]) because the concentration of several contaminants in tissues from our reference site sometimes exceeded those from the Harbor Island site. Without relating these exceedances to biological effects, one could develop erroneous concerns about the contaminants that might reasonably be associated with various sites. Moving the basis for evaluating effects of contaminants from elevation-above-reference values to toxicity-based values should improve sediment quality assessments. Shifting from estimating toxicity with established criteria to actual site-specific bioeffects measured *in-situ* should provide the necessary field validation for laboratory bioassays.

We agree with previous investigators in suggesting that more carefully designed studies are needed to relate bioaccumulation and toxicity (Cook et al. 1992; McKim and Schmieder 1991). Dose-response relationships for TBT, copper, and zinc based on field exposures of mussels in San Diego Bay (Salazar and Salazar this volume) suggest that the concentrations of these contaminants accumulated in adult mussels at the most contaminated sites around Harbor Island were not high enough to adversely affect mussel growth rates. This suggests that: (1) Dividing by the AWQC may have been reasonable to rank potential tissue toxicity, but dose-response data provide the best indicators; (2) It is important to develop these relationships from measuring dose and response in the same species and the same individuals (we used adults for bioaccumulation and juveniles for growth in this Puget Sound study); and (3) There are differences between juveniles and adults in bioaccumulation, growth, survival, and dose-response that should be considered in any assessment of this type (Salazar and Salazar this volume; data from this EPA pilot study not presented). A better normalization might be achieved by using a bioconcentration factor, along with a mussel-specific water quality criterion, to estimate maximum allowable tissue concentrations (MATC). Dividing the mussel tissue concentrations by this MATC could more closely approximate tissue toxicity.

Site-Specific Differences

Important information can be gained from our results that regulators could use in prioritizing cleanup. The highest sediment contamination, tissue contamination, and the lowest mussel growth rates were all found at N07 and justify a ranking of highest concern. Other work supports this conclusion. Previous studies have demonstrated high sediment toxicity around Harbor Island and near N07 in particular. For example, N07 is the only site where four different evaluation criteria were not met (i.e., less than 50% of reference abundance for polychaetes, crustaceans, and molluscs, and failure of the amphipod bioassays [Weston 1993]). In two separate laboratory bioassay studies with *Neanthes arenaceodentata* lasting 63 and 108 days, juvenile growth and reproductive success were significantly reduced in exposures to sediment from site N07 when compared to a Carr Inlet Control (Johns and Ginn 1990; Johns et al. 1991).

Improving Assessment Tools

This EPA pilot study conducted in Puget Sound has demonstrated how mussel transplants can supplement the chemical analysis of sediments to prioritize contaminated sites and emphasize the importance of biologically-based criteria. The concept that direct measurements of bioavailability and bioeffects provide information beyond routine analysis of contaminated sediments has been repeatedly emphasized by others. For example, the U.S. Army Corps of Engineers added a bioeffects component to their regulatory program in 1977 when they included a requirement for laboratory bioassays of dredge material for disposal (U.S. EPA 1990). This approach was improved with the development of a Sediment Quality Triad for the evaluation of contaminated sediments that combined bulk sediment chemistry, laboratory bioassays and assessment of benthic community structure (Chapman et al. 1985). Recently, the State of Washington adopted a regulatory program based on the Apparent Effects Threshold which combines bulk sediment chemistry with effects from laboratory bioassays and benthic effects measurements (Washington State Department of Ecology 1991; Barrick et al. 1988, 1989). The approach proposed here and tested in this pilot project can be used to supplement these other approaches.

We have shown how replication at some of the sites increased the discriminating power of the approach in detecting differences among sites. With replication, we were able to detect a statistically significant difference in juvenile mussel growth where sites were only separated by 23 mg/wk (K01=K09 > N07; see Table 5). Further, any statistically significant difference in growth could have effects at the population level (Bayne et al. 1985). Just as we have shown how increased replication can improve the ability to detect differences among sites based on growth, additional transplants at various depths and horizontal distances from suspected sources can identify and locate sources on a finer scale. Because the mussel transplant approach provides a great deal of experimental control, it could be used more intensively around Harbor Island to clarify pathways and exposure routes of contaminants. By transplanting mussels at various depths and distances from suspected sources (sediments, outfalls or landfills) the location of sources can be more clearly identified. This gradient approach, used in San Diego Bay showed that ship hulls rather than sediment were the primary of copper and TBT in the water column. The details of this approach are provided in a companion article in this volume (Salazar and Salazar) and elsewhere (Salazar and Salazar 1991, 1994).

Assessments of water overlying contaminated sediments have been conducted previously. Several other studies have transplanted bivalves near contaminated sediment and made various measurements, such as bioaccumulation and bioeffects (Widdows and Donkin 1992; Roesijadi et al. 1984). For example, in addition to the San Diego Bay study mentioned above, results from mussels transplants in the southern California Bight demonstrated that DDT in bottom sediment was the source of DDT in mussel tissues (Young et al. 1976). In Bermuda, TBT and PAHs in sediment were shown to accumulate in mussel tissues and cause reductions in scope for growth (Widdows et al. 1990). We believe, ours is the first study to use synoptic measurements of bioaccumulation and bioeffects in transplanted mussels to assess contaminated sediments in Puget Sound or at any EPA Superfund site.

CONCLUSIONS

By using transplanted mussels, we demonstrated that combining mussel growth, tissue chemistry, and sediment chemistry was effective in differentiating areas of contamination and potential bioeffects. Our limited synoptic measurements of mussel growth rates and tissue chemistry could only distinguish between the most contaminated and the least contaminated sites. However, we were able to show an association between toxicity-normalized tissue and sediment concentrations. There was a statistically significant relationship between mussel growth and both tissue and sediment chemistry, and mussels accumulated many of the contaminants measured in sediments.

Our original purpose was to determine the utility of measuring bioaccumulation and growth in transplanted mussels as a supplement to standard approaches used to evaluate contaminated sediments. When we attempted to rank the sediment and tissue concentrations, we were dissatisfied with approaches such as elevations above reference, so we normalized for toxicity. The normalization and ranking system presented here should be regarded as preliminary. We encourage continuing efforts to develop a method for normalizing based on toxicity.

More importantly, our results could be used as part of an ecological risk assessment. Assessments of sediment toxicity could benefit greatly from (1) using *in-situ* bioassays, (2) evaluating overlying water, and (3) measuring bioaccumulation and bioeffects. In the context of environmental toxicology and risk assessment, we believe that the sediment compartment should be viewed as a dynamic, interactive system. As such, sediments should be evaluated for potential bioaccumulation and bioeffects in the ecosystem. We have provided one approach that could be used for such an holistic assessment.

ACKNOWLEDGEMENTS

We thank Duane Karna and the EPA-Region 10 divers for transplanting the mussels, Gary Rosenthal and the EVS benthic sorting team for extracting the mussel tissues, Joe Cummins and the EPA-Region 10 chemists for analyzing the mussel tissues, and Kimberly Galimanis for creating Figures 1 and 2. We also thank Peter Chapman, Bob Dexter, Ed Long, and four anonymous reviewers, particularly Reviewer #2, for their comments on the manuscript. We thank Chris Mebane for continuous support and encouragement in all phases of the work (including mussel shucking until midnight).

REFERENCES

Barrick, R., S. Becker, L. Brown, H. Beller, and R. Pastorok, 1988, Sediment quality values refinement: 1988 update and evaluation of Puget Sound AET. Volume 1. Final Report, Prepared for Tetra Tech Inc. and U.S. Environmental Protection Agency, Region 10. PTI Environmental Services, Bellevue, WA. 74 pp + appendices.

Barrick, R., H. Beller, S. Becker, and T. Ginn, 1989, "Use of the apparent effects threshold approach (AET) in classifying contaminated sediments," In: Contaminated Marine Sediments -- Assessment and Remediation, Committee on Contaminated Marine Sediments, Marine Board, National Academy Press, pp. 64-77.

Bayne, B. L., D. A. Brown, K. Burns, D. R. Dixon, A. Ivanovici, D. R. Livingstone, D. M. Lowe, N. M. Moore, A. R. D. Stebbing, and J. Widdows, 1985, "The Effects of Stress and Pollution on Marine Animals," Praeger Special Studies, Praeger Scientific, New York. 384 pages.

Chapman, P.M., R.N. Dexter, R.M. Kocan, and E.R. Long, 1985, "An overview of biological effects testing in Puget Sound, Washington: Methods, results, and implications," ASTM Special Technical Publication 854, ASTM, Philadelphia, 1985.

Chapman, P. M. and E. R. Long, 1983, "The use of bioassays as part of a comprehensive approach to marine pollution assessment," Marine Pollution Bulletin, Vol. 14, No. 3, pp. 81-84.

Cook, P. M., A. R. Carlson, and H. Lee II, 1992, "Chapter 7: Tissue Residue Approach," In: Sediment Classification Methods Compendium, EPA 823-R-006, United States Environmental Protection Agency, Office of Water.

Ekelund, R., A. Granmo, M. Berggren, L. Renberg and C. Wahlberg, 1987, "Influence of suspended solids on bioavailability of hexachlorobenezene and lindane to the deposit-feeding marine bivalve *Abra nitida* Mueller," Bulletin of Environmental Contamination and Toxicology, Vol. 38, No. 3, pp. 500-508.

Hermsen, W., I. Sims, and M. Crane, 1994, "The bioavailability and toxicity to *Mytilus edulis* L. of two organochlorine pesticides adsorbed to suspended solids," Marine Environmental Research, Vol. 38, pp. 61-69.

Johns, D. M. and T. C. Ginn, 1990, Development of a *Neanthes* sediment bioassay for use in Puget Sound, PTI Environmental Services Technical Report. Prepared for U.S. Environmental Protection Agency, Seattle, Washington.

Johns, D. M., T. C. Ginn, and R. Ciammaichella, 1991, *Neanthes* long-term exposure experiment: Further evaluation of the relationship between juvenile growth and reproductive stress, PTI Environmental Services Technical Report. Prepared for U. S. Environmental Protection Agency, Seattle, Washington.

Kiorboe, T., F. Mohlenberg and O. Nohr, 1981, "Effect of suspended bottom material on growth and energetics in *Mytilus edulis*," Marine Biology, Vol. 61, pp. 283-288.

Laughlin, R. B., Jr., W. French, and H. E. Guard, 1986, "Accumulation of bis(tributyltin) oxide by the marine mussel *Mytilus edulis*," Environmental Science and Technology, Vol 20, pp. 884-890.

Lee, C.R., J.W. Simmers, D.L. Brandon, and B.L. Folsom, Jr., 1993, "The importance of biological testing in the assessment of metal contamination and site remediation: a case study," Environmental Toxicology and Risk Assessment: 2nd Volume, ASTM STP 1173, Joseph W. Gorsuch, F. James Dwyer, C.G. Ingersoll, and T.W. La Point, Eds., American Society for Testing and Materials, Philadelphia, 1993.

Lobel, P. B., S. P. Belkhode, S. E. Jackson, and H. P. Longerich, 1991, "Sediment in the intertidal tract: A potentially serious source of error in aquatic biological monitoring programs," Marine Environmental Research, Vol. 31, pp. 163-174.

Long, E. R. and P. M. Chapman, 1985, "A sediment quality triad: Measures of sediment contamination, toxicity and infaunal community composition in Puget Sound," Marine Pollution Bulletin, Vol. 16, No. 10, pp. 405-415.

Long, E. R. and D. D. MacDonald, 1992, "Chapter 14: National status and trends program approach," In: Sediment Classification Methods Compendium, EPA 823-R-006, United States Environmental Protection Agency, Office of Water.

Long, E. R. and L. G. Morgan, 1991, The potential for biological effects of sediment-sorbed contaminants tested in the National Status and Trends Program, NOAA Technical Memorandum NOS OMA 52.

Malins, D. C., B. B. McCain, M. S. Myers, D. W. Brown, M. M. Krahn, W. T. Roubal, M. H. Schiewe, J. T. Landahl, and S.-L. Chan, 1987, "Field and laboratory studies of the etiology of liver neoplasms in marine fish from Puget Sound," Environmental Health Perspectives, Vol. 71, pp. 5-16.

McCain, B. B., D. C. Malins, M. M. Krahn, D. W. Brown, W. D. Gronlund, L. K. Moore, and S-L. Chan, 1990, "Uptake of aromatic and chlorinated hydrocarbons by juvenile Chinook salmon (*Oncorhynchus tshawytscha*) in an urban estuary," Archives of Environmental Contamination and Toxicology, Vol. 19, pp. 10-16.

McCarty, L.S, 1991, "Toxicant Body Residues: Implications for Aquatic Bioassays with Some Organic Chemicals," Aquatic Toxicology and Risk Assessment: Fourteenth Volume, ASTM STP 1124, M.A. Mayes and M.G. Barron, Eds., American Society for Testing and Materials, Philadelphia.

McKim, J. M. and P. K. Schmieder, 1991, "Bioaccumulation: does it reflect toxicity?" In: R. Nagel and R. Loskill (Eds.), Bioaccumulation in Aquatic Systems: Contributions to the Assessment. Proceedings, International Workshop, Berlin. 1990. VCG Publishers, New York. pp. 161-188.

Metcalfe-Smith, J. L., J. C. Merriman, and S. P. Batchelor, 1992, "Relationships between concentrations of metals in sediment and two species of freshwater mussels in the Ottawa River," Water Pollution Research Journal of Canada, Vol. 27, No. 4, pp. 845-869.

Pastorok, R.A., and D.S. Becker, 1990, "Comparative Sensitivity of Sediment Toxicity Bioassays at Three Superfund Sites in Puget Sound," Aquatic Toxicology and Risk Assessment: Thirteenth Volume, ASTM STP 1096, W. G. Landis and W. H. van der Schalie, Eds., American Society for Testing and Materials, Philadelphia, 1990, pp. 123-139.

PTI and Tetra Tech 1988, Elliott Bay Action Program: Analysis of Toxic Problem Areas, Prepared for U.S. Environmental Protection Agency, Region 10.

Puget Sound Dredged Disposal Analysis (PSDDA), 1989, Management Plan Report — Unconfined Open-water Disposal of Dredged Material, Phase II (North and South Puget Sound), U.S. Army Corps of Engineers Seattle District, Washington State Department of Natural Resources, U.S. EPA Region 10, Washington State Department of Ecology.

Robinson, W. E., D. K. Ryan, and G. T. Wallace, 1993, "Gut contents: A significant contaminant of *Mytilus edulis* whole body metal concentrations," Archives of Environmental Contamination and Toxicology, Vol. 25, pp. 415-421.

Roesijadi, G., J. S. Young, A. S. Drum, and J. M. Gurtisen, 1984, "Behavior of trace metals in *Mytilus edulis* during a reciprocal transplant field experiment," Marine Ecological Progress Series, Vol. 18, pp. 155-170.

Salazar, M. H., 1986, "Environmental significance and interpretation of organotin bioassays," In: Proceedings, Oceans 1986 Conference, Washington D. C., 23-25 Sept 1986, Organotin Symposium, Vol. 4, pp. 1240-1245.

Salazar, M. H. and S. M. Salazar, 1991, "Assessing site-specific effects of TBT contamination with mussel growth rates," Marine Environmental Research, Vol. 32, pp. 131-150.

Salazar, M. H. and S. M. Salazar, 1994, "Mussels as bioindicators: effects of tributyltin on survival, bioaccumulation and growth under natural conditions", In: M. A. Champ and P. F. Seligman (Eds.), Tributyltin: Environmental Fate and Effects. Elsevier.

Stein, J. E., T. K. Collier, W. L. Reichert, E. Casillas, T. Hom, and U. Varanasi, 1992, "Bioindicators of contaminant exposure and sublethal effects: studies with benthic fish in Puget Sound, Washington," Environmental Toxicology and Chemistry, Vol. 11, pp. 701-714.

Tetra Tech, 1989, Recommended protocols for measuring metals in Puget Sound water, sediment, and tissue samples, Prepared for U.S. Environmental Protection Agency, Region X, Seattle, Washington. December 1989.

U.S. EPA, 1986, Quality Criteria for Water, U.S. Environmental Protection Agency. EPA/440/5-86-001.

U.S. EPA, 1992, Sediment Classification Methods Compendium, U.S. EPA 823-R-006, United States Environmental Protection Agency, Office of Water.

U.S. EPA/US Army Corps of Engineers, 1990, Draft Ecological Evaluation of Proposed Discharge of Dredged Material into Ocean Waters, U.S. EPA, Office of Marine and Estuarine Protection, EPA-503-8-90/002.

Varanasi, U., E. Casillas, M. R. Arkoosh, T. Hom, D. A. Misitano, D. W. Brown, S-L. Chan, T. K. Collier, B. B. McCain, and J. E. Stein, 1993, Contaminant exposure and associated biological effects in juvenile Chinook salmon (*Oncorhynchus tshawytscha*) from urban and nonurban estuaries of Puget Sound, NOAA Technical Memorandum NMFS-NWFSC-8, U.S. Department of Commerce, National Oceanic and Atmospheric Administration, National Marine Fisheries Service. 112 pp.

Varanasi, U., J. E. Stein, L. L. Johnson, T. K. Collier, E. Casillas, and M. S. Myers, 1992, "Evaluation of bioindicators of contaminant exposure and effects in coastal ecosystems," In: D. H. McKenzie, D. E. Hyatt, and V. J. McDonald, Ecological Indicators, Vol. 1, Proceedings, International Symposium, Fort lauderdale, Florida, October 16-19, 1990.

Waldock, M. J. and J. E. Thain, 1983, "Shell thickening in *Crassostrea gigas*: organotin antifouling or sediment induced?" Marine Pollution Bulletin, Vol. 14, No. 11, pp. 411-415.

Washington State Department of Ecology, 1991, Sediment Management Standards, Chapter 173-204, WAC.

Water Resources Control Board, California Inland Surface Waters Plan, 1991, Water Quality Control Plan for Inland Surface Waters of California, State of California. Water Resources Control Board. 91-13 WQ.

Weston R. F., Inc., 1991, Harbor Island Sampling and Analysis Project Plan, Seattle, Washington.

Weston R. F., Inc., 1993, Remedial Investigation Report Harbor Island, Part 2 - Sediment, Prepared for U.S. Environmental Protection Agency, Region X, Seattle, Washington. Contract No. 68-W9-0046. May 1993.

Widdows, J., Burns, K. A., Menon, N. R., Page, D. S., and Soria, S., 1990, "Measurement of Physiological Energetics (Scope of Growth) and Chemical Contaminants in Mussels (*Arca zebra*) Transplanted Along a Contamination Gradient in Bermuda," Journal of Experimental Marine Biology and Ecology, Vol. 138, pp. 99-117.

Widdows, J. and P. Donkin, 1992, "Mussels and environmental contaminants: bioaccumulation and physiological aspects," In: E. Gosling (Ed.), The Mussel Mytilus: Ecology, Physiology, Genetics and Culture. Elsevier Science Publishers B.V., Amsterdam. pp. 383-424.

Young, D. R., T. C. Heesen, and D. J. McDermott, 1976, "An offshore biomonitoring system for chlorinated hydrocarbons," Marine Pollution Bulletin, Vol. 7, No. 8, pp. 156-160.

Zar, J. H., Biostatistical Analysis, Prentice-Hall, Englewood Cliffs. 620 pp., 1974.

Fate and Effects of Chemicals

Jonathan E. H. Wilson,[1] Patricia A. Cunningham,[2] David W. Evans,[3] and John D. Costlow, Jr.[4]

USING GRASS SHRIMP EMBRYOS TO DETERMINE THE EFFECTS OF SEDIMENT ON THE TOXICITY AND PERSISTENCE OF DIFLUBENZURON IN LABORATORY MICROCOSMS

REFERENCE: Wilson, J.E.H., Cunningham, P.A., Evans, D.W., and Costlow, Jr. J.D., "**Using Grass Shrimp Embryos to Determine the Effects of Sediment on the Toxicity and Persistence of Diflubenzuron in Laboratory Microcosms,**" Environmental Toxicology and Risk Assessment - Third Volume, ASTM STP 1218, Jane S. Hughes, Gregory R. Biddinger, and Eugene Mones, Eds., American Society for Testing and Materials, Philadelphia, 1995.

ABSTRACT: Grass shrimp (*Palaemonetes pugio*) embryos were used to determine the effects of estuarine sediment on the toxicity and persistence of diflubenzuron (DFB) in two laboratory microcosm systems. The experimental microcosms contained DFB in seawater with sediment and DFB in seawater without sediment while the control microcosms contained seawater with sediment and seawater without sediment. Concentrations of DFB in seawater were determined by high performance liquid chromatography (HPLC) analysis of water samples collected from the DFB-treated microcosms. The estimated half-life of DFB in seawater was 18.7d in the microcosm without sediment compared to 5.2d in the system

---

[1]Associate Professor and Director, Marine Science Program, Department of Biology, Jackson State University, Jackson, MS 39217.

[2]Environmental Scientist, Center for Environmental Analysis, Research Triangle Institute, Research Triangle Park, NC 27709.

[3]National Marine Fisheries Service, NOAA Southeast Fisheries Center, Beaufort Laboratory, Beaufort, NC 28516.

[4]Retired Director, Duke University Marine Laboratory, Beaufort, NC 28516.

with sediment. The toxicity of aged DFB from the microcosms (initial nominal concentration = 10 µg/L) was determined by exposing 5-day old embryos of Palaemonetes pugio to 1 L of seawater (withdrawn from the microcosms) for 4d in a static system. Delayed toxicity was monitored at the larval stage. Toxicity end-points studied were: hatchability of the eggs, morphological abnormality of the larvae and larval viability. The results indicate that the presence of organic sediment in the DFB-treated microcosm significantly reduced the efficacy of DFB in seawater. The initial 10 µg/L DFB in the DFB-sediment microcosm aged for 30d before delayed toxicity was reduced to a non-significant level. By day 30, embryos reared in seawater from DFB-sediment microcosm produced larvae with no significant morphological abnormality and larval viability was comparable to the controls. Embryos reared in seawater from DFB-seawater microcosm (devoid of sediment) produced larvae with severe abnormalities and very low viability even after the solution aged for 65d. Hatchability of the eggs was not significantly affected by seawater from either of the DFB-treated microcosms.

KEYWORDS: Diflubenzuron, embryotoxicity, microcosms, aquatic toxicology, hazard assessment, grass shrimp, delayed toxicity, sediment.

Diflubenzuron (DFB), a benzoylphenylurea that is marketed under the tradename Dimilin®, is an insect growth regulator. This pesticide exhibits activity against arthropods by interfering with the molting process. DFB is presently being produced by Duphar, B.V., Amsterdam, Holland. It has been approved by the U.S. Environmental Protection Agency for control of the gypsy moth, boll weevil forest insect pests, foliar feeders on soybeans and cotton leaf perforator (Cunningham, 1986; Fisher and Lenwood, 1992). DFB is being considered for use on citrus crops and in mosquito control (Cunningham, 1986). Because of its toxicity to non-target aquatic invertebrates, direct application of DFB in water or wetlands is prohibited except in California, where it is used for control of mosquito larvae (Fischer and Lenwood, 1992).

The effects of DFB on non-target organisms (both freshwater and estuarine) have been well documented (Cunningham, 1986; Fischer and Lenwood, 1992). Despite the large volume of literature on the toxicity of DFB to marine and estuarine invertebrates, only a few have addressed the question of persistence and degradation of this compound. Using both static and flow through laboratory microcosms containing seawater and estuarine sediment, Pritchard et al.

(1979), studied the degradation of technical grade DFB. In that study only chemical analysis of DFB residue in the water and sediment was performed, no bioassay was conducted. The halflife of DFB in seawater with sediment present was reported as 17d (Pritchard et al., 1979). Christiansen and Costlow (1980) studied the persistence of DFB in a laboratory microcosm using the mud crab larval toxicity test. However, no sediment or organic matter was present. This exclusion of sediment is an unnatural condition and is not representative of the estuarine environment in which crustacean larvae are normally found (Cunningham et al. 1987). The only DFB study reported so far in which both bioassay and chemical residue analysis were performed using a laboratory microcosm with organic sediment present, is that of Cunningham, et al. (1987). It should be pointed out however, that continuous exposure of crustacean larvae to seawater from a DFB sediment microcosm is also unnatural. This is because results from field studies with DFB have shown that residues of this compound decrease rapidly from the water column (90% decline) within 24 h post application (Cunningham and Myers, 1986). Much of this decline was attributed to dilution, degradation and adsorption of DFB to sediment. This, together with the fact that these larvae are planktonic, make it very unlikely that they will be exposed to even sublethal concentrations of DFB in the estuary for more than 2 or 3 d after runoff or overspray.

This application and degradation information led to the development of a 4 day single pulse exposure method for grass shrimp embryos (Wilson, 1985). The embryo-larval stages have been shown to be the most sensitive life stages for fish (Macek and Sleight, 1977; and McKim, 1985) and invertebrates. Therefore tests using these stages should be very sensitive and also be predictive of long-term toxicity. Indeed Wilson (1985) has demonstrated that for DFB, when grass shrimp embryos were exposed to a single pulse sublethal nominal concentration and the effects measured at the larval stage, the calculated maximum acceptable toxicant concentration (MATC) was lower than that obtained in a 32 day subchronic test with the same species and compound in a flow through system (EG & G Bionomics, 1975).

The present study was designed to further test the delayed sublethal bioassay (DSB) described by Wilson (1985). The specific objective of this study was to evaluate the extent to which grass shrimp embryos could be used to determine the effects of sediment on the toxicity and persistence of DFB in laboratory microcosms. The no observable effects concentration (NOEC) obtained by the DSB method is compared with that from the chronic larval exposure method described by Cunningham, et al. (1987) and other tests. Our results indicate that the grass shrimp embryos are useful for determining the effects of sediment on the toxicity and persistence of DFB. Also the DSB method was found to be more sensitive than the chronic larval test with either grass shrimp or the mud crab (Rhithropanopeus harrisii).

MATERIALS AND METHODS

Preparation of Microcosms

The wettable powder - 25% (WP-25%) formulation of diflubenzuron (DFB) was used in this study. This formulation contains 25% active ingredient (i.e. DFB) and was selected for this study because: 1. it is the commercial or field formulation; 2. it has a much higher solubility in water than the technical grade formulation without the need for an organic solvent as carrier; and 3. a comparative toxicity study by Wilson and Costlow (1986) has shown that there is no significant difference in the efficacy of the technical grade and WP-25% formulations to the grass shrimp.

The method described by Christiansen and Costlow (1980) was modified for use in this study; details of which are given in Cunningham et al. (1987). Two sets of microcosm systems were prepared. The experimental microcosms contained DFB in seawater with sediment and DFB in seawater without sediment while the control microcosms contained seawater with sediment and seawater without sediment (Table 1). A stock suspension of 1 g/L active ingredient DFB was prepared by mixing the WP-25% in filtered (50 μM) natural seawater (20ppt) that was pumped from Taylor Creek in Beaufort, North Carolina. The 1 g/L stock suspension was diluted further with filtered seawater to 1 mg/L DFB. An appropriate amount of the 1 mg/L suspension was then added to a 20 L glass carboy to produce a final nominal concentration of 10 μg/L DFB in seawater. A similar procedure was followed in preparing the DFB sediment microcosm except that 2 kg of autoclaved marsh sediment was added to the carboy containing filtered seawater. The sediment was allowed to settle for 24 h before the DFB was introduced into the system. The control microcosms contained only filtered seawater or seawater and 2 kg of autoclaved marsh sediment. All four microcosms were aerated with one airstone each and maintained at room temperature (24 - 26^0 C) under natural light conditions. The microcosms were allowed to age for 10 days prior to the start of embryo toxicity tests because the results of prior studies indicated that percent survival to postlarvae was 0% when grass shrimp embryos were exposed to nominal DFB concentration of 2.5 ppb (Wilson, 1985). HPLC determination of DFB residue in seawater started on day 7.

Determination of DFB residue in seawater

As the microcosms aged, water samples were collected periodically from the DFB microcosms for DFB residue

Table 1--Summary of experimental conditions in the four microcosm systems.

Microcosm Systems	Contents of Carboys		
	Filtered seawater[a]	Autoclaved saltmarsh sediment	Initial DFB seawater concentrations (nominal)
Control Seawater	18 L	0	0
DFB Seawater	18 L	0	10 μg/L
Control Sediment	18 L	2 kg	0
DFB Sediment	18 L	2 kg	10 μg/L

[a]Seawater was filtered to remove all suspended particles larger than 50 μM.

analysis. Duplicate water samples were collected in clean Nalgene polyethylene bottles on days 7, 10, 14, 21, 25, 35, 43, 49 and 65. The water samples were frozen and stored immediately after collection at -20°C until required for analysis. Quantitative determination of DFB in all water samples was performed by high performance liquid chromatography (HPLC).

The procedure followed for concentrating DFB from seawater and preparation for HPLC analysis was that described by Cunningham et al. (1987). The water samples were allowed to thaw completely then vacuum-filtered through a 47-μM glass-fiber filter (Gelman A/E) to remove suspended particles. The filtrate (200 ml) was drawn through a Sep-Pak cartridge by vacuum at a flow rate of 30 ml/min. The cartridge was then washed with 10 ml deionized water followed by elution of DFB with 2 ml HPLC-grade methanol. The eluent was collected in a clean glass vial, sealed with parafilm® and stored for no more than 2 days at 10°C for HPLC analysis.

A Waters HPLC system consisting of a model U6K injector, model 6000A pump, model 440 uv-vis detector, and model M730 data module/recorder, was used for analysis of DFB. The column used was a 10 cm C-18 (Waters) in a Radial Compression Module (RCM); mobile phase: Methanol + water (90 + 10 by volume); flow rate: 1.0 ml/min; wavelength: 254 nm with 0.005 absorbance full scale. The detection limit was 0.75 ng DFB and recovery of 2 μg DFB spikes added to 200 ml seawater was 103 ± 6%.

Sediment Analysis

The organic content and grain size distribution of the estuarine sediment used in the microcosms were analyzed. The method used is discussed in Cunningham et al. (1987). Organic content was determined by loss on ignition of preweighed oven-dried samples in a muffle furnace at 500°C for 12 h. Ten replicate samples were analyzed for organic content. Following organic content analysis, the samples were pooled into three groups for determination of grain size distribution. Five sieves with screen sizes ranging from 45 to 710 μM were used to separate the particles by size after which they were classified using the Wentworth particle size classification system (Folk, 1974).

Embryotoxicity test

Feral ovigerous grass shrimp, *Palaemonetes pugio* collected from Callico Creek in Morehead City, NC were used throughout this study. Once in the laboratory, the shrimp were kept in holding tanks (38 L all-glass aquariums) to acclimate for 24-48 h before sorting according to the stage of embryonic development (based on yolk consumption and eye development) as described by Wilson (1985). All shrimp carrying 5.5 day-old embryos (i.e. stage IV or body segmentation stage), were placed in large Carolina culture bowls (20 cm inside diameter) containing solutions siphoned from the four microcosm systems. Each bowl contained 1 L of solution and 5 shrimp which were randomly introduced following the stratified randomized method outlined in Wilson and Costlow (1987). The animals were maintained in the test solutions for four days (static test) during which time they were fed, ad libitum, newly hatched *Artemia salina* nauplii once a day. The *A. salina* cysts were from the Great Salt Lake region.

Although Wilson and Costlow (1987) successfully (hatchability > 90%) reared excised grass shrimp embryos in seawater from stages III - VII until hatching, simultaneous exposure of females and eggs during this toxicity test was preferred because: a. it represented a more "natural situation" and b. it was quicker and therefore reduced the setup time required for the exposure tests. Following the 4-day exposure, the shrimp were transferred into clean seawater (20 ppt) which was changed daily until the eggs hatched. The shrimp were kept in a culture chamber set at 25°C and a 12-h photoperiod throughout the embryonic and larval development. After the eggs hatched, the larvae were monitored (in clean seawater) for delayed toxic effects as detailed in Wilson et al. (1985). The criteria used to assess toxicity were: hatchability, occurrence and severity of morphological malformations and percent survival of the larvae (larval viability). The duration of larval development was also noted.

Morphological malformations -- Although several morphological abnormalities were observed by us in larvae that hatched from embryos exposed to a single pulse nominal concentration of DFB, only the degree of stuntedness (stunting) and degree of ballooning (swelling) were used in the present study. The degree of stuntedness is the abnormality index that measures the extent to which the larvae from DFB exposed embryos were stunted when compared to larvae from seawater controls. The degree of ballooning is the abnormality index that measures the extent to which the larvae from DFB exposed embryos were swollen when compared to larvae from seawater controls. Photomicrographs of the larvae were taken at selected intervals during the course of the study. The length and width of the telson and standard length of the larvae were measured just after hatching using a microscope fitted with a calibrated eyepiece micrometer (American Optics). Measurements were first recorded in optical divisions and later converted to millimeters (Wilson, 1985). The abnormalities were quantified using the method described by Wilson (1985). This involved morphometric measurements of the larvae ≤ 1 day after hatching from embryos that were exposed to aged seawater and DFB solutions. Using the length and width of telson data, abnormality indices were computed as follows:

1. Degree of stuntedness (DS) -- The equation for this is $DS = (1 - LT_d \div LT_w)100$, where LT_d is the telson length (mm) of larvae from DFB exposed embryos and LT_w is the length (mm) of the telson for larvae from unexposed embryos.

2. Degree of ballooning (DB) -- The equation for this is $DB = (WT_d - WT_w)100$, where WT_d is the telson width of larvae from DFB exposed embryos and WT_w is the width of the telson for larvae from unexposed embryos.

Larval viability -- Larval viability was determined following the procedure outlined in Wilson (1985). Fifty first stage larvae from each ovigerous female were reared 10 per small culture bowl (8 cm inside diameter) containing 50 ml seawater (20 ppt) in a culture cabinet set at 25^{0}C and a 12-h photoperiod. The seawater was changed and the larvae were fed excess of freshly hatched Artemia nauplii daily. This procedure was repeated daily and for larvae hatched from all exposed ovigerous shrimp until the larvae metamorphosed to the post larval stage. Mortality was recorded daily. Each larval rearing experiment was conducted at least two times for each day the solutions were withdrawn from the microcosms.

Statistical analyses -- Statistical analyses were performed on the data using one way analysis of variance (ANOVA) followed by Sums of Squares Simultaneous Test Procedure (SSSTP) to determine significant differences between treatments (Sokal and Rohlf, 1981). Unless otherwise stated, the level of significance was set at $p < 0.05$. The survival data were arcsine transformed before statistical analyses but are reported as percent survival.

RESULTS

DFB Residue Analysis

The results of HPLC analysis of DFB residue in seawater from DFB microcosms during the test period (day 7 - day 65) are shown in Fig. 1. The semi-log transformation of this data is presented as an insert in Fig. 1. The rate of loss of DFB from the seawater in the DFB microcosms was determined from linear regression equations. For the DFB sediment microcosm, the rate of loss is described by the equation: $\ln Y = -0.12X + 2.232$ with $r = 0.954$. Regression analysis was performed only on data from day 7 to day 30. DFB loss in the DFB sediment microcosm was apparently due to both adsorption of DFB to the sediment and to degradation of the compound (Cunningham, et al. 1987). It should be noted that after aging for about 15 days, this microcosm had a rich growth of algae on the walls of the carboy and on the sediment. The estimated halflife for DFB in this system was 5.2d. In the DFB seawater microcosm, the rate of DFB loss was primarily associated with chemical degradation (Cunningham et al. 1987). The regression equation describing this loss is given as: $\ln Y = -0.042X + 2.387$ ($r = 0.974$). All DFB residues from day 7 to day 65 were used in the regression analysis. The estimated half-life for the DFB seawater microcosm was 18.7d.

The regression equations were used to compute the DFB residues for each day the embryonic exposure tests started. This was necessary because seawater for residue analyses were not always collected on the day embryonic exposure tests started. Arrows in Fig. 1 indicate the age of the solutions when no significant difference was observed between controls and DFB sediment exposed test species. It is apparent from this graph (and in later sections of this paper) that the grass shrimp embryo test described as Delayed Sublethal Bioassay (DSB) by Wilson (1985) is much more sensitive to DFB than either the grass shrimp or the mud crab larval bioassays reported by Cunningham et al. (1987).

Sediment analysis

The results of sediment composition analysis show that the estuarine sediment used in this study contained 87% sand

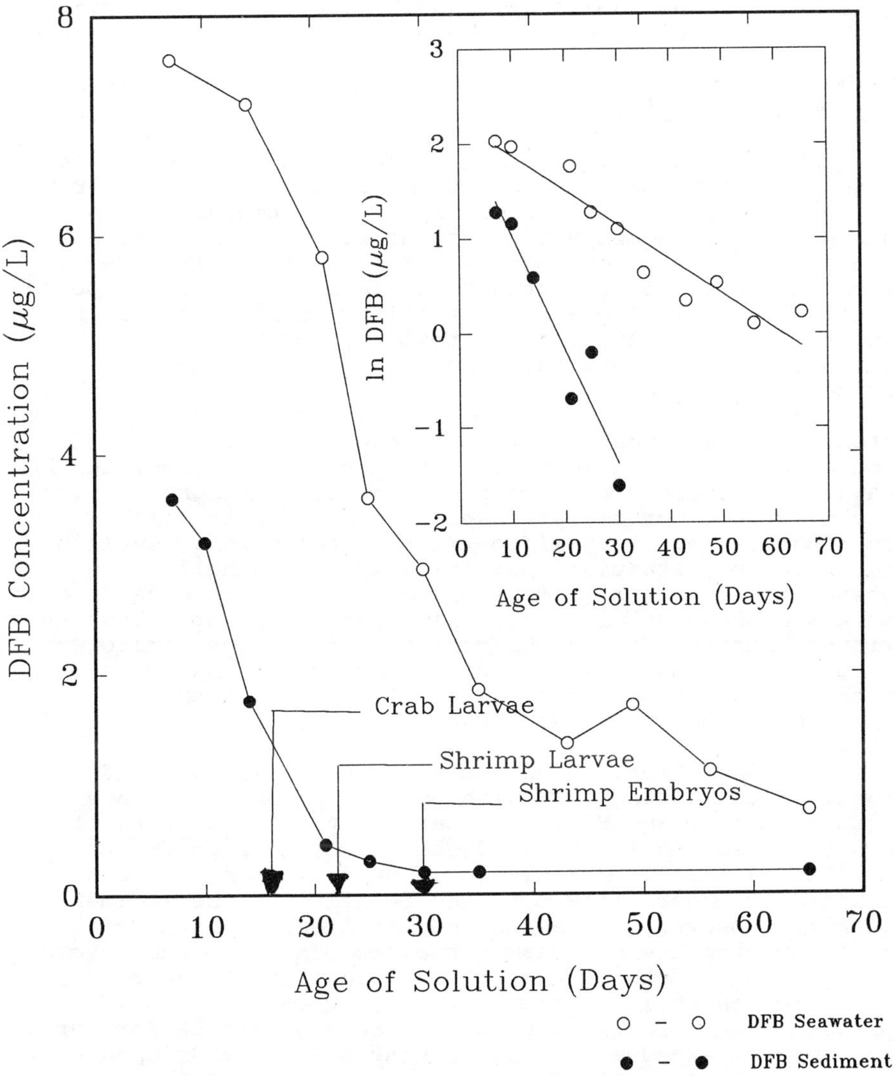

Figure 1 -- Loss of DFB from seawater in the DFB sediment and DFB seawater microcosms as a function of age of solution. Data points are means of 2 or 3 replicates. Insert is the semi-log transformation of the data. Arrows indicate the age of solution when no significant difference in toxicity endpoint (see text) was observed between controls and DFB sediment exposed test species.

(grain size range 90-710 μM) and 7% silt/clay (grain size ≤ 45 μM). The organic content determined by weight loss on ignition was 5.8%.

Embryotoxicity tests

Embryo lethality was not observed in this study when ovigerous shrimp were exposed to solutions from seawater and DFB sediment microcosms, even on day 10. Embryonic development proceeded upto hatching with hatchability ≥ 98% in all the DFB exposed embryos. This is to be expected since Wilson (1985) reported that grass shrimp eggs exposed directly to nominal DFB concentrations as high as 5 μg/L resulted in 100% hatch. This toxicity end-point (hatchability) is apparently not the most sensitive indicator of DFB exposure.

Photomicrographs of 1-day old larvae of P. pugio that hatched from embryos that were exposed for 4 days to a single dose of aging solutions from the DFB sediment and DFB seawater microcosms are shown in Fig. 2. The morphological abnormalities (terata) observed were similar to that described in detail by Wilson (1985); these were: swelling or ballooning, stunting (particularly the cephalic appendages and telson); loss of parts of the appendages e.g. setae and abdominal flexture which includes bent telson and twisted abdomen. As is apparent in Fig. 2, the teratogenic expressions became less severe as the age of the solutions in the DFB microcosms increased. A summary of the morphometric measurements (Mean ± S.D.) made is given in Table 2.

The variations in degree of stuntedness (DS) and degree of ballooning (DB) with age of DFB solutions are given in Fig. 3 and Fig. 4 respectively. The severity of both of these abnormality indices decreased significantly as the DFB sediment microcosm aged. By day 30 there was no significant abnormality observed relative to the sediment control. However, larvae hatched from embryos exposed to solutions from the DFB seawater microcosm exhibited severe malformations (both DS and DB) up to day 65. Even on day 65, there was no indication that either DS or DB would approach a non-significant level. Both DS and DB for larvae from embryos exposed to DFB sediment solutions dropped by 92% and 100% respectively by day 30. For the DFB seawater exposed embryos, the abnormality indices of the larvae decreased by only 21.5% and 48% for DS and DB, respectively, after the microcosm had aged for 65 days.

Larval viability (survival from hatching to the postlarval stage) was not significantly different between the control sediment and the control seawater groups for the duration of the experiment (Fig. 5). Thus larvae hatched from embryos exposed to seawater from microcosm containing sediment were equally viable as those hatched from embryos exposed to seawater only. Viability of larvae from DFB sediment and DFB seawater-exposed embryos varied

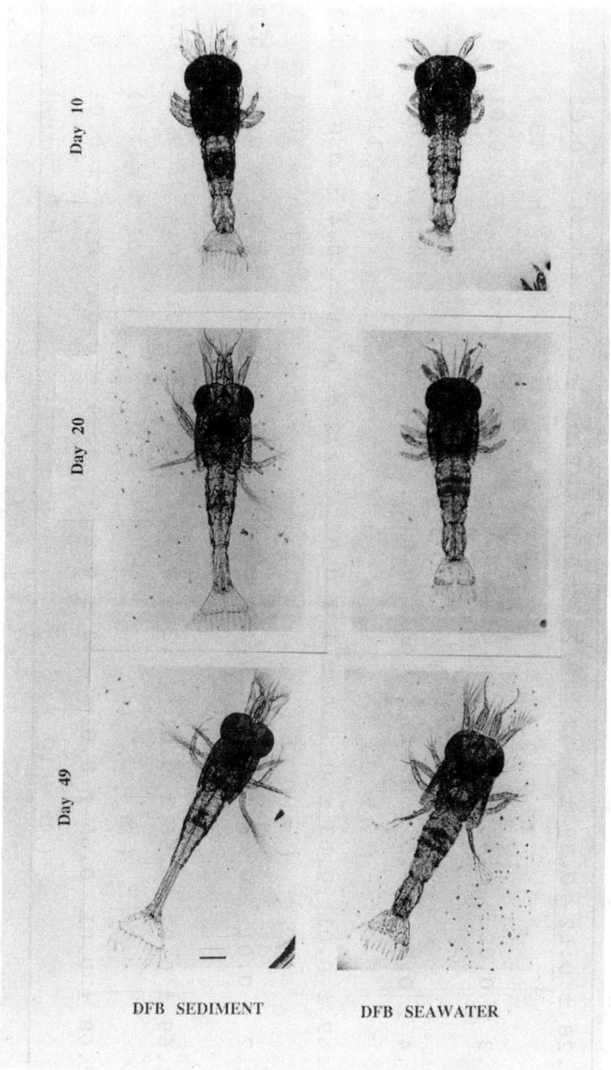

Figure 2 -- Photomicrographs of 1-day old larvae of <u>Palaemonetes pugio</u> hatched from embryos that were treated for 4 days with a single dose of seawater from aging DFB microcosms. Scale bar = 0.3mm.

Table 2--Morphometric measurements (mm) for 24-h old P. pugio larvae hatched from embryos exposed to seawater from DFB microcosm systems. Data represent Mean ± S.D. Figures in parentheses = number of larvae measured.

Age of Solution (Days)	DFB Sediment			DFB Seawater		
	SL[a]	LT[b]	WT[c]	SL	LT	WT
10	2.28 ± 0.02	0.39 ± 0.02 (n = 10)	0.28 ± 0.02	2.03 ± 0.03	0.31 ± 0.02 (n = 15)	0.3 ± 0.0
15	2.3 ± 0.02	0.45 ± 0.01 (n = 11)	0.21 ± 0.01	1.82 ± 0.02	0.37 ± 0.01 (n = 11)	0.29 ± 0.01
20	2.4 ± 0.01	0.5 ± 0.01 (n = 11)	0.2 ± 0.01	2.1 ± 0.02	0.4 ± 0.01 (n = 11)	0.3 ± 0.01
30	2.69 ± 0.01	0.63 ± 0.1 (n = 12)	0.1 ± 0.01	2.2 ± 0.01	0.4 ± 0.0 (n = 10)	0.3 ± 0.01
41	2.7 ± 0.01	0.66 ± 0.01 (n = 10)	0.1 ± 0.01	2.4 ± 0.01	0.43 ± 0.01 (n = 10)	0.25 ± 0.01
49	2.69 ± 0.02	0.66 ± 0.01 (n = 12)	0.1 ± 0.01	2.47 ± 0.01	0.45 ± 0.01 (n = 12)	0.28 ± 0.0
65	2.68 ± 0.01	0.65 ± 0.01 (n = 10)	0.1 ± 0.0	2.39 ± 0.01	0.45 ± 0.01 (n = 10)	0.2 ± 0.01

[a]SL = standard length
[b]LT = length of 6th abdominal segment
[c]WT = Width of 6th abdominal segment

For seawater and sediment controls, days 10 and 65 combined.
SL = 2.7 ± 0.01; LT = 0.7 ± 0.01;
WT = 0.1 ± 0.00; (n = 30)

significantly with age of the solution. In the DFB sediment-exposed group, larval viability exhibited a gradual increase with age of the solution at time of embryonic

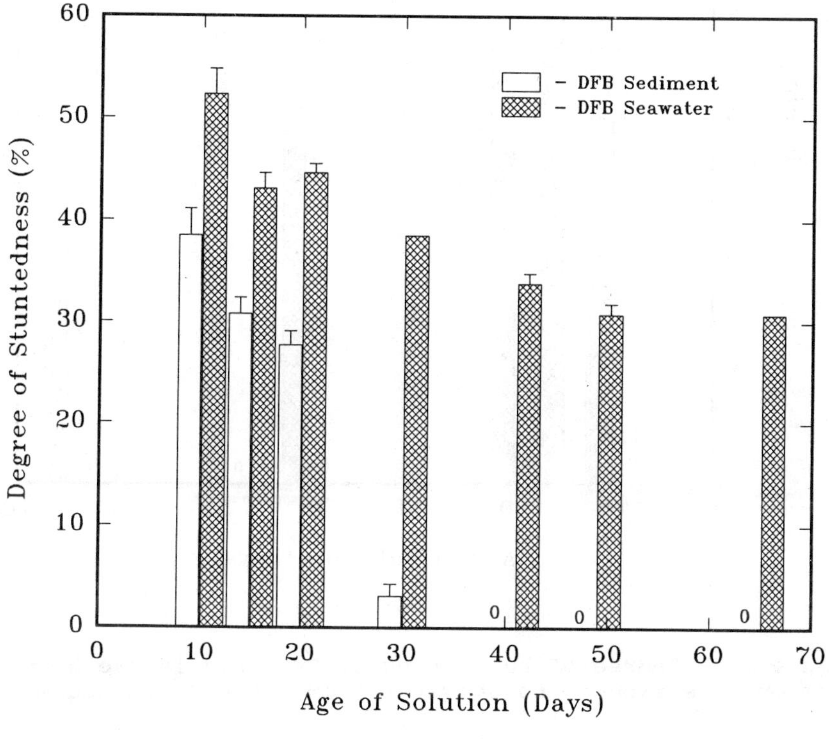

Figure 3 -- Degree of stuntedness of 24-h old larvae hatched from embryos exposed to seawater from the DFB microcosms.

exposure, up to day 30 when the larval viability became comparable to the controls. With the DFB seawater-exposed group however, larval viability increased only to 32% after the solution had aged for 65 days. There is no clear correlation between the age of the microcosm solution to which the embryos were exposed and the duration of larval development (Table 3). However, when the duration of larval development for embryos exposed to DFB seawater is compared with the seawater control (for days 30-65) it is clear that the DFB seawater larvae developed in a significantly ($p < 0.05$, chi square) shorter time. No such difference in developmental time was observed between the DFB sediment and control sediment groups.

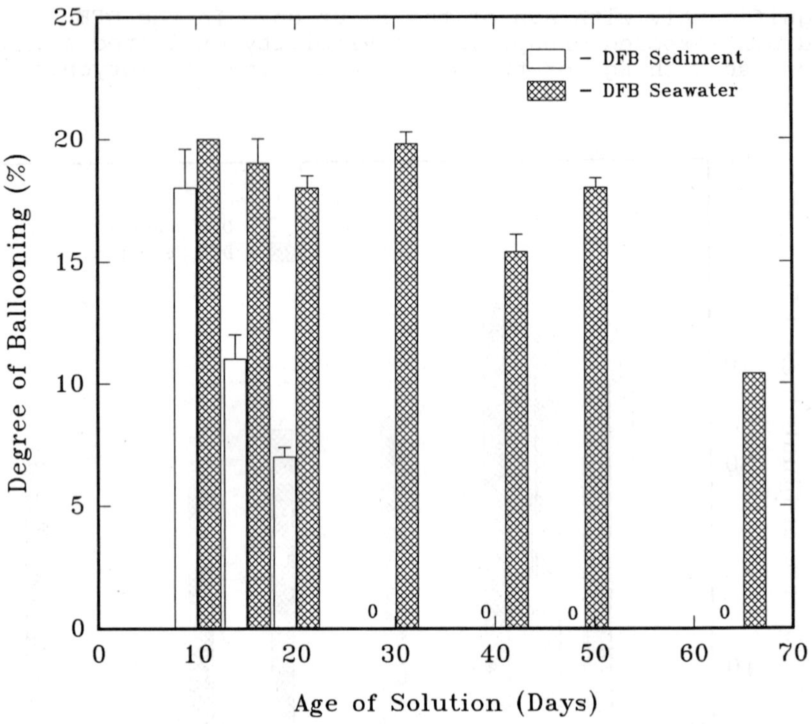

Figure 4 -- Degree of ballooning of 24-h old larvae hatched from embryos exposed to seawater from the DFB microcosms.

The age of the solutions from the DFB sediment microcosm that resulted in no observable effects on the test organisms using different toxicity tests is given in Table 4. This table also compares the calculated NOEC (no observable effect concentrations) for the various tests. With the grass shrimp embryo test, the DFB sediment microcosm aged the longest (30 days) before the solution became non-toxic. The calculated DFB concentration (measured) for 30-day old DFB sediment solution is 0.3 μg/L compared to 0.9 μg/L obtained for the crab and grass shrimp larval bioassays in a similar study by Cunningham et al. (1987).

DISCUSSION

The results of our study clearly indicate that the delayed sublethal bioassay protocol described by Wilson (1985) was used successfully to determine the effects of estuarine sediment on the persistence and toxicity of DFB in laboratory microcosms. Exposing 5-d old grass shrimp embryos for 4 days to single dose of solutions from the DFB microcosms with and without sediment did not have any effect on embryonic development and hatching success (hatchability). However, after hatching, the larvae were

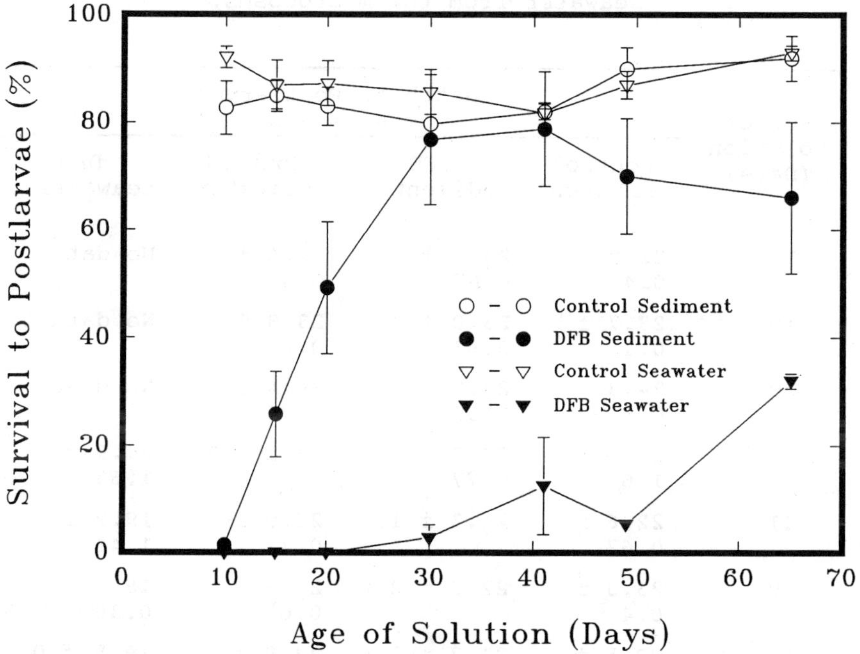

Figure 5 -- Survival to the postlarval stage of P. pugio larvae hatched from embryos exposed to seawater from the microcosm systems. Data plotted are the Mean ± S.D.

malformed and the larval viability was reduced. As the microcosms aged, the severity of the terata in the larvae decreased and larval viability increased. Larvae hatched from embryos exposed to DFB sediment solution exhibited significant decreases in morphological abnormalities up to day 30 when no abnormalities were observed. Similarly, the viability of the larvae increased steadily with the age of the DFB sediment microcosm up to day 30 when the viability of larvae from exposed embryos was similar to that from control embryos. The calculated DFB concentration(from measured values) in the water on day 30 was 0.3 μg/L (Table 4). This concentration is the same as the NOEC determined from various parameters (swimming speeds, phototaxis, larval viability, occurrence and severity of abnormality) measured as delayed toxicity endpoints at the larval stage following embryonic exposure to nominal concentrations of DFB (Wilson, 1985, Wilson et al. 1985, Wilson et al. 1987).

Table 3--Mean (± S.D.) duration of development (days) of P. pugio larvae hatched from embryos exposed to seawater from the microcosms.

Age of Solution (Days)	Hatch to Postlarvae Mean ± S.D.			
	Control Sediment	DFB Sediment	Control Seawater	DFB Seawater
10	22.9 ± 0.4	24.5 ± 0.87	22.6 ± 0.8	No data
15	23.7 ± 0.1	23.0 ± 0.93	23.8 ± 0.2	No data
20	24.3 ± 0.5	23.9 ± 1.53	26.4 ± 0.06	No data
30	23.7 ± 1.6	22.2 ± 0.77	28 ± 0.2	24.9 ± 1.63
41	22.6 ± 0.67	21.3 ± 1.6	25.9 ± 0.4	19.9 ± 1.48
49	23.3 ± 0.4	22.3 ± 2.0	23.9 ± 0.07	18.3 ± 0.35
65	22.5 ± 0.4	21.3 ± 0.0	23.8 ± 0.5	19.5 ± 0

The Delayed Sublethal Bioassay (DSB) appears to be the most sensitive indicator of the effects of DFB on estuarine macrocrustaceans as it degrades in the presence of sediment. Adverse effects were observed up to day 30, compared to day 19 for crabs and day 22 for shrimp larvae determined by Cunningham, et al. (1987) in routine chronic bioassays. Also, while the larvae were chronically exposed to DFB residues throughout development (23-26 days) in Cunningham et al. (1987), the embryos in the present study were exposed only to a single dose of the DFB residue. It should be pointed out that the measured concentration of DFB residues in the glass bowls (measured by HPLC) decreased by 60-70%

Table 4--Comparison of age of solution from DFB sediment microcosm that resulted in no observable effects on the test organisms using different toxicity tests. The calculated NOEC values (from measured DFB concentrations) are also given.

Toxicity Test	Age of Solution (Days)	NOEC (μg/L) Calculated
Crab larvae[c]	19	0.9
Grass shrimp larvae [c]	22	0.7
Grass shrimp embryos:		
1. Larval viability[a]	30	0.3
2. Abnormal indices[b]	30	0.3
Grass shrimp chronic larval exposure[d]	--	0.5
Grass shrimp 35d subchronic[e]	--	0.63

[a]Larval viability = Percent survival of larvae from hatching until the post larval stage (Wilson, 1985)

[b]Abnormality indices = Degree of stunting and degree of swelling/ballooning, see text for details (Wilson, 1985).

[c]Age of solution for crab and grass shrimp larval toxicity tests obtained from data in Cunningham et al. (1987)

[d]Grass shrimp larvae are chronically exposed to DFB in a static renewal system (no microcosm used) from hatching until the postlarval stage (Wilson and Costlow, 1986)

[e]A 35-day subchronic test in a flowthrough system (without microcosm) using grass shrimp larvae (EG & G Bionomics, 1975).

during the 4 day single exposure of the ovigerous grass shrimps. Much of this decline could be attributed to adsorption of DFB to the walls of the glass bowls and uptake by the shrimps. Thus it is reasonable to assume that the test organisms experience the measured DFB concentrations for an even shorter period (less than 2 days). This exposure regime is more closely representative of the natural situation in a salt marsh or estuary following DFB use. For example, Cunningham and Myers (1986) reported that the measured concentration of DFB in the water column at a supratidal saltmarsh lagoon declined from more than 10 µg/L to less than 1.0 µg/L within 24-h post application. Similarly within 2 d of application of DFB to a shallow salt marsh pool, the measured concentration in the water column declined by 74% (Hester et al. 1986).

When larvae of P. pugio were chronically exposed to DFB in a static renewal system (without sediment), a NOEC of 0.3 µg/L (nominal concentration) was obtained (Wilson and Costlow, 1986). Similarly, EG & G Bionomics (1975) reported a NOEC of 0.7 µg/L DFB for a 35-day subchronic toxicity test using P. pugio larvae in a flow through system. These findings support the speculation by Wilson (1985) that delayed sublethal bioassay (DSB) using the frequency and severity of morphological abnormalities in grass shrimp larvae, can be predictive of chronic toxicity of DFB and similar compounds. It is interesting to note that, in the present study, the same NOEC (0.3 µg/L, DFB) was obtained for both larval abnormalities (DS and DB) and larval viability (Table 4). Thus the degree of abnormality (which is determined 1 day after the eggs hatch) can adequately predict the viability of the larvae which takes up to 30 day post hatch to estimate. We therefore conclude that DSB is potentially useful as a short term indicator of chronic toxicity for DFB and similar compounds. The test could be terminated following measurements of the larvae, thereby reducing duration and cost.

ACKNOWLEDGEMENTS

This research was supported in part by a grant from Duphar B.V., The Netherlands to Dr. John D. Costlow, an AFGRAD Fellowship from the African American Institute to J.E.H. Wilson and a DOE Special Programs grant No. DE-FG05-86ER75274 to Jackson State University. The technical assistance of S. Taylor, A. Wilson and V. Repaka is greatfully acknowledged.

REFERENCES

Christiansen, M. E. and Costlow, J. D. Jr., 1980., "Persistence of the Insect Growth Regulator Dimilin® in Brackish Water: A Laboratory Evaluation using Larvae of an Estuarine Crab as Indicator," Helgolander Meeresunters, Vol. 33, pp. 327-332.

Cunningham, P.A., 1986, "A review of toxicity testing and degradation studies used to predict the effects of Diflubenzuron (Dimilin) on estuarine crustaceans," Environ. Pollut. Series A, Vol. 40, pp. 63-86.

Cunningham, P. A., Wilson, J. E. H., Evans, D. W., and Costlow, J. D. Jr., 1987, "Effects of Sediment on the Persistence and Toxicity of Diflubenzuron (Dimilin ®) in Estuarine Waters: A Laboratory Evaluation using Larvae of Two Estuarine Crustaceans," pp. 299-331 In: Pollution Physiology of Estuarine Organisms, W. B. Vernberg, A. Calabrese, F. P. Thurberg and F. J. Vernberg, eds., University of South Carolina Press, Columbia, SC.

Cunningham, P. A. and Myers, L. E., 1986, "Dynamics of diflubenzuron (Dimilin) concentrations in water and sediment of a supratidal salt marsh site following repetitive aerial applications for mosquito control," Environ. Pollut. Series A. 41(1), pp. 63-88.

EG & G Bionomics Marine Research Laboratory, 1975, "The acute and subchronic toxicity of R-20458, Altosid and TH 6040 to the grass shrimp, Palaemonetes pugio," A Final Report to Zoecon Corporation, 36 pp.

Fischer, S. A., and Lenwood, H. W. Jr., 1992, "Environmental Concentrations and Aquatic Toxicity Data on Diflubenzuron (Dimilin)", Critical Reviews in Toxicology, Vol. 22(1), pp. 45-79.

Folk, R. L., 1974, Petrology of sedimentary rocks, Hamphill Publishing Co. pp. 182.

Hester, P. G., Floore, T. G., and Olson, M. A., 1986, "Efficacy of diflubenzuron on three estuarine decapods Callinectes sp., Palamonetes pugio and Uca pugilator." J. Fla. Anti-Mosquito Ass., Vol. 9, pp. 227-232.

Macek, K. J. and Sleight, B. H. III., 1977, "Utility of toxicity tests with embryos and fry of fish in evaluating hazards associated with chronic toxicity of chemicals to fishes." Aquatic Toxicology and Hazard Evaluation. ASTM STP 634. F. L. Mayer and J. L. Hamelink, eds., American Society for Testing and Materials, pp. 137-146.

McKim, J. M. 1985, "Early life stage toxicity tests." In: Fundamentals of Aquatic Toxicology, G. M. Rand and S. R. Paetrocelli, eds., Hemisphere Publishing Corporation, Washington, pp. 58-95.

Pritchard, P. H., Bourquin, A. W., Fredrickson, H. L., and Maziarz, T., 1979, "System design factors affecting environmental fate studies in microcosms." In: Microbial Degradation of Pollutants in Marine Environments, A. W. Bourquin and P. H. Pritchard, eds., U.S. Environmental Protection Agency, Washington, DC. pp. 251-272.

Sokal, R. R., and Rohlf, F. J., 1981, Biometry, 2nd edition. Freeman and Company, Sanfrancisco. pp. 859.

Wilson, J. E. H., and Costlow, J. D., 1987, "Acute toxicity of diflubenzuron (DFB) to various life stages of the grass shrimp, Palaemonetes pugio," Water, Air and Soil Pollution, 33, pp 411-417.

Wilson, J. E. H., 1985, "Sublethal Effects of Diflubenzuron (Dimilin) on the reproduction and photobehavior of the grass shrimp, Palaemonetes pugio Holthuis (Caridea, Palaemonidae). Ph.D. Dissertation, Duke University, 211 pp.

Wilson, J. E. H., Forward, R. B. and Costlow, J. D., 1985, "Effects of embryonic exposure to sublethal concentrations of Dimilin on the photobehaivor of grass shrimp larvae," pp 377-396. In: Marine Pollution and Physiology - Recent Advances, F. J. Vernberg, F. P. Thurberg, A. Calabrese and W. Vernberg, eds., University of South Columbia Press, Columbia, SC.

Wilson, J. E. H. and Costlow, J. D., 1986, "Comparative Toxicity of Two Dimilin Formulations to the Grass Shrimp Palaemonetes pugio," Bull. Environ. Contam. Toxicol., Vol. 36, pp 858-865.

Wilson, J. E. H., Forward, R. B. Jr. and Costlow, J. D., 1987, "Delayed effects of diflubenzuron on the swimming and vertical distribution of Palaemonetes pugio," pp 351-317. In: Pollution Physiology of Estuarine Organisms, W. B. Vernberg, A. Calabrese, F. P. Thurberg and F. J. Vernberg, eds., University of South Columbia Press, Columbia, SC.

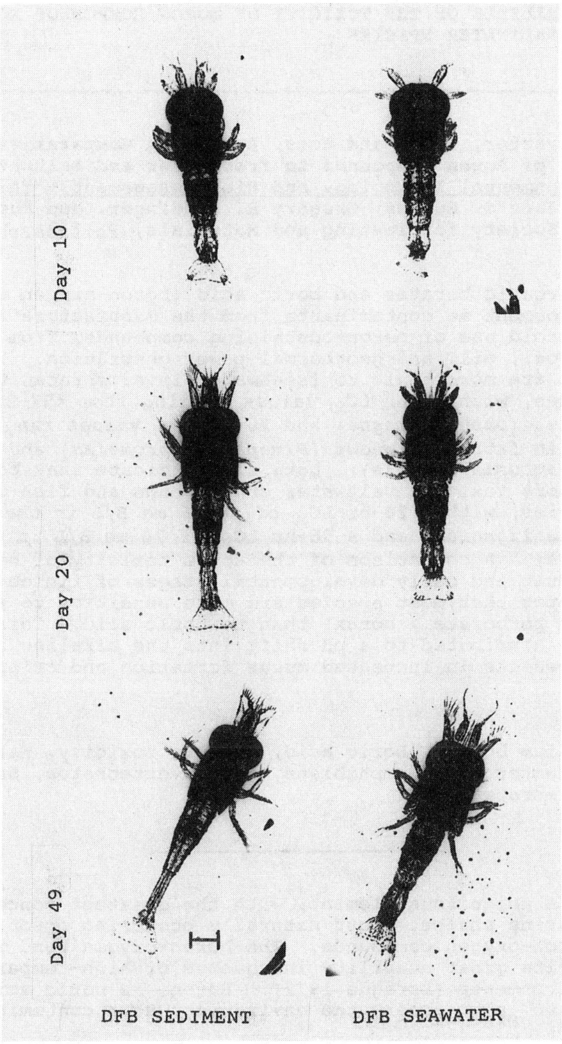

Figure 2 -- Photomicrographs of 1-day old larvae of <u>Palaemonetes pugio</u> hatched from embryos that were treated for 4 days with a single dose of seawater from aging DFB microcosms. Scale bar = 0.3mm.

Patricia S. Hovatter[1] and Robert H. Ross[2]

A COMPARATIVE ANALYSIS OF THE TOXICITY OF BORON COMPOUNDS TO FRESHWATER AND SALTWATER SPECIES

REFERENCE: Hovatter, P. S. and Ross, R. H., "**A Comparative Analysis of the Toxicity of Boron Compounds to Freshwater and Saltwater Species,**" Environmental Toxicology and Risk Assessment - Third Volume, ASTM STP 1218, Jane S. Hughes, Gregory R. Biddinger, and Eugene Mones, Eds., American Society for Testing and Materials, Philadelphia, 1995.

ABSTRACT: Inorganic borates and boric acid (boron-oxygen compounds) enter the environment as contaminants from the manufacture and industrial and household use of boron-containing compounds; from borax mining; and from coal, oil, and geothermal power generation. In general, boron compounds are more toxic to freshwater invertebrates than to freshwater fishes, with 48-hr LC_{50} values ranging from <52-226 mg B/L in the water flea (*Daphnia magna*) and 96-hr LC_{50} values ranging from 332-979 mg B/L in fathead minnows (*Pimephales promelas*) and mosquitofish (*Gambusia affinis*). Data also indicate that boron compounds are more toxic to saltwater crustaceans and fish than to freshwater species, with a 24-hr LC_{50} of 28.35 mg B/L in the saltwater isopod (*Limnoria lignorum*) and a 96-hr LC_{50} of 74 mg B/L in dab (*Limanda limanda*). A comparison of the acute toxicity of boron-oxygen compounds to adult and early developmental stages of fishes and invertebrates indicates that most species are more sensitive to sodium borates (sodium perborate > borax) than to boric acid. This increased toxicity may be attributed to a pH shift into the alkaline range, which in fish results in increased mucus formation and crippling behavior.

KEYWORDS: Sodium borate, Boric acid, Aquatic toxicity, Water quality criteria, Freshwater fish, amphibians, and invertebrates, Saltwater fish and invertebrates

---

Boron is a ubiquitous element, with the greatest concentrations occurring in marine shales. Most naturally occurring boron exists in the form of boron-oxygen compounds. The boron-oxygen bond in these chemicals exhibits great stability in aqueous or high-temperature oxygenated environments (Sprague 1972). Boron, as boric acid and inorganic borates, also enters the environment as a contaminant,

---

[1]Chemical Hazard Evaluation Group, Health and Safety Research Division, Oak Ridge National Laboratory, Oak Ridge, Tennessee 37831-6050.

[2]Chemical Hazard Evaluation Group, Group Leader, Health and Safety Research Division, Oak Ridge National Laboratory, Oak Ridge, Tennessee 37831-6050.

primarily from the manufacture and industrial and household use of boron-containing compounds; the mining and processing of borax (sodium borate); coal, oil and geothermal power generation; and sewage and sludge disposal. Monitoring data from various sources in the U.S. indicate that boron exists in surface waters at concentrations ranging from 0.1-15.0 mg/L in freshwaters and at 4.5 mg/L in the oceans; in groundwater at concentrations up to 100 mg/L; in drinking water at concentrations ranging from 0.4-4.9 mg/L; in soils at concentrations ranging from 10-300 mg/kg; in sewage at concentrations ranging from 0.4-4.05 mg/L; and in coal fly ash at concentrations as high as 1 900 mg/kg.

Boron does not appear to persist in the atmosphere. As a particulate, boron would be removed from the atmosphere by either dry deposition or by wet deposition due to its relatively high water solubility (Gladney et al. 1978). In natural waters, boron does not appear to be chemically or biologically degraded, but exists primarily either as a negatively charged borate ion or as undissociated boric acid, depending on the concentration and pH. A direct relationship exists between the solubility of boric acid and sodium borate and water temperature (Bodek et al. 1988). The adsorption of boron in the sediments of natural aquatic systems could provide a long-term sink as a result of the continual adsorption-desorption processes at the sediment-water interface. In soils, boron persists by either physical or chemical adsorption, with the degree of adsorption directly related to soil type, pH, salinity, organic matter content, iron and aluminum oxide content, and clay content. An equilibrium exists between adsorbed and dissolved boron in soils. Boron is relatively mobile in sand and gravel aquifers, with retardation occurring as a result of adsorption to clay or organic matter.

Human exposure to boron could result from the following sources: the consumption of drinking water from natural or municipal sources that contain boron; the consumption of crops either grown in boron-enriched soils, irrigated with boron-enriched waters, or contaminated with airborne boron particles; the consumption of aquatic organisms inhabiting natural waters high in boron; the dermal application of cosmetic products; or the inhalation and dermal absorption of boron compounds during mining, manufacturing, and industrial processing.

Based on the potential human and environmental exposure of boron compounds, an analysis of the toxicity data for these compounds was undertaken in order to calculate Water Quality Criteria for the protection of human health and aquatic life from exposure to the boron compounds. In the process of reviewing the data, several aquatic toxicity trends were observed between and among species; between life stages within species; and between the boron-oxygen compounds, the form in which most boron occurs in the environment.

TRENDS IN TOXICITY OF BORON-OXYGEN COMPOUNDS TO AQUATIC ORGANISMS

Toxic Responses Among Freshwater Invertebrates, Fish and Algae

Table 1 presents median response concentrations for freshwater fauna exposed to boron compounds. The data were compiled from studies performed following approved ASTM or USEPA toxicity testing procedures. In general, boron compounds are more toxic to freshwater invertebrates than to freshwater fishes, with 48-hour LC_{50} values ranging from <52-226 mg B/L for the water flea (*Daphnia magna*) (Gersich 1984; Lewis and Valentine 1981; Anderson 1946) and 96-hour LC_{50} values ranging from 332-979 mg B/L for fathead minnows (*Pimephales promelas* and mosquitofish (*Gambusia affinis*) (NAPM 1974; Wallen et al.

TABLE 1--Median respones concentrations for freshwater fauna exposed to boron compounds[a]

Organism	Chemical	Test Method[b]	Median Response Concentration (as mg B/L) 24-hour	48-hour	96-hour	Other	Comments	Reference
ARTHROPODA								
Crustacea								
Daphnidae								
Daphnia magna	**boric acid**	**S, N**	...	**133.0**	...	...		**Gersich 1984**
Daphnia magna	**boric acid**	**S, N**	...	**226.0**	...	...		**Lewis and Valentine 1981**
Daphnia magna	borax	S, N	73.0	...	...	...		Bringmann and Kuhn 1977
Daphnia magna	**anhydrous borax**	**S, N**	...	**<52.0**	...	...	**threshold concentration based on immobilization**	**Anderson 1946**
CHORDATA								
Osteichthyes								
Salmonidae								
Onchorhynchus kisutch	sodium metaborate	S, N	...	...	...	113.0	alevins, 283-hour exposure	Thompson et al. 1976
Onchorhynchus mykiss	borax	S, N	602.0	387.0	...	...		Alabaster 1969
Cyprinidae								
Pimephales promelas	**sodium tetraborate, pentahydrate**	**S, N**	...	...	**332.0**	...		**NAPM 1974**
Poeciliidae								
Gambusia affinis	**borax**	**S, N**	**1361.0**	**930.0**	**408.0**	...		**Wallen et al. 1957**
Gambusia affinis	**boric acid**	**S, N**	**3146.0**	**1835.0**	**979.0**	...		**Wallen et al. 1957**

[a] Bolded entries represent values that could be used in the derivation of a freshwater quality criterion.
[b] S = Static test; N = Nominal concentration

1957). Rainbow trout (*Onchorhynchus mykiss*) appear to be more sensitive to boron (as borax) than mosquitofish, based on 24- and 48-hour LC_{50} values (Alabaster 1969; Wallen et al. 1957) (see Table 1). Alabaster (1969) reported a 48-hour LC_{50} value of 387 mg B/L for rainbow trout and Wallen et al. (1957) reported a 48-hour LC_{50} value of 930 mg B/L for mosquitofish. Fathead minnows were slightly more sensitive to sodium borates than mosquitofish, with 96-hour LC_{50} values of 332 mg B/L for fathead minnows (NAPM 1974) and 408 mg B/L for mosquitofish (Wallen et al. 1957).

The only chronic toxicity data available for boron indicates that boric acid affects growth and reproduction of *Daphnia magna* (Gersich 1984; Lewis and Valentine 1981). The mean number of broods per daphnid, mean total young per daphnid, mean brood size per daphnid and mean size were significantly reduced at concentrations of ≥13.6 mg B/L ($\alpha = 0.05$, two-sided Dunnett's test). The maximum acceptable toxicant concentration (MATC) for boric acid lies approximately between 6 and 13 mg B/L in these studies.

Freshwater algae appear to be somewhat more sensitive to boron than freshwater fish. Table 2 presents effective concentrations for freshwater and saltwater algae exposed to boron. NAPM (1974) observed a slight lag in growth in the green alga, *Selenastrum capricornutum* following 7 days exposure to 100 mg B/L. Concentrations >50 mg B/L result in the formation of giant cells in the green alga, *Chlorella pyrenoidosa*, probably as a direct effect on cytokinesis (Maeso et al. 1985). Growth rates are adversely affected in blue-green algal species (*Microcystis aeruginosa* and *Anacystis nidulans*) at concentrations ranging from 73-100 mg B/L, with photosynthetic pigments completely disappearing after 72 hours of exposure (Martinez et al. 1986; Bringmann and Kuhn 1978).

TABLE 2--Effective concentrations for freshwater and saltwater algae exposed to boron compounds

Organism	Effective Concentration (as mg B/L) Effective Concentration	Effect	Reference
FRESHWATER			
Chlorophyta *Chlorella pyrenoidosa*	>50	Formation of giant cells from cytokinesis	Maeso et al. 1985
Selenastrum capricornutum	100	Slight lag in growth	NAPM 1974
Cyanophyta *Anacystis nidulans*	73-100	Growth rate, photosynthetic pigments disappeared after 72 hours	Martinez et al. 1986; Bringmann and Kuhn 1978
Microcystis aeruginosa	73-100	Growth rate, photosynthetic pigments disappeared after 72 hours	Martinez et al. 1986; Bringmann and Kuhn 1978
SALTWATER			
5 of 19 species tested	50	Growth strongly inhibited	Antia and Cheng 1975
12 of 19 species tested	100	Growth strongly inhibited	Antia and Cheng 1975
7 of 19 species tested	100	Lethal	Antia and Cheng 1975

Toxic Responses of Freshwater versus Saltwater Invertebrates, Fish and Algae

Table 3 presents median response concentrations for saltwater fauna exposed to boron compounds. The saltwater fish, *Limanda limanda*, was more sensitive than freshwater fish to boron, as borax, with a 96-hour LC_{50} of 74 mg B/L (Taylor et al. 1985) compared to values ranging from 332-979 mg B/L for freshwater fishes (see Table 1). A comparison of 24-hour LC_{50} values for freshwater and saltwater crustaceans also indicate that the saltwater isopod (*Limnoria lignorum*) (28.35 mg B/L, Robinson and Perkins 1977) was more sensitive to boron, as borax, than the freshwater water flea (73 mg B/L, Bringmann and Kuhn 1977, see Table 1). Thompson et al. (1976) observed an order of magnitude difference in the sensitivities of two life stages of the coho salmon (*Onchorhynchus kisutch*), freshwater alevins and saltwater underyearlings. The 283-hour LC_{50} for the freshwater alevins was 113 mg B/L (see Table 1) and the 283-hour LC_{50} for the saltwater underyearlings was 12.2 mg B/L. Mann (1973) observed that increases in salinity can result in increased toxicity of both boric acid and borax. In the common eel (*Anguilla anguilla*), the 24-hour LC_{100} values were ≥1 748 mg B/L at a salinity of 12.39 ppt and 1 311 mg B/L at a salinity of 25.05 ppt for both compounds.

In tests with nineteen species of marine phytoplankton, Antia and Cheng (1975) found that growth was strongly inhibited in 26% of the species at 50 mg B/L and in 63% of the saltwater species at 100 mg B/L. In addition, 100 mg B/L was lethal to 37% of the species. At 100 mg B/L, NAPM (1974) observed only a slight lag in growth in the freshwater algae, *Selenastrum capricornutum*. Antia and Cheng (1975) concluded that higher boron concentrations would be expected to cause species redistribution, favoring growth of some forms and suppressing growth of others.

Toxic Responses Between Early Developmental and Adult Stages of Freshwater Fish

Table 4 presents median response concentrations for early developmental stages of freshwater fauna exposed to boron-oxygen compounds. In general, early developmental stages of freshwater fish appear to be more sensitive to boron compounds than adult forms. The 24-hour LC_{50} values for rainbow trout embryos ranged from 65-150 mg B/L (Birge and Black 1977); whereas, the 24-hour LC_{50} value for adult rainbow trout was 602 mg B/L (Alabaster 1969) (see Table 1). The 72-hour LC_{50} values for goldfish (*Carassius auratus*) embryos ranged from 68-178 mg B/L and 120-hour LC_{50} values for catfish (*Ictalurus punctatus*) embryos ranged from 102-235 mg B/L (Birge and Black 1977). The 96-hour LC_{50} values for some adult fish species ranged from 332-979 mg B/L (NAPM 1974; Wallen et al. 1957) (see Table 1).

Comparison of Toxicity of Sodium Borates versus Boric Acid in Freshwater and Saltwater Species

The disparity in toxic responses between exposure to sodium borates (predominantly borax) versus boric acid was observed in various invertebrate, fish, and amphibian species. As can be seen in Figure 1, sodium borates are more toxic than boric acid to a variety of aquatic species, with early developmental stages of fish and amphibian species being the most sensitive.

Mann (1973) determined 24-hour LC_{100} values for tubificid worms of 227 mg B/L for borax and 1 748 mg B/L for boric acid. The minimum lethal doses determined by LeClerc (1960) for minnows was 340-374 mg B/L for borax and 3 145-3 321 mg B/L for boric acid. This difference

TABLE 3--Median response concentrations for saltwater fauna exposed to boron compounds[a]

Organism	Chemical	Test Method[b]	Median Response Concentration (as mg B/L) 24-hour	48-hour	96-hour	Other	Comments	Reference
ARTHROPODA								
Crustacea								
Limnoriidae								
Limnoria lignorum	borax	S, N	28.35	...	...	...	after 5-day recovery period	Robinson and Perkins 1977
MOLLUSCA								
Gastropoda								
Onchidiidae								
Onchidoris fusca	borax	S, N	>28.35	...	...	...	after 5-day recovery period	Robinson and Perkins 1977
CHORDATA								
Osteichthyes								
Salmonidae								
Onchorhynchus kisutch	sodium metaborate	S, N	...	...	...	12.2	underyearlings, 283-hour exposure, salinity 28±1°/₀₀	Thompson et al. 1976
Pleuronectidae								
Limanda limanda	**anhydrous borax**	**semi-Static, N**	...	...	**74.0**	...		**Taylor et al. 1985**

[a] Bolded entries represent values that could be used in the derivation of a freshwater quality criterion.
[b] S = Static test; N = Nominal concentration

TABLE 4--Median response concentrations for early developmental stages of fauna exposed to boron compounds

Organism	Chemical	Test Method[a]	Median Response Concentration (as mg B/L) 24-hour	48-hour	96-hour	Other	Comments	Reference
CHORDATA								
Osteichthyes Salmonidae								
Onchorhynchus mykiss	borax	FT, N	65.0	...	...	...	embryo, hardness of 50 ppm $CaCO_3$	Birge and Black 1977
Onchorhynchus mykiss	boric acid	FT, N	150.0	...	...	...	embryo, hardness of 50 ppm $CaCO_3$	Birge and Black 1977
Onchorhynchus mykiss	borax	FT, N	88.0	...	...	...	embryo, hardness of 200 ppm $CaCO_3$	Birge and Black 1977
Onchorhynchus mykiss	boric acid	FT, N	100.0	...	...	...	embryo, hardness of 200 ppm $CaCO_3$	Birge and Black 1977
Onchorhynchus mykiss	borax	FT, N	...	...	...	27.0	alevin, 28-day exposure, hardness of 50 ppm $CaCO_3$	Birge and Black 1977
Onchorhynchus mykiss	boric acid	FT, N	...	...	...	100.0	alevin, 28-day exposure, hardness of 50 ppm $CaCO_3$	Birge and Black 1977
Onchorhynchus mykiss	borax	FT, N	...	...	...	54.0	alevin, 28-day exposure, hardness of 200 ppm $CaCO_3$	Birge and Black 1977
Onchorhynchus mykiss	boric acid	FT, N	...	...	...	79.0	alevin, 28-day exposure, hardness of 200 ppm $CaCO_3$	Birge and Black 1977

[a] FT = Flow-through test; N = Nominal concentration

TABLE 4, continued

Median response concentrations for early developmental stages of fauna exposed to boron compounds

Organism	Chemical	Test Method[a]	Median Response Concentration (as mg B/L) 24-hour	48-hour	96-hour	Other	Comments	Reference
Cyprinidae								
Carassius auratus	borax	FT, N	...	...	...	71.0	embryo, 72-hour exposure, hardness of 50 ppm $CaCO_3$	Birge and Black 1977
Carassius auratus	boric acid	FT, N	...	...	...	178.0	embryo, 72-hour exposure, hardness of 50 ppm $CaCO_3$	Birge and Black 1977
Carassius auratus	borax	FT, N	...	...	...	68.0	embryo, 72-hour exposure, hardness of 200 ppm $CaCO_3$	Birge and Black 1977
Carassius auratus	boric acid	FT, N	...	...	...	170.0	embryo, 72-hour exposure, hardness of 200 ppm $CaCO_3$	Birge and Black 1977
Carassius auratus	borax	FT, N	...	...	...	65.0	fry, 7-day exposure, hardness of 50 ppm $CaCO_3$	Birge and Black 1977
Carassius auratus	boric acid	FT, N	...	...	...	46.0	fry, 7-day exposure, hardness of 50 ppm $CaCO_3$	Birge and Black 1977
Carassius auratus	borax	FT, N	...	...	...	59.0	fry, 7-day exposure, hardness of 200 ppm $CaCO_3$	Birge and Black 1977
Carassius auratus	boric acid	FT, N	...	...	...	75.0	fry, 7-day exposure, hardness of 200 ppm $CaCO_3$	Birge and Black 1977

[a] FT = Flow-through test; N = Nominal concentration

TABLE 4, continued
Median response concentrations for early developmental stages of fauna exposed to boron compounds

Organism	Chemical	Test Method[a]	Median Response Concentration (as mg B/L) 24-hour	48-hour	96-hour	Other	Comments	Reference
Ictaluridae								
Ictalurus punctatus	borax	FT, N	...	...	...	235.0	embryo, 120-hour exposure, hardness of 50 ppm $CaCO_3$	Birge and Black 1977
Ictalurus punctatus	boric acid	FT, N	...	...	...	220.0	embryo, 120-hour exposure, hardness of 50 ppm $CaCO_3$	Birge and Black 1977
Ictalurus punctatus	borax	FT, N	...	...	...	120.0	embryo, 120-hour exposure, hardness of 200 ppm $CaCO_3$	Birge and Black 1977
Ictalurus punctatus	boric acid	FT, N	...	...	...	102.0	embryo, 120-hour exposure, hardness of 200 ppm $CaCO_3$	Birge and Black 1977
Ictalurus punctatus	borax	FT, N	...	...	...	155.0	fry, 9-day exposure, hardness of 50 ppm $CaCO_3$	Birge and Black 1977
Ictalurus punctatus	boric acid	FT, N	...	...	...	155.0	fry, 9-day exposure, hardness of 50 ppm $CaCO_3$	Birge and Black 1977
Ictalurus punctatus	borax	FT, N	...	...	...	71.0	fry, 9-day exposure, hardness of 200 ppm $CaCO_3$	Birge and Black 1977
Ictalurus punctatus	boric acid	FT, N	...	...	...	22.0	fry, 9-day exposure, hardness of 200 ppm $CaCO_3$	Birge and Black 1977

[a] FT = Flow-through test; N = Nominal concentration

TABLE 4, continued
Median response concentrations for early developmental stages of fauna exposed to boron compounds

Organism	Chemical	Test Method[a]	Median Response Concentration (as mg B/L) 24-hour	48-hour	96-hour	Other	Comments	Reference
Amphibia								
Ranidae								
Rana pipiens	borax	FT, N	...	...	...	54.0	embryo, 84-hour exposure, hardness of 50 ppm $CaCO_3$	Birge and Black 1977
Rana pipiens	boric acid	FT, N	...	...	...	157.0	embryo, 84-hour exposure, hardness of 50 ppm $CaCO_3$	Birge and Black 1977
Rana pipiens	borax	FT, N	...	...	...	60.0	embryo, 84-hour exposure, hardness of 200 ppm $CaCO_3$	Birge and Black 1977
Rana pipiens	boric acid	FT, N	...	...	...	145.0	embryo, 84-hour exposure, hardness of 200 ppm $CaCO_3$	Birge and Black 1977
Rana pipiens	borax	FT, N	...	...	...	47.0	fry, 7.5-day exposure, hardness of 50 ppm $CaCO_3$	Birge and Black 1977
Rana pipiens	boric acid	FT, N	...	...	...	130.0	fry, 7.5-day exposure, hardness of 50 ppm $CaCO_3$	Birge and Black 1977
Rana pipiens	borax	FT, N	...	...	...	54.0	fry, 7.5-day exposure, hardness of 200 ppm $CaCO_3$	Birge and Black 1977
Rana pipiens	boric acid	FT, N	...	...	...	135.0	fry, 7.5-day exposure, hardness of 200 ppm $CaCO_3$	Birge and Black 1977

[a] FT = Flow-through test; N = Nominal concentration

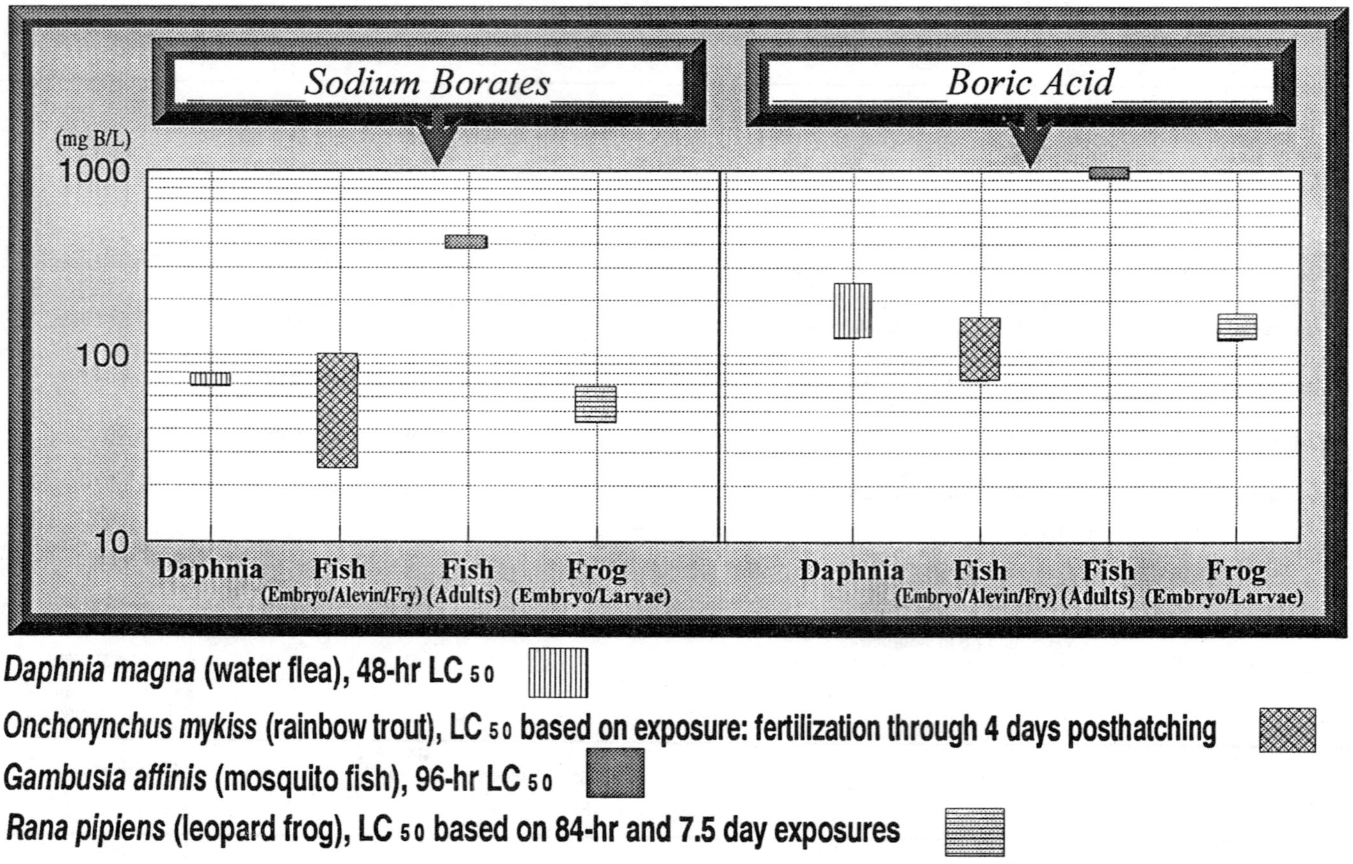

FIG. 1--Toxicity of sodium borates and boric acid to invertebrates, fish, and amphibians.

is also clearly demonstrated using LC_{50} data for a representative invertebrate test species (*Daphnia magna*) and a representative vertebrate test species (*Gambusia affinis*). LC_{50} values (48-hour) for *Daphnia magna* exposed to borax ranged from <52-73 mg B/L (Anderson 1946; Bringmann and Kuhn 1977); whereas, LC_{50} values (48-hour) from exposure to boric acid ranged from 133-226 mg B/L (Gersich 1984; Lewis and Valentine 1981). LC_{50} values (96-hour) for *Gambusia affinis* exposed to sodium borates ranged from 332-408 mg B/L (NAPM 1974; Wallen et al. 1957); whereas the LC_{50} value (96-hour) reported for exposure to boric acid was 979 mg B/L (Wallen et al. 1957). Sodium perborate is even more toxic to both freshwater and saltwater fishes than borax (Mann 1973). The LC_{100} value for both freshwater rainbow trout and guppies was 66.1 mg B/L. The LC_{100} value for the saltwater common eel was 99.2 mg B/L. The authors attributed the increased toxicity of sodium perborate to a pH shift into the alkaline range (up to 9.1), which resulted in increased mucus formation with the fish exhibiting a crippling effect, reacting only slightly when touched or pushed. Perhaps, this ph shift could also explain the differences in toxicity between boric acid and the other sodium borate compounds (borax, anhydrous borax, sodium tetraborate pentahydrate), which occur as alkaline salts.

Early developmental stages of freshwater fish and amphibians exhibited the same increased sensitivity to borax versus boric acid. This difference in toxicity was observed in rainbow trout embryo and alevin, goldfish embryo and fry, and leopard frog (*Rana pipiens*) embryo and larvae (Birge and Black 1977) (see Table 4). In this study, exposure to the fish was initiated subsequent to fertilization (embryo) and continued through four days posthatching (alevin/fry). Frog embryos were exposed to the boron compounds for 3.5 days. Frog larvae were exposed for 7.5 days. LC_{50} values ranged from 27-88 mg B/L and from 59-71 mg B/L for rainbow trout and goldfish, respectively, following borax exposure; and, from 70-150 mg B/L for rainbow trout and from 46-178 mg B/L for goldfish following boric acid exposure. The LC_{50} values for the leopard frog ranged from 47-60 mg B/L for borax and from 130-157 mg B/L for boric acid.

Based on limited data, boron trifluoride appears to be intermediate in toxicity between borax and boric acid, with 24-hour LC_{50} values of 1 361 mg B/L in mosquitofish exposed to borax (Wallen et al. 1957), 2 391 mg B/L in bluegill (*Lepomis macrochirus*) exposed to boron trifluoride (Turnbull et al. 1954), and 3 146 mg B/L in mosquitofish exposed to boric acid (Wallen et al. 1957).

CALCULATION OF WATER QUALITY CRITERIA

According to the methodology proposed by U.S. EPA (Stephan et al. 1985), toxicity data are presently insufficient to calculate water quality criteria for boron for the protection of either freshwater or saltwater aquatic organisms and their uses. The aquatic criteria consist of two values, a Criterion Maximum Concentration (CMC) and a Criterion Continuous Concentration (CCC). The CMC is equal to one-half the Final Acute Value and represents a one-hour average concentration not to be exceeded more than once every three years. The CCC is equal to the lowest of the Final Chronic Value, the Final Plant Value, or the Final Residue Value and represents the four-day average concentration not to be exceeded more than once every three years.

The only acceptable data available for calculating a criterion for saltwater organisms is an acute LC_{50} for one fish species: *Limanda limanda* (family in Phylum Chordata). Aquatic toxicity data are presently unavailable for the following taxonomic categories required for derivation of a criterion: another family in the Phylum Chordata; family in phylum other than Arthropoda or Chordata; family Mysidae or Penaeidae; three other families not in Phylum Chordata; and any other family. Consequently, a water quality criterion for boron for the protection of saltwater aquatic organisms and their uses cannot be established.

Acceptable acute LC_{50} values are available for only three of the eight freshwater taxa required for the derivation of the Final Acute Value: *Daphnia magna* (planktonic crustacean), *Pimephales promelas* (second family in Class Osteichthyes), and *Gambusia affinis* (third family in Phylum Chordata). Data are presently unavailable for the following taxonomic categories: family Salmonidae; benthic crustacean; insect species; family in phylum other than Arthropoda or Chordata; and any phylum not already represented. Consequently, a CMC for boron for the protection of freshwater aquatic organisms cannot be established.

Chronic toxicity data are available for only one (*Daphnia magna*: invertebrate) of the three freshwater families required for derivation of a Final Chronic Value. Chronic data are currently unavailable for a fish species and an acutely sensitive species. Results of acceptable tests with freshwater vascular plants are available. Nobel (1981) determined LC_{50} values for three macrophytes: 5 mg B/L for *Elodea canadensis* and *Myriophyllum alterniflorum*, and 10 mg B/L for *Ranunculus penicillatus*. Therefore, the Final Plant Value for boron would be 5 mg B/L. Information concerning the bioaccumulation of boron by freshwater organisms is contradictory and; therefore, of questionable use in the derivation of a Final Residue Value. A BCF of 0.3 in fathead minnows and green sunfish was reported by Suloway et al. (1983) in tests conducted with coal fly ash extracts. In contrast, Tsui and McCart (1981) determined enrichment ratios (ratio of concentration of metal in tissue to concentration in water) ranging from 51.52-198.41 for five freshwater fish species. The required maximum permissible tissue concentration, either an FDA action level or dietary intake based on a long-term feeding study, is not available at this time. Therefore, a Final Residue Value cannot be determined.

Since a Final Chronic Value and Final Residue Value cannot be calculated, the CCC for boron for the protection of freshwater aquatic organisms cannot be established.

REFERENCES

Alabaster, J. S., 1969, "Survival of Fish in 164 Herbicides, Insecticides, Fungicides, Wetting Agents and Miscellaneous Substances," International Pest Control, Vol. 11, No. 2, pp. 29-35.

Anderson, B. G., 1946, "The Toxicity Thresholds of Various Sodium Salts Determined by the Use of *Daphnia magna*," Sewage Works Journal, Vol. 18, No. 1, pp. 82-87.

Antia, N. J. and Cheng, J. Y., 1975, "Culture Studies on the Effects from Borate Pollution on the Growth of Marine Phytoplankters," Journal of the Fisheries Research Board of Canada, Vol. 32, pp. 2487-2494.

Birge, W. J. and Black, J. A., 1977, "Sensitivity of Vertebrate Embryos to Boron Compounds," EPA-560/1-76-008, Prepared by University of Kentucky, Lexington, KY, under Contract No. 68-01-3920, Office of Toxic Substances, United States Environmental Protection Agency, Washington, DC.

Bodek, I., Ehntholt, E. J., Glazer, A. E., Loreti, C. P., and Lyman, W., 1988, "10. Chemical Classes, 10.9. Boron-containing compounds," Environmental Inorganic Chemistry: Properties, Processes, and Estimation Methods, Pergamon Press, New York.

Bringmann, G. and Kuhn, R., 1977, "The Toxicity of Waterborne Contaminants towards *Daphnia magna*," Z. Wasser Abwasser Forsch., Vol. 10, No. 5, pp. 161-166.

Bringmann, G. and Kuhn, R., 1978, "Testing of Substances for their Toxicity Threshold: Model Organisms *Microcystis* (*Diplocystis*) *aeruginosa* and *Scenedesmus quadricauda*," Mitt. Internat. Verein. Limnol., Vol. 21, pp. 275-284.

Gersich, F. M., 1984, "Evaluation of a Static Renewal Chronic Toxicity Test Method for *Daphnia magna* Straus Using Boric Acid," Environmental Toxicology and Chemistry, Vol. 3, pp. 89-94.

Gladney, E. S., Wangen, L. E., Curtis, D. B., and Jurney, E. T., 1978, "Observations on Boron Release from Coal-fired Power Plants," Environmental Science and Technology, Vol. 12, No. 9, pp. 1084-1085.

Lewis, M. A. and Valentine, L. C., 1981, "Acute and Chronic Toxicities of Boric Acid to *Daphnia magna* Straus," Bulletin of Environmental Contamination and Toxicology, Vol. 27, pp. 309-315.

Maeso, E. S., Fernandez-Valiente, E., Bonilla, I., and Mateo, P., 1985, "Accumulation of Proteins in Giant Cells, Induced by High Boron Concentrations in *Chlorella pyrenoidosa*," Journal of Plant Physiology, Vol. 121, pp. 301-311.

Mann, H., 1973, "Study of the Effect of Boron Compounds on Fish and Other Aquatic Organisms," Arch. Fischerei Wiss., Vol. 24, No. 1-3, pp. 171-175.

Martinez, F., Mateo, P., Bonila, I., and Fernandez-Valiente, E., 1986, "Cellular Changes Due to Boron Toxicity in the Blue-green Alga *Anacystis nidulans*," International Journal of Experimental Botany, Vol. 46, No. 2, pp. 145-152.

NAPM (National Association of Photographic Manufacturers), 1974, Environmental Effect of Photoprocessing Chemicals, Vol. 1., Prepared by NAPM, Inc., in cooperation with Hydroscience, Inc., Harrison, NY. [Also publ. on microfiche as EPA/OTS Doc #40-8469216.]

Nobel, W., 1981, "The Effect of Boron on Submerged Soft-water Macrophytes," Angew. Botany, Vol. 55, pp. 501-514.

Robinson, D. J. S. and Perkins, E. J., 1977, "The Toxicity of Some Wood Pulp Effluent Constituents," Scientific Report No. 74/1, Cumbria Sea Fish. Comm., The Courts, Carlisle, England.

Sprague, R. W., 1972, The Ecological Significance of Boron, United States Borax Research Corporation, Anaheim, California.

Stephan, C. E., Mount, D. I., Hansen, D. J., Gentile, J. H., Chapman, G. A., and Brungs, W. A., 1985, "Guidelines for Deriving Numerical National Water Quality Criteria for the Protection of Aquatic Organisms and Their Uses," Final Report, PB85-227049, United States Environmental Protection Agency Office of Research and Development, Washington, DC.

Suloway, J. J., Roy, W. R., Skelly, T. M., Dickerson, D. R., Schuller, R. M., and Griffin, R.A., 1983, Chemical and Toxicological Properties of Coal Fly Ash, Illinois State Geological Survey, Champaign, Illinois.

Taylor, D., Maddock, B. G., Mance, G., 1985, "The Acute Toxicity of Nine "Gray List" Metals (Arsenic, Boron, Chromium, Copper, Lead, Nickel, Tin, Vanadium and Zinc) to Two Marine Fish Species: Dab (*Limanda limanda*) and Gray Mullet (*Chelon labrosus*)," Aquatic Toxicology, Vol. 7, No. 3, pp. 134-144.

Thompson, J. A. J., Davis, J. C., and Drew, R. E., 1976, "Toxicity, Uptake and Survey Studies of Boron in the Marine Environment," Water Research, Vol. 10, No. 10, pp. 869-875.

Tsui, P. T. P. and McCart, P. J., 1981, "Chlorinated Hydrocarbon Residues and Heavy Metals in Several Fish Species from the Cold Lake Area in Alberta, Canada," International Journal of Environmental and Analytical Chemistry, Vol. 10, pp. 277-285.

Turnbull, H., Demann, J. G., and Weston, R. F., 1954, "Toxicity of Various Refinery Materials to Freshwater Fish," Industrial Engineering and Chemistry, Vol. 46, pp. 324-333.

Wallen, I. E., Greer, W. C., and Lasater, R., 1957, "Toxicity to *Gambusia affinis* of Certain Pure Chemicals in Turbid Waters," Sewage Industrial Wastes, Vol. 29, No. 6, pp. 695-711.

W. James Fleming,[1] M. Stephen Ailstock,[2] and Jeffrey J. Momot[3]

NET PHOTOSYNTHESIS AND RESPIRATION OF SAGO PONDWEED (*POTAMOGETON PECTINATUS*) EXPOSED TO HERBICIDES

REFERENCE: Fleming, W. J., Ailstock, M. S., and Momot, J. J. **"Net Photosynthesis and Respiration of Sago Pondweed (*Potamogeton pectinatus*) Exposed to Herbicides."** Environmental Toxicology and Risk Assessment: Third Volume ASTM STP1218, Jane S. Hughes, Greg R. Biddinger, and Eugene Mones, Eds., American Society for Testing and Materials, Philadelphia, 1995.

ABSTRACT: We determined net photosynthesis and respiration rates for sago pondweed (*Potamogeton pectinatus*) exposed to various concentrations of 11 herbicides widely used in Maryland during the past decade. Net photosynthesis and respiration were determined by measuring changes in the oxygen content of solutions containing dilutions of technical grade herbicides. At 20-22° C and 58 $\mu mol/m^2/sec$ of photosynthetically active radiation (PAR), oxygen production of undosed plants averaged 0.72-2.03 mg/g fresh wt/h. Respiration rates of undosed plants averaged 0.46-0.60 mg O_2/g fresh wt/h. Nominal herbicide concentrations (ng/L) that reduced net photosynthesis by 50 percent (IC_{50}) were: metribuzin, 8; atrazine, 29; cyanazine, 32; linuron, 70; simazine, 164; and paraquat, 240. IC_{50} values for 2,4-D, acifluorfen, glyphosate and metolachlor exceeded the maximum test concentration of 10,000 ng/L. The IC_{50} value for alachlor was estimated to be between 1,000 and 10,000 ng/L. None of the herbicides tested had a significant effect on dark respiration.

KEYWORDS: aquatic plants, sago pondweed, *Potamogeton pectinatus*, herbicides, toxicity testing, photosynthesis, respiration.

---

[1]Leader, North Carolina Cooperative Fish and Wildlife Research Unit, National Biological Survey, N.C. State University, Box 7617, Raleigh, NC 27695-7617, USA.

[2]Associate Professor, Environmental Center, Anne Arundel Community College, 101 College Parkway, Arnold, MD 21012, USA.

[3]Contaminant Specialist, U.S. Fish and Wildlife Service, 3704 Griffin Lane, SE, Suite 102, Olympia, WA 98501-2192, USA

During the past 3 decades, some submersed aquatic vascular plant populations have declined in localized areas throughout the world (Den Hartog and Polderman 1975; Peres and Picard 1975; Stuckey 1978). Notable examples in North America include the Chesapeake Bay (Orth and Moore 1983) and the Upper Mississippi River in the United States and Whitewater Lake in Canada (Dale and Miller 1978). A number of factors have been implicated in the reductions of these plant populations. These include natural population fluctuations, reduced light availability (caused by suspended particulate materials andphytoplankton blooms and epiphytic growth enhanced by eutrification), and toxic substances. Of the toxic substances, the potential influences of herbicides have frequently been questioned.

Most research supports the hypothesis that herbicides have not played a role in the decline of submersed aquatic plant populations (Kemp et al. 1982; 1985). However, it is clear that herbicides contaminate many surface waters (e.g. Richard et al. 1975; Hollister and Walsh 1973; Glotfelty et al. 1984). Glotfelty et al. (1984) concluded that as much as 2 percent of the triazine herbicides may be transported from agricultural fields, golf courses, recreational areas and lawns, and by the unintentional direct drift of herbicides during application. Transport in fogwater has also been reported (Glotfelty et al. 1986). These data suggest that some aquatic plant populations may be unintentionally exposed to herbicides. With exposure comes the potential for adverse effects.

The potential for aquatic plants to be exposed to herbicides would seem to be increased as greater quantities of herbicides are used. Herbicide use has increased during the last decade. For example, herbicide use in Maryland increased from 935,365 kg in 1982 to 3,752,386 kg in 1985 (Table 1; Maryland Dept. of Agriculture 1985, 1986). In 1988, the Maryland Department of Agriculture (1990) reported that 2,913,668 kg of herbicides were applied in the state. This is an amount equivalent to the application of 1.13 kg to every ha of surface area in the state.

To predict and evaluate the potential for herbicides to affect submersed aquatic macrophyte populations, scientists and natural resource managers use information of herbicide solubilities, degradation and adsorption characteristics, transport, toxicity, and plant resistance. In this report, we summarize the results of several short-term experiments in which we determined the toxicities of selected herbicides to sago pondweed *(Potamogeton pectinatus)*, a submersed aquatic macrophyte. To assess toxicity, we determined the relative abilities of herbicides to affect photosynthesis and respiration of clonal lines of sago pondweed.

EXPERIMENTAL METHODS

Plant Stock

Sago pondweed was propagated by micropropagation to produce clonal lines of healthy, intact plants free of epiphytes and other microorganisms (Ailstock et al. 1991). Plants used in these studies were established from native plants collected in Wisconsin and the Chesapeake Bay. The Wisconsin plant line was established from a single plant and was used in all experiments unless otherwise noted. Cultured plants exhibited vigorous growth and vegetative features characteristic of natural populations.

Photosynthesis and Respiration Determinations

To determine apparent (net) photosynthesis, intact plants were placed into 300-mL clear BOD (Winkler) bottles filled with the test solutions (distilled water with or without herbicide added) which had been purged with nitrogen to reduce the dissolved oxygen (DO) content to 2-3 mg/L. $NaHCO_3$ was then added to achieve 10 g $NaHCO_3$/L. Test solutions containing plants were immediately incubated for 3 h in a 20-22° C waterbath under full spectrum fluorescent lighting which produced an average illumination of 58 μmol/m^2/sec of photosynthetically active radiation (PAR). DO concentrations of solutions were measured at the beginning and end of the 3-h test period using an Orion model 97-08-00 air-calibrated oxygen electrode coupled to an Orion model 901 ion analyzer (Cambridge, MA). Net photosynthesis, presented as mg O_2/g fresh weight/h, is the difference in DO content of test solutions, adjusted for changes in DO content of concurrently run control solutions without plants added, divided by the length of incubation.

Apparent (net) respiration was determined in a similar fashion with two exceptions: oxygen was not purged from the test solutions and light was not provided (plants were placed in opaque BOD bottles in a dark room). The decrease in DO concentration during the test period was interpreted as oxygen consumption during respiration.

Test Solutions

The herbicides examined in this study primarily were those that were used in greatest quantities in Maryland during the past decade (Table 1). These herbicides represent a variety of mechanisms of actions (Table 2).

Stock solutions were prepared by dissolving technical grade herbicides at the highest concentrations tested in either distilled water or small amounts of acetone. If acetone was used, the solution of acetone and herbicide was added to distilled water and the acetone evaporated by gently heating the solution for

TABLE 1--Maryland herbicide use estimates for 1982, 1985 and 1988, as published by the Maryland Department of Agriculture (1985, 1986, 1990).

Pesticide Common Name	1988 Kg Active Ingredient Applied	1988 Rank in Maryland	1988 % of Total Herbicides Applied	1985 Kg Active Ingredient Applied	1985 Rank in Maryland	1985 % of Total Herbicides Applied	1982 Kg Active Ingredient Applied	1982 Rank in Maryland	1982 % of Total Herbicides Applied
Metolachlor	821,011	1	28.2	861,834	1	23.0	212,165	2	22.7
Atrazine	530,709	2	18.3	725,755	2	19.4	219,654	1	23.5
Alachlor	258,097	3	8.9	458,133	3	12.2	107,041	3	11.5
Linuron	161,027	4	5.5	194,139	6	5.2	14,359	9	1.5
2, 4-D	156,491	5	5.4	159,439	8	4.3	48,290	6	5.2
Simazine	133,811	6	4.6	211,376	4	5.6	33,811	7	3.6
Paraquat	113,399	7	3.9	132,904	9	3.5	26,983	8	2.9
Cyanazine	102,059	9	3.5	206,976	5	5.5	78,673	5	8.4
Glyphosate	88,451	11	3.0	62,778	11	1.7	8,055	11	0.9
Acifluorfen	13,154	21	0.5	29,030	18	0.8	9,085	10	1.0
Metribuzin	4,082	33	0.1	11,657	23	0.3	1,029	21	0.1
TOTAL USE OF ALL HERBICIDES	2,907,589		100.0	3,744,557		100.0	933,414		100.0

TABLE 2--Names and modes of action for herbicides used in photosynthesis tests with sago pondweed. Information based on data summarized by the Weed Society of America (1989).

Trade Name	Chemical Name	Primary Mechanism of Action
Acifluorfen	Sodium 5-(2-chloro-4-(trifluoromethyl)-phenoxy)-2-nitrobenzoate	Light activated contact herbicide, may inhibit photosynthesis
Alachlor	2-chloro-2',-6' -diethyl-N-(methoxymethyl) acetanilide	Inhibits protein synthesis
Atrazine	2-Chloro-4-ethylamino-6-isopropylamino-s-triazine	Inhibits photosynthesis, may have additional effects
Cyanazine	2-(4-chloro-6-ethylamino-s-triazine-2-ylamino)-2-methylproprionitrile	Inhibits photosynthesis
Glyphosate	N-(phosphonomethyl) glycine	Inhibits the biosynthesis of aromatic amino acids
Linuron	N-(3,4-Dichlorophenyl)-N-methoxy-N-methylurea	Inhibits photosynthesis, strong inhibitor of the Hill reaction
Metolachlor	2-Chloro-N-(2-ethyl-6-methylphenyl)-N-(2-methoxy-1methylethyl)acetamide	General growth inhibitor, disruption of plant cell membranes
Metribuzin	4-Amino-6-(1,1-dimethylethyl)-3-(methylthio)-1,2,4-triazine-5-(4H)-one	Inhibits photosynthesis
Paraquat	1:1-Dimethyl-4,4'-Bipyridinium (cation) dichloride	Free radical formation with light and molecular oxygen
Simazine	2-Chloro-4,6-bis(ethylamino)-s-triazine	Inhibits photosynthesis, may have additional effects
2,4-D	2,4-Dichlorophenoxyacetic acid	Affects respiration, food reserves, and cell division

about 30 minutes in an uncapped flask. The total dissipation of the acetone was not confirmed analytically. Test solutions of lower concentration were prepared by vol/vol dilutions of this stock. All herbicide values reported in this paper are nomimal concentrations that were not confirmed by analytical chemistry. Test solutions were used within 24 hours of stock preparation.

Herbicide Tests

Unless otherwise noted, 5 to 9 plants of a single clonal were used per experimental group. All plants weighed between 0.4 and 1.7 g fresh weight. Plants were exposed to herbicides for the 3 h, during which changes in the DO concentration of the test solution were measured.

Preliminary range finding tests were conducted for all herbicides. Test concentrations were 0, 1,000 or 5,000, and 10,000 ng/L. If photosynthesis was not inhibited by 50 percent or more at 1,000 ng/L, no further tests were conducted.

When an effect on photosynthesis was produced in the range finding tests, definitive toxicity tests were conducted. Test concentrations were derived from a range of concentrations (Table 3) estimated to bracket the concentration that would inhibit net photosynthesis by 50 percent (IC_{50}). This procedure optimized the identification of an IC_{50} value for each herbicide.

Net photosynthesis was measured in plants exposed to each of the herbicides listed in Table 2. Respiration rates were determined for plants exposed to six of these herbicides (acifluorfen, glyphosate, linuron, metolachlor, paraquat, and 2,4-D).

Net photosynthesis and respiration rates of herbicide treatment groups were compared to untreated plants (controls) tested concurrently. In instances where several chemicals were tested simultaneously, several groups of concurrently run controls were pooled into a single, larger control group. For each chemical, the effect of test concentrations were examined by analysis of variance with mean separation by Bonferroni's test of means where alpha = 0.05. Where treatment effects were observed at test concentrations $\leq$ 1,000 ng/L, an IC_{50} value was calculated by linear regression of net photosynthesis (expressed as a percent of undosed plants) versus the log of herbicide concentrations >0 with r^2 for the least-square fit line (Neter et al. 1985). IC_{50} values and confidence intervals (CI) were expressed as antilogs of values obtained.

RESULTS

Net photosynthesis of control plants averaged 0.72-2.03 mg O_2/g fresh plant wt/h. Dry weights averaged 10 to 13 percent of the wet weights. Thus, photosynthesis on a dry weight basis can be approximated by multiplying fresh weight values by 10.

Within the range of concentrations tested, metribuzin was the most phototoxic herbicide, significantly inhibiting photosynthesis at 4 ng/L. All triazine herbicides (atrazine, cyanazine, metribuzin and simazine) significantly inhibited photosynthesis at concentrations of 30 ng/L or less (Table 3). Linuron (a urea compound) and paraquat (a bipyridylium compound) significantly decreased photosynthesis at 125 ng/L. Metolachlor (an acetamide herbicide) inhibited photosynthetic oxygen evolution by 25 percent at 5,000 ng/L and alachlor inhibited photosynthesis by 62 percent at 10,000 ng/L. Acifluorfen, glyphosate and 2,4-D had no inhibitory effect on photosynthesis in sago pondweed at concentrations up to 10,000 ng/L (Table 3).

We were able to determine IC_{50} values for six of the eleven herbicides (Table 4). The ranking of LC_{50} values for these chemicals from most phototoxic to least was: metribuzin> atrazine > cyanazine > linuron > simazine > paraquat. Differences in toxicity between some herbicides were small with overlapping confidence intervals. Overall, triazine herbicides were more phototoxic than other classes of herbicides.

Net respiration rates for sago pondweed averaged 0.46 to 0.60 mg O_2/g fresh plant weight/h. None of the herbicides tested significantly reduced respiration rates over the 3-h test period (Table 5).

DISCUSSION

Herbicide studies with submersed aquatic macrophytes have generally not employed protocols that are standardized among experiments (Fleming et al. 1991; Bowmer 1986). This severely complicates the interpretation and application of results. Bowmer (1986) reported that exposure time, dose, and plant resilience are all critical in determinations of deleterious effects of contaminants on aquatic plants. The application of laboratory data to field situations is further complicated by the complexity and heterogeneity of natural systems and characteristics of individual chemicals and chemical mixtures. However, if standardized testing protocols are used, the relative toxicity of different herbicides can be determined. Comparison of relative toxicities, in combination with other information, such as environmental transport, degradation, and herbicide use, can be used by resource managers to evaluate the potential effect of herbicides on submersed aquatic plants.

TABLE 3--Net photosynthesis (mg O_2/g fresh weight/h) of sago pondweed exposed to herbicides at about 58 µmol/ m^2/sec photosynthetically active radiation and 20-22° C. Means followed by different letters within rows were significantly different ($P \leq 0.05$).

Aciflurofen	Conc. (ng/L)	0	1,000	10,000				
	Mean	0.68(A)	0.88(A)	0.96(A)				
	SD	0.45	0.38	0.69				
	N	6	6	6				
Alachlor	Conc. (ng/L)	0	1,000	10,000				
	Mean	1.73(A)	1.35(B)	0.63(C)				
	SD	0.35	0.22	0.21				
	N	15	9	9				
Atrazine	Conc. (ng/L)	0	30	60	120	240	480	2,000
	Mean	1.34(A)	0.83(B)	0.52(B)	0.11(C)	-0.15(CD)	-0.25(D)	-0.4(D)
	SD	0.24	0.23	0.21	0.09	0.02	0.14	0.07
	N	5	5	5	5	5	5	5
Cyanazine	Conc. (ng/L)	0	5	25	125	625	3,125	
	Mean	2.03(A)	1.93(A)	1.18(B)	0.02(C)	-0.26(C)	-0.39(C)	
	SD	0.37	0.29	0.13	0.14	0.04	0.07	
	N	5	5	5	5	5	5	
Glyphosate	Conc. (ng/L)	0	1,000	10,000				
	Mean	0.87(A)	0.97(A)	1.03(A)				
	SD	0.52	0.37	0.46				
	N	12	6	6				
Linuron	Conc. (ng/L)	0	20	50	125	312	780	1,950
	Mean	0.68(A)	0.64(A)	0.42(AB)	0.14(BC)	-0.01(BC)	-0.12(C)	-0.12(C)
	SD	0.45	0.4	0.23	0.08	0.1	0.05	0.1
	N	6	6	6	6	6	6	6

TABLE 3--(Cont.)

Metolachlor	Conc. (ng/L)	0	5000	10,000				
	Mean	1.46(A)	1.1(B)	0.91(B)				
	SD	0.29	0.18	0.24				
	N	15	9	9				
Metribuzin	Conc. (ng/L)	0	4	12	36	108	324	2,000
	Mean	1.34(A)	0.88(B)	0.76(B)	0.18(C)	-0.18(D)	-0.3(D)	-0.48(D)
	SD	0.24	0.17	0.24	0.07	0.1	0.13	0.06
	N	5	5	5	5	5	5	5
Paraquat	Conc. (ng/L)	0	8	31	125	500	2,000	8,000
	Mean	0.72(A)	0.54(AB)	0.84(A)	0.38(BC)	0.37(BC)	0.08(CD)	-0.09(D)
	SD	0.24	0.16	0.18	0.14	0.11	0.08	0.05
	N	21	6	6	6	6	6	6
Simazine	Conc. (ppm)	0	30	120	480	1,920	2,680	
	Mean	2.03(A)	1.56(B)	0.91(C)	0.03(D)	-0.17(D)	-0.64(E)	
	SD	0.37	0.3	0.15	0.08	0.05	0.11	
	N	5	5	5	5	5	5	
2,4-D	Conc. (ppm)	0	1,000	10,000				
	Mean	0.87(A)	0.89(A)	0.84(A)				
	SD	0.52	0.52	0.53				
	N	12	6	6				

TABLE 4--Relative effects of herbicides on net photosynthesis in sago pondweed. The IC_{50} is the predicted concentration that inhibits photosynthesis by 50%. Photosynthesis was determined by measuring O_2 production by plants over 3 h at 20-22°C and about 58 μmol/m^2/sec of photosynthetically active radiation from full spectrum fluorescent lighting.

Herbicide	Range of Conc. Tested (ng/L)	N	IC_{50}	95% Confidence Interval	Slope	r^2
Acifluorfen	1,000 - 10,000		>10,000			
Alachlor	1,000 - 10,000		1,000<IC_{50}<10,000			
Atrazine	30 - 2,000	30	29	20 - 42	-50.97	0.81
Cyanazine	5 - 3,125	25	32	21 - 48	-42.91	0.88
Glyphosate	1,000 - 10,000		>10,000			
Linuron	20 - 1,950	36	70	43 - 112	-59.14	0.64
Metolachlor	5,000 - 10,000		>10,000			
Metribuzin	4 - 13	30	8	5 - 12	-41.25	0.86
Paraquat	8 - 8,000	36	240	130 - 420	-36.04	0.68
2,4-D	1,000 - 10,000		>10,000			

TABLE 5--Net respiration (mg O_2/g fresh weight/h) of sago pondweed exposed to herbicides. Tests were conducted at 20-22° C and 58 mmol/m^2/sec of photosynthetically active radiation. There were no differences in respiration among test concentrations for each herbicide ($P \leq 0.05$)

Aciflurofen	Conc. (ng/L)	0	1,000	10,000
	Mean	0.52	0.49	0.32
	SD	0.16	0.21	0.04
	N	6	6	6
Glyphosate	Conc. (ng/L)	0	1,000	10,000
	Mean	0.46	0.41	0.44
	SD	0.12	0.19	0.14
	N	6	6	6
Linuron	Conc. (ng/L)	0	780	1,950
	Mean	0.52	0.38	0.53
	SD	0.16	0.09	0.18
	N	6	6	6
Metolachlor	Conc. (ng/L)	0	5000	10,000
	Mean	0.60	0.74	0.64
	SD	0.12	0.13	0.12
	N	15	6	6
Paraquat	Conc. (ng/L)	0	1,000	10,000
	Mean	0.59	0.61	0.75
	SD	0.48	0.13	0.21
	N	15	6	6
2,4-D	Conc. (ng/L)	0	1,000	10,000
	Mean	0.46	0.41	0.36
	SD	0.12	0.14	0.13
	N	6	6	6

Oxygen evolution is a commonly employed method to determine phytoplankton productivity and aquatic macrophyte responses to toxic compounds (Dawes 1981; Correll and Wu 1982; Cunningham et al. 1984; Kemp et al. 1982, 1985; Jones and Winchell 1984, Jones et al. 1986). In part, this is because of the ease and simplicity of the assay. Assessment of photosynthesis by use of carbon assimilation techniques have received widespread acceptance and can be used as an alternative method for measuring photosynthesis (American Public Health Association 1989). Regardless of the technique, examination of photosynthesis is especially useful for assessing the relative toxicities of herbicides that inhibit the Hill reaction. Kemp et al. (1985) reported that plant biomass production generally paralleled that of plant photosynthetic activity. Likewise, we have found that biomass production of sago pondweed begins to decrease significantly at triazine herbicide concentrations that inhibit photosynthesis by 30 to 50 percent (unpublished data). In contrast, the toxicity of compounds that have alternative modes of action (e.g., affecting growth or morphological development) may be difficult to assess by monitoring photosynthesis. Further, it is also difficult to detect the actual toxicity of compounds whose primary mode of action may be photosynthetic inhibition but which also show adverse effects on secondary plant metabolism.

Although the precise mechanisms of action for many herbicides are not completely known, most herbicides are developed to operate primarily on metabolic pathways unique to plants. This specificity minimizes toxic effects on animals. Of the 11 herbicides evaluated in this study, five (the triazines and linuron) inhibit photosynthesis as the primary mechanism of action (Table 2; Weed Society of America 1989). All five of these inhibited photosynthesis at concentrations less than 125 ng/L. Paraquat, like the triazines, inhibited photosynthesis. However, unlike the triazines, which exert a direct effect on photosynthetic pathways, paraquat's mechanism of action is more general. Other herbicide groups that we tested did not inhibit photosynthesis, which is as expected based on known modes of action (Table 2). 2,4-D has been reported to affect respiration in plants (Table 2), something that we did not observe in our study.

The estimated IC_{50} values that we generated compare favorably with those reported for a variety of test conditions and aquatic plant species. Reported IC_{50} values for atrazine range from 55 to 117 ng/L, compared to our estimate of 29 ng/L (Jones and Winchell 1984; Kemp et al. 1982; Kemp et al. 1986). Kemp et al. (1985) reported IC_{50} values for linuron of 45 and 80 ng/L wherease we report an IC_{50} value of 70. Differences in sensitivities between species may account for some of the variability in reported IC_{50} values. The data of Kemp et al. (1985) suggest that*Myriophyllum spicatum,* is about half as sensitive to both linuron and atrazine as is *Potamogeton perfoliatus* .

The herbicides evaluated in this study are widely used in Maryland (Table 1). The 11 herbicides tested have consistently accounted for 81 percent of the quantity of herbicides applied. In most studies designed to evaluate whether herbicides may be implicated in the loss of submersed aquatic vegetation, the herbicides considered are those used in the greatest quantity in a particular watershed. This approach is not without merit, but also bears a certain risk. For example, metribuzin was ranked 33rd in the quantity of active ingredients applied in Maryland in 1988 at 4091 kg. Yet, it exhibited the highest phytotoxicity (IC_{50} = 8 ng/L). In contrast, metolachlor was ranked number one, with 822,727 kg applied during 1988, and has a IC_{50} value that is greater than

10,000 ng/L. In comparing the two herbicides, about 200 times more metolachlor was applied in Maryland than metribuzin, but when the IC_{50} values of the two herbicides are compared, metribuzin is 1250 times more phototoxic.

Assessing the potential effects of herbicides on aquatic systems is extremely difficult. One evaluation approach is to simplify the system by isolating individual components and examining them separately. This can provide a better understanding of individual species' responses to contaminants. If such tests are conducted under standardized conditions, responses of individuals or groups of organisms can be compared. This information, coupled with data on chemical properties, environmental persistence, application rates, and total amount used per geographic area, etc., can be used to prioritize environmental concerns. Use of any one of these factors, by itself, is not likely to be sufficient for evaluating potential environmental consequences. Toxicity values, such as IC_{50} data, obtained from standardized testing protocols, should not be directly extrapolated to field situations. The complexity of natural system components and their interactions may mediate plant responses to specific herbicides.

Our review of the literature indicates that there have been no successful attempts to standardize protocols for phytotoxicity tests with submersed aquatic plants. We recommend that the scientific community proceed with the development and adoption of such protocols. These tests should emphasize biologically significant endpoints or bioindicators of those endpoints such as photosynthesis, growth, or seed germination.

ACKNOWLEDGMENTS: This work was conducted while Fleming and Momot were employed at the U.S. Fish and Wildlife Service's Patuxent Wildlife Research Center, Laurel, MD which supported this work. Dr. Stratford Kay and Dr. Sally Hornor provided helpful reviews of this manuscript. We appreciate the help of Mrs. Dorothy Wright for typing and proofreading the manuscript.

REFERENCES

Ailstock, M. S., Fleming, W. J., and Cooke, T. J., 1991, "The characterization of axenic culture systems suitable for plant propagation and experimental studies of the submersed aquatic angiosperm *Potamogeton pectinatus* (sago pondweed)," Estuaries, Vol. 14, pp. 57-64.

American Public Health Association, 1989, Standard Methods for the Examination of Wastewater, 17th Edition, American Public Health Association, Washington, D.C.

Bowmer, K. H., 1986, "Rapid biological assay and limitations in macrophyte ecotoxicology: A review," Australian Journal of Marine Freshwater Research, Vol. 37, pp. 297-308.

Correll, D. L. and Wu, T. L., 1982, "Atrazine toxicity to submersed vascular plants in simulated estuarine microcosms," Aquatic Botany, Vol. 14, pp. 151-158.

Cunningham, J. J., Kemp, W. M., Lewis, M. R., and Stevenson, J. C., 1984, "Temporal responses of the macrophytes," Estuaries, Vol. 7, pp. 519-530.

Dale, H. M. and Miller, G. E., 1978, "Changes in aquatic macrophyte flora of Whitewater Lake near Sudbury, Ontario from 1947-1977," Canadian Field Naturalist, Vol. 92, pp. 264-270.

Dawes, C. J. 1981. "Marine Botany," John Wiley and Sons, Inc., NY.

Den Hartog, C. and Polderman, P. J. G., 1975, "Changes in seagrass populations of the Dutch Waddenzee," Aquatic Botany, Vol. 1, pp. 14-17.

Fleming, W. J., Ailstock, M. S., and Momot, J. J., 1991, "Response of sago pondweed, a submersed aquatic macrophyte, to herbicides in three laboratory culture systems," Pages 267-275, In J. W. Gorsuch, W. R. Lower, W. Wang, and M. A. Lewis (eds.), Plants for Toxicity Assessment: Second Volume, ASTM STP 1115, American Society for Testing and Materials, Philadelphia, PA.

Glotfelty, D. E., Taylor, A. W., Isensee, A. R., Jersey, J., and Glenn, S., 1984, "Atrazine and simazine movement to Wye River estuary," Journal of Environmental Quality, Vol. 13, pp. 115-121.

Glotfelty, D. E., Seiber, J. N., and Liljedahl, L. A., 1986, "Pesticides and other organics in fog," Pages 168-175 in Proceedings of the Symposium of the Measurement of Toxic Air Pollutants, U. S. Environmental Protection Agency/Air Pollution Control Association.

Hollister, T. A. and Walsh, G. E., 1973, "Differential responses of marine phytoplankton to herbicides: Oxygen evolution," Bulletin of Environmental Contamination and Toxicology, Vol. 9, pp. 291-295.

Jones, T. W., Kemp, W. M., Estes, P. S., and Stevenson, J. C., 1986, "Atrazine uptake, photosynthetic inhibition, and short-term recovery for the submersed vascular plant, *Potamogeton perfoliatus* L.," Archives of Environmental Contamination and Toxicology, Vol. 15, pp. 277-283.

Jones, T. W. and Winchell, L., 1984, "Uptake and photosynthetic inhibition by atrazine and its degradation products on four species of submerged aquatic plants," Journal of Environmental Quality, Vol. 13, pp. 243-247.

Kemp, W. M., Boynton, W. R., Cunningham, J. J., Stevenson, J. C., Jones, T. W., and Means, J. C., 1985, "Effects of atrazine and linuron on photosynthesis and growth of the macrophytes, *Potamogeton perfoliatus* L. and *Myriophyllum spicatum* L. in an estuarine environment," Marine Environmental Research, Vol. 16, pp. 255-280.

Kemp, W. M., Means, J. C., Jones, T. W., and Stevenson, J.C., 1982, "Herbicides in Chesapeake Bay and their effects on submerged aquatic vegetation," Pages 503-567 in Chesapeake Bay Program Technical Studies: a synthesis, U.S. Environmental Protection Agency, Washington, D.C.

Maryland Department of Agriculture, 1990, Maryland pesticide statistics for 1988, 50 Harry S. Truman Parkway, Annapolis, MD.

Maryland Department of Agriculture, 1986, Maryland pesticide statistics for 1985, 50 Harry S. Truman Parkway, Annapolis, MD.

Maryland Department of Agriculture, 1985, Maryland pesticide statistics for 1982, 50 Harry S. Truman Parkway, Annapolis, MD.

Neter, J., Wasserman, W., and Kutner, M. H., 1985, Applied linear statistical models, 2nd Edition, Irwin, Homewood, IL.

Orth, R. J. and Moore, K. A., 1983, "Chesapeake Bay: An unprecedented decline in submerged aquatic vegetation," Science, Vol. 222, pp. 51-53.

Peres, J. M. and Picard, J., 1975, "Causes de la rarefaction et de la disparition de herbiers de *Posidonia oceanica* sur les cotes Francaises de la Mediterranean," Aquatic Botany, Vol. 1, pp. 133-139.

Richard, J. J., Junk, G. A., Avery, M. J., Nehring, W. L., Fritz, J. S., and Svec, H. J., 1975, "Analysis of various Iowa waters for selected pesticides: Atrazine, DDE, and dieldrin - 1974," Pesticide Monitoring Journal, Vol. 9, pp. 117-123.

Stuckey, R. L., 1978, "The decline of lake plants," Natural History, Vol. 87, pp. 6-69.

Weed Society of America, 1989, "Herbicide Handbook," 6th edition, Weed Society of America, Champaign, IL.

Karl F. Moschner[1] and Anthony Cece[2]

DEVELOPMENT OF A GENERAL QSAR FOR PREDICTING OCTANOL-WATER PARTITION COEFFICIENTS AND ITS APPLICATION TO SURFACTANTS

REFERENCE: Moschner, K. F., and Cece, A., **"Development of a General QSAR for Predicting Octanol-Water Partition Coefficients and its Application to Surfactants,"** Environmental Toxicology and Risk Assessment - Third Volume, ASTM STP 1218, Jane S. Hughes, Gregory R. Biddinger, and Eugene Mones, Eds., American Society for Testing and Materials, Philadelphia, 1995.

ABSTRACT: Octanol-water partition coefficients (log P) are key parameters for estimating toxicological and pharmacological properties of organic compounds. The significance of log P and the difficulty in experimentally measuring log P has led to the development of several Log P estimation techniques. Methods based on group contributions, such as CLOGP and CHEMICALC2, are widely used. While very fast, their reliability is highly dependent on the availability of experimental log P values for representative compounds. Quantitative structure-activity relationships (QSARs) have also been used to estimate log P and address the limitations of other methods. While QSARs also depend on a set of compounds with reliable log P values, use of general structural descriptors rather than specific fragments promises to provide more broadly applicable predictive models. A number of QSARs have been reported for predicting log P values, however these are limited to specific compound classes. This paper presents an approach to develop a broadly applicable QSAR for log P based on general molecular structural parameters. Examples are given for a variety of compound classes including those containing mixed functional groups. Emphasis is placed on compounds relevant to the household and personal products industries. Limitations and pitfalls in developing reliable predictive correlations are identified and strategies for extending the model are discussed.

KEYWORDS: Hydrophobicity, Octanol-Water Partition Coefficients, Log P, Surfactants, QSAR

[1]Senior Group Leader, Unilever Research U.S., 45 River Road, Edgewater, NJ 07020, USA

[2]Principal Research Chemist, Unilever Research U.S., 45 River Road, Edgewater, NJ 07020, USA

INTRODUCTION

The hydrophobicity of a chemical compound as measured by its octanol-water partition coefficient or its logarithm, log P, has been demonstrated to be a key predictor of its pharmaceutical and envirotoxicological properties (Leo et. al. 1971; Leo 1983). The importance of log P combined with the difficulty in obtaining reliable experimental measurements has prompted extensive research aimed at developing accurate predictive models using two general approaches, group contribution methods (GCM) and quantitative structure-activity relationships (QSARs). Efforts to develop accurate models for log P have focused almost exclusively on compounds for the pharmaceutical and agrichemical industries or bulk chemical feedstocks. Little has been reported on developing reliable log P predictions for common household chemicals such as surfactants.

Group contribution methods have found the broadest use for predicting log P owing to the ready availability of computer programs and the speed and accuracy of the estimations. The most notable computerized implementations of this method for predicting log P are CLOGP (Daylight Chemical Information Systems, Inc. 1992), CHEMICALC (Suzuki and Kudo 1990) and CASE (Klopman and Wang 1991). These programs are expert systems which apply predetermined correction terms to key functional groups and general structural features identified from an analysis of specific chemical structure line notations. Additional correction terms may also be applied (Leo 1983, 1989) for electronic interactions, hydrogen bonding, flexibility, branching, aromatic substitution patterns, and compound class types such as aliphatic hydrocarbon and amino acids. Since GCM require only connectivity information, less than a second is typically required to predict log P with average errors <±0.5 units for well characterized compounds. Larger errors may be introduced by ambiguities in identifying fragments and approximations applied to special cases. GCM may also fail completely on encountering urecognized substrutures. Some of these shortcomings may be addressed by deriving contribution coefficients for new groups from correlations against extensive experimental measurements (Lipinski et. al. 1991). But poor transferability of group contribution values may also give rise to large errors which may be difficult to detect as in the prediction of log P of polyethoxylated nonionic surfactants (Roberts 1991).

Quantitative structure-activity relationships, like GCM, require a large, diverse set of well characterized compounds from which a linear correlation may be derived between the known log P and a series of molecular descriptors. However, in addition to group counts and class indices, QSARs usually also consider descriptors computed using molecular modeling techniques. Good correlations have been reported between log P and graph theoretical descriptors (Niemi et. al. 1992; Malihot and Peters 1988), molecular volume and molecular surface area (de Bruijn and Hermens 1990; Fumasaki et. al. 1985; Camilleri et. al. 1988) and, more recently, descriptors derived from semiempirical molecular orbital calculations (Nakagawa et. al. 1992; Sasaki et. al. 1992; Bodor and Huang 1992, 1991, 1989; Famini et. al. 1992). Graph theoretical descriptors have been useful in a variety of chemiophysical property estimates (Mihalic and Trinajstic 1992) since, like GCM, they depend solely on connectivity and therefore may be computed very quickly. Other geometry dependent QSAR descriptors, particularly those derived from quantum mechanical calculations, require significantly greater computational resources and have thus been applied to a more limited range of compounds.

This study evaluates the use of molecular modeling methods to develop a general predictive model for log P by coupling the demonstrated benefits of both GCM and QSAR methods through exploitation of the capabilities of readily available molecular modeling software. Particular attention is paid to identifying more broadly applicable models which reliably predict the log P of surfactants, an important class of compounds poorly predicted by current methods.

COMPUTATIONAL METHODS

The Sybyl software suite (Tripos Associates, Inc.) was used for all molecular modeling and QSAR computations. One hundred ninety-three compounds (Appendix 1), including twenty-seven surfactants (166-193), were selected from the open literature as a training set. Starting conformations were retrieved from the standard fragment library or drawn using the sketch facility. Amino acids, including 3-hydroxypiccolinic acid (127), were represented as zwitterions and salts as ion pairs. For each compound, atom-type assignments were verified by visual inspection; atom-centered charges were assigned using the Gasteiger-Hückel method; and, then, a single low-energy conformation was identified by repeated dynamic annealing. Subsequently, QSAR tables were prepared with fifty molecular descriptors computed using built-in functions, when available, custom macros for atom-type counts and summed charges, and manual assignments for compound class indices and reported log P values. Partial least-squares (PLS) with cross-validation was then used to identify the best linear correlation between the tabulated molecular descriptors and the reported log P values. For comparison, CLOGP3 values were computed using PCmodels (Daylight Chemical Information Systems, Inc.) accessed through the Sybyl interface. All computations were performed on a Silicon Graphics 4D/35 or Crimson UNIX workstation.

RESULTS AND DISCUSSION

A good correlation (Fig. 1) was obtained for 191 of 193 compounds in the training set. The derived model (Eq. 1) uses only twelve general terms (Table 1). Two outliers, 1-methoxy-2,3,4,5,6-pentachlorocyclohexane (120) and sodium dodecylsulfate (166), were excluded from development of the model because of their large residuals and inconsistent impact on the regression detected during cross-validation runs. Other compounds with residuals significantly greater than the standard deviation were retained because they did not alter the final model.

The predictive ability of Eq. 1 is demonstrated by the good agreement with the reported log P values (Table 2) and the consistent performance for the diverse compound classes represented. The QSAR also compares favorably with CLOGP3 (Table 2) for this set of compounds and an

Figure 1. Correlation of Predicted Verses Experimental Log P

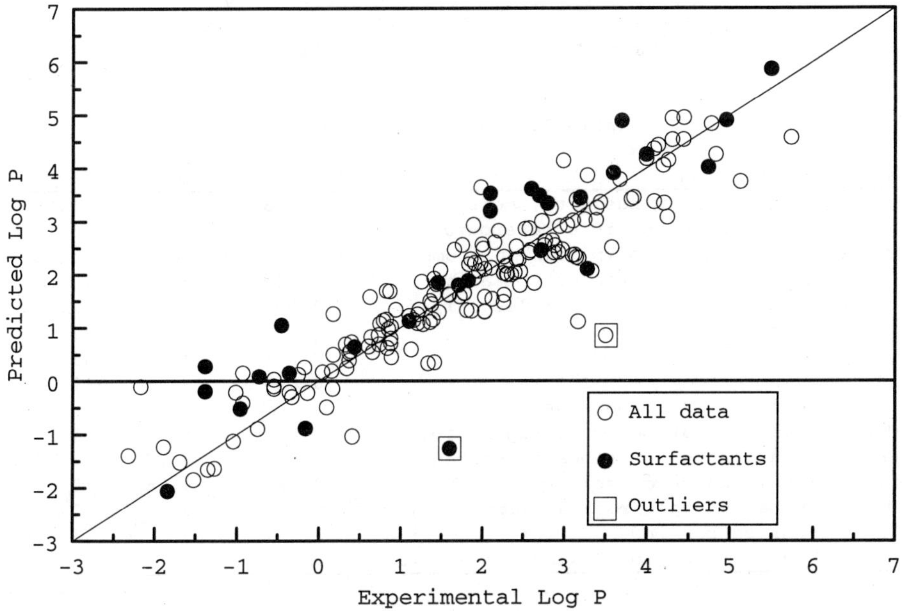

Figure 2. Correlation of CLOGP3 Verses Experimental Log P

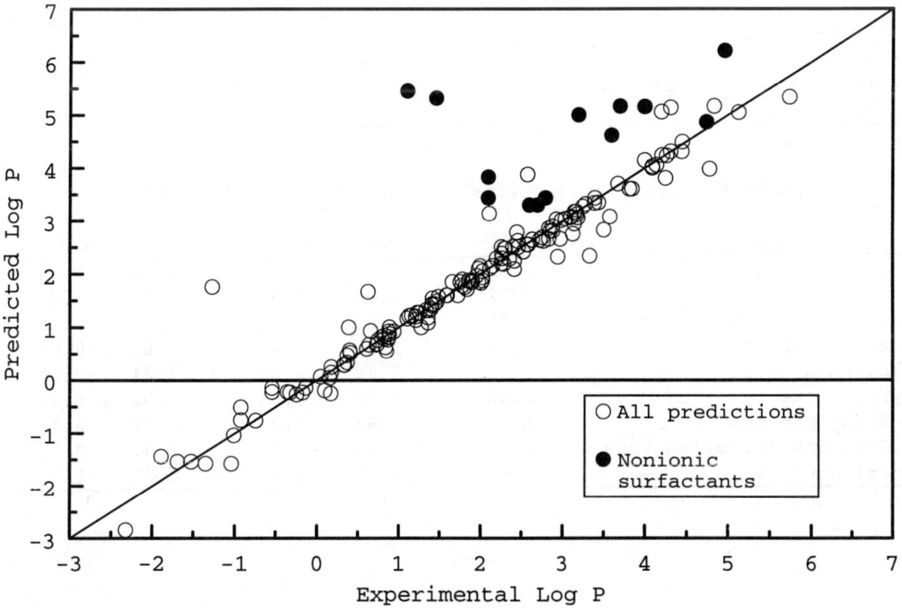

$$\log P = -1.926 + 5.564 * B - 2.985 * cC3 + 0.170 * nCar + 2.415 * \log MW - 0.150 * \mu + 0.007 * V - 2.639 * iAA - 0.896 * nNar + 1.589 * cCar + 0.688 * cO3 - 0.866 * nN3 - 0.612 * iCH \quad (1)$$

Table 1. Terms in the QSAR

Term	Description	Fraction	Low	High
B	Electrostatic basicity, most negative charge on a heteroatom	0.193	-1.00	-0.04
cC3	Total charge on sp^3 carbon atoms	0.121	-0.90	0.92
nCar	Number of aromatic carbon atoms	0.110	0	17
log MW	Base 10 logarithm of molecular weight	0.095	1.42	2.81
μ	Dipole moment	0.093	0.00	19.70
V	Molecular volume in $Å^3$	0.081	27.2	541.1
iAA	Amino acid index; 1 for amino acids, otherwise 0	0.080	0	1
nNar	Number of aromatic nitrogen atoms	0.043	0	1
cCar	Total charge on aromatic carbons	0.054	-0.72	0.44
cO3	Total charge on sp^3 oxygen atoms	0.054	-4.06	0
nN3	Number of sp^3 nitrogen atoms	0.039	0	1
iCH	Hydrocarbon index; 1 for hydrocarbons, otherwise 0	0.037	0	1

Table 2. Summary Statistics for Predicted Log P Values

	This work	CLOGP3
N	191	176
Outliers	2	17
R^2	0.85	0.85
Standard deviation of residuals	0.61	0.63
Standard error	0.60	0.60

Table 3. Log P Predictions for Selected Test Compounds

Compound Name	Log P[a]	Pred.	Resid.	CLOGP3	Resid.
Lactic acid	-0.62	0.02	-0.64	-0.76	0.14
Citric acid	-1.72	0.12	-1.84	-2.07	0.35
Tetrahydrofuran	0.46	0.21	0.25	0.33	0.13
Phenyl benzoate	3.59	3.31	0.28	3.62	-0.03
Benzophenone	3.18	2.49	0.69	3.21	-0.03
Pyrrolidine	0.46	0.52	-0.06	0.00	0.46
3-Phenylpropanol	1.88	1.83	0.05	1.71	0.17
2,2-Dimethylpropylbenzene	4.11	4.13	-0.02	3.97	0.14
Acrylonitrile	-0.92	1.18	-2.10	0.23	-1.15

a) Leo and Hansch 1971.

additional separate set of nine test structures (Table 3). More importantly, the model provides estimates for many surfactants. Very good agreement was obtained for the log P of polyethoxylated nonionic surfactants (180-183) and for cationic surfactants (171-179). However, poorer predictions were obtained for sodium hexanoate (18) and anionic surfactants (166-170). In comparison CLOGP3 predicts polyethoxylated compounds poorly (Roberts 1991) and cannot predict log P for disconnected structures.

The derived predictive model is surprisingly simple and reflects many previously reported Log P correlations. The terms in the equation include two compound class indices, three atom-type counts, two general molecular descriptors, and five terms dependent on charge distribution. Interestingly, only 2 of 12 terms, μ and V, depend on the molecular conformation which suggests that the model is very general and may not demand time-consuming conformational searching used in this study.

Molecular class indices have been used in both GCM and QSAR approaches for saturated aliphatic hydrocarbons (Klopman and Wang 1991; Bodor and Huang 1992, 1991) and amino acids (Klopman and Wang 1991). These corrections apply a systematic correction for compound classes which are otherwise modeled well by non-class-specific terms. The large negative correction for amino acids, -2.639 log P units, indicates that the model otherwise significantly overpredicts the log P of these compounds. This hydrophylic correction may be rationalized by the preference of the amino acids for their zwitterionic tautomers. A smaller but significant and surprisingly hydrophilic correction, -0.612 log P units, is also applied to hydrocarbons, both saturated and unsaturated. Visual inspection of the results suggest that the correlation may be improved by employing correction terms for other classes of compounds, e.g., nitro compounds (115-117 and 135-139). However, in this study, an arbitrary minimum of ten representative compounds was established for consideration of a compound class index to reduce the risk of introducing a unique correction term.

Atom-type counts are the simplest groups used in GCM methods (Klopman 1991) and are employed here to mimic these techniques. Values were computed for all atom-types present in ten or more compounds in the training set. Significant hydrophilic corrections are applied for nNar and nN3 which, since the corrections are nearly equal, may be combined. Note that the training set contained only one example of a compound with more than one nitrogen, phenylurea (119). Therefore, in this case, nN3 and nNar act as compound class corrections rather than true atom-type counters and a further evaluation of their validity is warranted. By comparison, compounds with nCar values up to seventeen were considered for which a proportional hydrophobic correction was applied.

High correlations have been reported between log P and molecular volume (de Bruijn 1990, Famini 1992) or molecular surface area (Bodor and Huang 1992, 1991, 1989; Camilleri et. al. 1988; Famini et. al. 1992; Fumasaki et. al. 1985) which are also highly cross-correlated (Pearlman 1986). The molecular volume is principally dependent on the elemental composition since all computational methods rely on assigned atomic radii, and, to a lesser extent, on the connectivity and conformation.

However, a 10% change in the volume of the largest molecule considered would result in a change of ±0.4 log P units, within the standard deviation of the residuals. The relative insensitivity of the model to reasonable variations in molecular volume therefore suggests that exhaustive conformational searching is unnecessary.

Charge dependent terms, B, cC3, μ, cCar, and cO3, together account for 51.5% of the predicted log P. Various charge-dependent terms have been reported in log P QSARs including B (Famini et. al. 1992), μ and atom-centered charges (Bodor and Huang 1992), and surface point charges (Sasaki et. al. 1991). This study employed the far more rapid empirical Gasteiger-Hückel method to compute atom-centered charges rather than the more computationally demanding semiempirical quantum mechanical methods used previously. A discussion of the merits of one approach over another is beyond the scope of this report. Here, the selection addresses a key requirement for computational speed with the expectation that the predicted atom-centered charges are qualitatively reliable, i.e., oxygen and nitrogen atoms will have larger negative charges than carbon atoms, and that quantitative differences are compensated by the scale factors in the derived model. More troubling is the potential impact of molecular conformation on the dipole moment. Larger residuals might therefore be expected for more polarized and charge-separated compounds such as amino acids and anionic and cationic surfactants. This effect is observed for sodium and potassium 4-dodecylbenzene-sulfonates (167 and 168) and octanoates (169 and 170) in which the differences in the predicted log P for both pairs of salts is wholly due to differences in the dipole moments with the largest difference of 0.89 log P units for the the 4-dodecylbenzenesulfonates.

Predictions of log P must be fast as well as reliable. Since most of the terms in the QSAR are insensitive to differences in molecular conformation, log P estimates for most neutral organic compounds may be computed in a few seconds. However, more complex structures and those possessing high dipole moments may necessitate a conformational search which typically requires less than one hour of CPU time. In practice, most of the user's time is spent entering and verifying structures which are subsequently processed using automated routines. An additional advantage of this approach is that it greatly simplifies expansion of the training set and evaluation of new terms thus speeding development of improved QSARs.

CONCLUSIONS

Reliable estimates of log P may be rapidly computed from a QSAR derived from molecular modeling descriptors. The model may be applied to a wide range of compounds including nonionic and cationic surfactants which are poorly modeled by other methods. The log P of anionic surfactants may also be predicted but with a much larger uncertainty. Expansion of the training set is expected to improve the predictive ability of the model and extend its application to a wider range of compounds. This approach does not replace but augments existing methods, such as CLOGP3.

REFERENCES

Bodor, N., and Huang, M.-J., 1992, "An Extended Version of a Novel Method for Estimation of Partition Coefficients," J. Pharm. Sci., Vol. 81, No. 3, pp. 272-281.

Bodor, N., and Huang, M.-J., 1991, "Predicting Partition Coefficients for Isomeric Diasteriomers of Some Tripeptide Analogs," J. Comput. Chem., Vol. 12, No. 10, pp. 1182-1186.

Camilleri, P., Watts, S. A., and Boraston, J. A., 1988,"A Surface Area Approach to Determination of Partition Coefficients," J. Chem. Soc. Perkin Trans II, pp. 1699-1707.

Caux, P. Y., 1988, "A Physiological Study of the Effects of Triton Surfactants on Lemna Minor L," Environ. Tox. Chem., Vol. 7, pp. 671-676.

Daylight Chemical Information Systems, Inc.,1992, PCmodels User's Guide V.4.2, 18500 Von Karman Ave., #450, Irvine, CA 92715.

de Bruijn, J., and Hermens, J., 1990, "Relationships Between Octanol/Water Partition Coefficients and Total Molecular Surface Area and Total Molecular Volume of Hydrophobic Organic Chemicals," Quant. Struct.-Act. Relat., Vol. 9, pp. 11-21.

Famini, G. R., Penski, C. A., and Wilson, L. Y., 1992, "Using Theoretical Descriptors in Quantitative Structure-Activity Relationships: Some Physiochemical Properties," J. Phys. Org. Chem., Vol. 5, pp. 395-408.

Fumasaki, N; Hada, S., and Neya, S., 1985, "Partition Coefficients of Aliphatic Ethers - Molecular Surface Area Approach", J. Phys. Chem., Vol. 89, No. 14, pp. 3046-3049.

Klopman, G., and Wang, S., 1991, "A Computer Automated Structure Evaluation (CASE) Approach to Calculation of Partition Coefficient," J. Comput. Chem., Vol. 12, No. 8, pp. 1025-1032.

Leo, A., Hansch, C., and Elkins, D., 1971, "Partition Coefficients and Their Uses," Chem. Rev., Vol. 71, No. 6, pp. 525-616.

Leo, A., 1983, "The Octanol-Water Partition Coefficient of Aromatic Solutes: the Effect of Electronic Interactions, Alkyl Chains, Hydrogen Bonds, and ortho-Substitution," J. Chem. Soc. Perkin Trans. II, pp. 825-838.

Leo, A. J., 1989, "Increasing the Accuracy of Computer Calculated log P(oct/water) Values," QSAR: Qunatitative Structure-Activity Relationships in Drug Design, Alan R. Liss, Inc., pp. 53-58.

Lipinski, C. A., Frese, E. F, and Korst, R. J., 1991, "pKa, Log P and MedChem CLOGP Fragment Values for Acidic Heterocyclic Potential Bioisosteres," Quant. Struct.-Act. Relat., Vol. 10, pp. 109-117.

McLeese, D. W., Zitko, V., Sergeant, D. B., Burridge, L., and Metcalfe, C. D., 1981, "Lethality and Accumulation of Alkylphenols in Aquatic Fauna," Chemosphere, Vol. 10, No. 7, pp. 723-730.

Malihot, H. and Peteres, R. H., 1988, "Empirical Relationships between the 1-Octanol/Water Partition Coefficient and Nine Physiochemical Properties," Environ. Sci. Technol., Vol. 22, No. 12, pp. 1479-1488.

Mihalic, Z., and Trinajstic, N., 1992, "A Graph-Theoretical Approach to Structure-Property Relationships," J. Chem. Ed., Vol. 69, No. 9, pp. 701-712.

Nakagawa, Y., Izumi, K., Oikawa, N., Sotomatsu, T., Shigemura, M., and Fujita, T., 1992, "Analysis and Prediction of Hydrophobicity Parameters of Substituted Acetanilides, Benzamides and Related Aromatic Compounds," Environ. Tox. Chem., Vol. 11, pp. 901-916.

Niemi, G. J., Basak, S. C., Vieth, G. D., and Grunwald, G., 1992, "Prediction of Octanol/Water Partition Coeffient (K_{OW}) with Algorithmically Derived Variables," Environ. Tox. Chem., Vol. 11, pp. 893-900.

Pearlman, R. S., 1986, "Molecular Surface Area and Volume: Their Calculation and Use in Predicting Solubilities and Free Energies of Desolvation," Partition Coefficients Determination and Estimation, W. J. Dunn III, J. H. Block , and R. S. Pearlman, Eds., Pergamon Press, New York, pp. 1-20.

Roberts, D. W., 1991, "QSAR issues in aquatic toxicity of surfactants," Sci. Total Environ., Vol. 109/110, pp. 557-568.

Sasaki, Y., Kubodera, H., Matuszaki, T., and Umeyama, H., 1991, "Prediction of Octanol/Water Partition Coefficients Using Parameters Derived from Molecular Structures," J. Pharmacobio-Dyn., Vol. 14, pp. 207-214.

Schüürmann, G., 1990, "QSAR Analysis of Acute Toxicity of Ethoxylated Surfactants," Chemosphere, Vol. 212, No. 4-5, pp. 467-478.

Suzuki, T., and Kudo, Y., 1990, "Automatic log P estimation based on combined additive modeling methods," J. Comput.-Aided Mol. Des., Vol. 4, pp. 155-198.

Tripos Associates, Inc., 1699 South Hanley Road, Suite 303, St. Louis, MO 63144.

Appendix I. Training Set for Development of the Log P QSAR

No.	Compound Name	Log P[a]	Pred.	Resid.	CLOGP3	Resid.
1	Methanol	-0.74	-0.90	0.16	-0.76	0.02
2	Ethanol	-0.32	-0.30	-0.02	-0.23	-0.08
3	1-Propanol	0.34	0.24	0.10	0.29	0.05
4	1-Butanol	0.88	0.71	0.17	0.82	0.06
5	1-Pentanol	1.40	1.15	0.25	1.35	0.05
6	1-Hexanol	2.03	1.57	0.46	1.88	0.15
7	1-Dodecanol	5.13	3.74	1.39	5.05	0.08
8	2-Methyl-2-propanol	0.37	0.53	-0.16	0.47	-0.10
9	2-Butanol	0.61	0.65	-0.04	0.60	0.01
10	2-Methyl-1-propanol	0.74	0.69	0.05	0.69	0.05
11	3-Methyl-1-butanol	1.16	1.14	0.02	1.22	-0.06
12	2,2-Dimethyl-1-propanol	1.36	1.10	0.26	1.09	0.27
13	Cyclohexanol	1.23	1.33	-0.10	1.27	-0.04
14	1,5-Hexadiene	2.45	2.28	0.17	2.78	-0.33
15	2-Hexanone	1.38	1.44	-0.06	1.32	0.06
16	Dipropyl ether	2.03	1.29	0.74	1.93	0.10
17	Dipropylamine	1.73	1.58	0.15	1.60	0.13
18	Sodium hexanoate	-2.17	-0.11	-2.06	c	
19	Hexanoic acid	1.90	1.93	-0.03	1.88	0.02
20	Aniline	0.94	1.33	-0.39	0.92	0.02
21	Anthracene	4.45	4.94	-0.49	4.49	-0.04
22	Formic acid	-0.54	0.02	-0.56	c	
23	Bromobenzene	2.99	4.14	-1.15	3.01	-0.02
24	Chlorobenzene	2.84	3.24	-0.40	2.86	-0.02
25	Fluorobenzene	2.27	2.33	-0.06	2.29	-0.02
26	Iodobenzene	3.25	3.03	0.22	3.27	-0.02
27	Naphthalene	3.28	3.86	-0.58	3.32	-0.04
28	Nitrobenzene	1.86	2.28	-0.42	1.88	-0.02
29	Phenol	1.47	1.28	0.19	1.48	0.00
30	Acetic acid	-0.17	0.25	-0.42	-0.23	0.06
31	Propyl formate	0.83	1.15	-0.32	0.79	0.04
32	Methyl acetate	0.18	0.49	-0.31	0.14	0.04
33	Ethyl acetate	0.73	0.86	-0.13	0.67	0.06
34	Butyric acid	0.79	1.13	-0.34	0.82	-0.03
35	Decanoic acid	4.09	3.37	0.72	4.00	0.09
36	Dodecanoic acid	4.20	4.05	0.15	5.06	-0.86
37	Methyl 4-phenylbutyrate	2.77	2.63	0.14	2.62	0.15
38	1-Naphthanoic acid	3.10	2.36	0.74	3.06	0.04
39	4-Phenylbutyric acid	2.42	2.52	-0.10	2.24	0.18
40	Benzoic acid	1.87	1.31	0.56	1.88	-0.01
41	Ethyl benzoate	2.64	1.83	0.81	2.64	0.00
42	Phenyl acetate	1.49	2.08	-0.59	1.57	-0.08
43	4-Methylbenzoic acid	2.27	1.61	0.66	2.38	-0.11
44	4-Methylbenzyl acetate	2.11	2.12	-0.01	3.14	-1.03
45	Propionic acid	0.33	0.69	-0.36	0.29	0.04
46	3-Phenylpropionic acid	1.84	2.19	-0.35	1.71	0.13
47	Methyl benzoate	2.12	1.53	0.59	2.11	0.01
48	Phenylacetic acid	1.41	1.92	-0.51	1.41	0.00
49	Phenyl formate	1.26	1.86	-0.60	1.27	-0.01
50	2-Phenylethyl acetate	2.42	2.28	0.14	2.09	0.33

Appendix I. Continued.

No.	Compound Name	Log P[a]	Pred.	Resid.	CLOGP3	Resid.
51	Ethyl propionate	1.21	1.24	-0.03	1.20	0.01
52	Benzyl benzoate	2.58	2.87	-0.29	3.88	-1.30
53	Benzyl acetate	1.96	2.06	-0.10	1.96	0.00
54	Allyl alcohol	0.17	-0.15	0.32	-0.25	0.42
55	2-Propanol	0.05	0.17	-0.12	0.07	-0.02
56	3-Methyl-2-butanol	1.28	1.06	0.22	1.00	0.28
57	3-Pentanol	1.21	1.08	0.13	1.13	0.08
58	2-Methyl-2-butanol	0.89	1.01	-0.12	1.00	-0.11
59	3-Methylbenzyl alcohol	1.60	1.61	-0.01	1.60	0.00
60	Octanol	3.15	2.32	0.83	2.94	0.21
61	4-Ethylphenol	2.26	2.02	0.24	2.50	-0.24
62	4-Methylbenzyl alcohol	1.59	1.62	-0.03	1.60	-0.01
63	3-Ethylphenol	2.40	2.03	0.37	2.50	-0.10
64	2-Ethylphenol	2.47	2.05	0.42	2.50	-0.03
65	2-Propylphenol	2.93	2.42	0.51	3.03	-0.10
66	2-Isopropylphenol	2.88	2.41	0.47	2.90	-0.02
67	1-Naphthalenol	2.98	2.47	0.51	2.65	0.33
68	2-Naphthalenol	2.84	2.34	0.50	2.65	0.19
69	2,4-Dimethylphenol	2.30	2.00	0.30	2.47	-0.17
70	3,5-Dimethylphenol	2.31	1.99	0.32	2.47	-0.16
71	2-Phenylethanol	1.36	1.49	-0.13	1.18	0.18
72	Ethane	1.81	1.32	0.49	1.75	0.06
73	Propane	2.36	1.99	0.37	2.28	0.08
74	Butane	2.89	2.54	0.35	2.81	0.08
75	2-Methylpropane	2.76	2.54	0.22	2.68	0.08
76	2,2-Dimethylpentane	3.11	3.01	0.10	3.08	0.03
77	Pentane	3.39	3.02	0.37	3.34	0.05
78	2,2-Dimethylbutane	3.82	3.42	0.40	3.61	0.21
79	2,3-Dimethylbutane	3.85	3.45	0.40	3.61	0.24
80	Cyclohexene	2.86	2.64	0.22	2.81	0.05
81	Ethylene	1.13	0.59	0.54	1.21	-0.08
82	Acetylene	0.37	0.39	-0.02	0.34	0.03
83	Cyclohexane	3.44	3.36	0.08	3.35	0.09
84	Benzene	2.15	2.60	-0.45	2.14	0.01
85	Toluene	2.73	3.00	-0.27	2.64	0.09
86	Phenylacetylene	2.53	2.86	-0.33	2.41	0.12
87	Ethylbenzene	3.15	3.41	-0.26	3.17	-0.02
88	1,2-Dimethylnaphthalene	4.31	4.53	-0.22	4.31	0.00
89	1,7-Dimethylnaphthalene	4.44	4.53	-0.09	4.31	0.13
90	Hexamethylbenzene	4.31	4.93	-0.62	5.14	-0.83
91	1,2,4,5-Tetramethylbenzene	4.00	4.18	-0.18	4.14	-0.14
92	Butylbenzene	4.26	4.15	0.11	4.23	0.03
93	Propylbenzene	3.68	3.78	-0.10	3.70	-0.02
94	Biphenyl	4.09	4.36	-0.27	4.03	0.06
95	Diphenylmethane	4.14	4.43	-0.29	4.06	0.08
96	Diphenylacetylene	4.78	4.83	-0.05	3.98	0.80
97	Dimethyl ether	0.10	-0.50	0.60	-0.19	0.29
98	Furan	1.34	0.33	1.01	1.32	0.02
99	Diphenyl ether	4.21	3.34	0.87	4.24	-0.03
100	Propoxybenzene	3.18	2.30	0.88	3.12	0.06

Appendix I. Continued.

No.	Compound Name	Log P[a]	Pred.	Resid.	CLOGP3	Resid.
101	1-Ethoxybutane	2.03	1.30	0.73	1.93	0.10
102	1-Phenyl-2-propanone	1.44	1.81	-0.37	1.43	0.01
103	Phenylacetaldehyde	1.78	1.65	0.13	1.78	0.00
104	Acetone	-0.24	0.12	-0.36	-0.27	0.03
105	Hexaldehyde	1.78	1.64	0.14	1.89	-0.11
106	9-Fluorenone	3.58	2.50	1.08	3.08	0.50
107	2,2,2-Trichloroethanol	1.42	0.35	1.07	1.54	-0.12
108	2,2,2-Trifluoroethanol	0.41	-1.04	1.45	0.52	-0.11
109	2-Fluoroethanol	-0.92	-0.42	-0.50	-0.51	-0.41
110	2-Ethoxyethanol	-0.54	-0.10	-0.44	-0.22	-0.32
111	2,3-Butanediol	-0.92	0.15	-1.07	-0.75	-0.17
112	D-Ribose	-2.32	-1.40	-0.92	-2.85	0.53
113	Diethoxymethane	0.84	0.62	0.22	0.62	0.22
114	2-Amino-3-methylpentanoic acid	-1.69	-1.52	-0.17	-1.54	-0.15
115	p-Nitrophenol	1.91	2.21	-0.30	1.85	0.06
116	2,4-Dinitrotoluene	1.98	3.64	-1.66	1.85	0.13
117	4-Nitrobenzoic acid	1.89	2.93	-1.04	1.84	0.05
118	2-Hydroxybenzoic acid	2.26	1.47	0.79	2.19	0.07
119	Phenylurea	0.83	1.69	-0.86	0.85	-0.02
120	1-Methoxy-2,3,4,5,6-penta-chloro cyclohexane	3.51	0.85	2.66[b]	2.83	0.68
121	Isophthalic acid	1.66	2.46	-0.80	1.85	-0.19
122	2-Bromophenyl acetate	2.20	2.82	-0.62	2.29	-0.09
123	2-Flurophenyl acetate	1.76	2.55	-0.79	1.85	-0.09
124	Methyl 2-hydroxybenzoate	2.46	1.79	0.67	2.62	-0.15
125	Phenylalanine	-1.35	-1.66	0.31	-1.58	0.23
126	3-Ethoxyphenol	1.98	2.21	-0.23	2.10	-0.12
127	3-Hydroxypiccolinic acid	-1.27	-1.64	0.37	1.76	-3.03
128	4-Iodoanaline	3.34	2.06	1.28	2.34	1.00
129	Leucine	-1.52	-1.85	0.33	-1.54	0.02
130	Triflurometho xybenzene	3.17	1.11	2.06	3.17	0.00
131	4-Flourophenylalanine	-1.89	-1.24	-0.65	-1.44	-0.45
132	Propyl 4-hydroxybenzoate	3.04	2.93	0.11	3.04	0.00
133	Tryptophan	-1.04	-1.13	0.09	-1.58	0.54
134	Heptyl 4-hydoxybenzoate	4.83	4.25	0.58	5.16	-0.33
135	Nitroethane	0.18	1.25	-1.07	0.25	-0.06
136	Nitropropane	0.87	1.68	-0.81	0.77	0.10
137	Nitropentane	2.01	2.48	-0.47	1.83	0.18
138	1,3-Dimethyl-2-nitrobenzene	2.95	2.91	0.04	2.32	0.63
139	1-Nitronaphthalene	3.19	3.31	-0.12	3.06	0.13
140	Indole	2.00	2.56	-0.56	2.14	-0.14
141	9-Azaanthracene	3.40	3.25	0.15	3.43	-0.03
142	1-Azanaphthalene	2.03	2.10	-0.07	2.05	-0.02
143	1,2,3,4-Tetrahydroxy-1-azanaphthalene	2.29	2.16	0.13	2.18	0.11
144	N,N-Dimethylformamide	-1.01	-0.22	-0.79	-1.04	0.03
145	Ethylamine	-0.13	-0.23	0.10	-0.14	0.01
146	2-Methyl-2-aminopropane	0.40	0.72	-0.32	0.57	-0.17
147	Butylamine	0.88	0.79	0.09	0.92	-0.04
148	Piperidine	0.85	0.97	-0.12	0.56	0.30

Appendix I. Continued.

No.	Compound Name	Log P[a]	Pred.	Resid.	CLOGP3	Resid.
149	Pyridine	0.64	0.82	-0.18	0.67	-0.03
150	2-Methylpyridine	1.11	1.22	-0.11	1.16	-0.05
151	2,5-Dimethylpyridine	0.63	1.57	-0.94	1.66	-1.03
152	Trimethylamine	0.16	0.19	-0.03	0.05	0.11
153	Pyrrole	0.75	1.07	-0.32	0.76	-0.01
154	Triphenylamine	5.74	4.57	1.17	5.34	0.39
155	4-Hexylpyridine	4.25	3.08	1.17	3.81	0.44
156	4-Butylpyridine	3.13	2.37	0.76	2.75	0.38
157	2-Methyl-1-azanaphthalene	2.59	2.45	0.14	2.55	0.04
158	6-Methyl-1-azanaphthalene	2.57	2.41	0.16	2.55	0.02
159	Cinnamamide	1.41	1.62	-0.21	1.43	-0.02
160	Diethyl ether	0.89[a1]	0.45	0.44	0.87	0.02
161	3,6-Dioxaoctane	0.66[a1]	0.54	0.12	0.93	-0.27
162	3,6,9-Trioxaundecane	0.39[a1]	0.56	-0.17	1.00	-0.61
163	3-Oxa-1-pentanol	-0.35[a1]	-0.22	-0.13	-0.22	-0.13
164	3,6-Dioxaoctanol	-0.54[a1]	-0.15	-0.39	-0.15	-0.39
165	Dodecanol	5.13	3.74	1.39	5.05	0.08
166	Sodium dodecylsulfate	1.60	-1.26	2.86[b]	[c]	
167	Sodium 4-dodecylbenzene-sulfonate	-0.45	1.04	-1.49	[c]	
168	Potassium 4-dodecylbenzene-sulfonate	-0.35	0.15	-0.50	[c]	
169	Sodium octanoate	-1.38	-0.20	-1.18	[c]	
170	Potassium octanoate	-1.38	0.27	-1.65	[c]	
171	Decyltrimethylammonium iodide	-0.16	-0.89	0.73	[c]	
172	1-Decylpyridinium bromide	-0.72	0.08	-0.80	[c]	
173	1-Dodecylpyridinium bromide	0.44	0.64	-0.20	[c]	
174	Benzyldimethylhexadecyl-ammonium bromide	3.28	2.10	1.18	[c]	
175	Hexyltrimethylammonium iodide	-1.84	-2.06	0.22	[c]	
176	1-Octylpyridinium bromide	-0.95	-0.53	-0.42	[c]	
177	1-Hexadecylpyridinium bromide	1.83	1.88	-0.05	[c]	
178	1-Hexadecylpyridinium chloride	1.71	1.79	-0.08	[c]	
179	1-Octadecylpyridinium bromide	2.72	2.45	0.27		
180	5-[4-(1-Methylheptyl)phenoxy]-3-oxa-1-pentanol	4.74[a2]	4.01	0.73	4.87	-0.13
181	11-[4-(1-Methylheptyl)phenoxy]-3,6,9-trioxa-1-undecanol	3.20[a2]	3.44	-0.24	5.00	-1.80
182	29-[4-(1-Methylheptyl)phenoxy]-3,6,9,12,15,18,24,27-octaoxa-1-nonaeicosanol	1.46[a2]	1.84	-0.38	5.32	-3.86
183	35-[4-(1-Methylheptyl)phenoxy]-3,6,9,12,15,18,24,27,30,33-decaoxa-1-pentatricontanol	1.11[a2]	1.12	-0.01	5.45	-4.34

Appendix I. Continued.

No.	Compound Name	Log P[a]	Pred.	Resid.	CLOGP3	Resid.
184	4-Nonylphenol	4.96[a2]	4.90	0.06	6.21	-1.25
185	4-Hexylphenol	3.60[a3]	3.91	-0.31	4.62	-1.02
186	4-Heptylphenol	4.00[a3]	4.25	-0.25	5.15	-1.15
187	4-Dodecylphenol	5.50[a3]	5.86	-0.36		c
188	2-(1,1-Dimethylethyl)phenol	2.70[a3]	3.48	-0.78	3.30	-0.60
189	3-(1,1-Dimethylethyl)phenol	2.60[a3]	3.61	-1.01	3.30	-0.70
190	4-(1-Methylheptyl)phenol	3.70[a3]	4.89	-1.19	5.16	-1.46
191	2-(1-Methylpropyl)phenol	2.80[a3]	3.34	-0.54	3.43	-0.63
192	4-(1-Methylpropyl)phenol	2.10[a3]	3.20	-1.10	3.43	-1.33
193	4-(1-Methylbutyl)phenol	2.10[a3]	3.52	-1.42	3.83	-1.73

a) Reported by Hansch (1971); a1) Schüürmann (1990); a2) Caux (1988); and, a3) McLeese (1981). b) Not included in the summary statistics. c) CLOGP3 failed to provide a reliable prediction.

Dennis Postlethwaite[1]

RECENT DEVELOPMENTS IN LCA AND CRITICAL ISSUES

REFERENCE: Postlethwaite, D, "Recent Developments in LCA and Critical Issues," Environmental Toxicology and Risk Assessment - Third Volume, ASTM STP 1218, Jane S. Hughes, Gregory R. Biddinger, and Eugene Mones, Eds., American Society for Testing and Materials, Philadelphia, 1995.

ABSTRACT: Lifecycle Assessment (LCA) is a fast growing technique which is now being widely applied. The methodology for conducting LCA's is being developed and refined and attempts are underway to set up agreed working procedures and standards. Foremost amongst these are the activities of ISO, in developing formal standards, and SETAC, in resolving methodological issues, such as energy accounting and co-product allocation, and, especially, in deriving an agreed Code of Practice. SETAC has also established, by means of consensus workshops, key bases for further necessary work on impact assessment (the relation of chemical emissions to actual environmental impacts) and data quality. Data availability is still a major factor limiting more widespread application of LCA, although some progress is being achieved, notably on raw material data for plastics and surfactants.

KEYWORDS: Lifecycle, Assessment, Inventory, Environment, Impact, SETAC, Database, Standard(isation)

---

[1] Lifecycle Analysis Manager, Unilever Research Port Sunlight Laboratory, England, and Chairman of the SETAC European LCA Task Group.

INTRODUCTION

Lifecycle Assessment (LCA) is increasingly being used and advocated as a tool for assessing the environmental implications of product manufacture and use and of service industry operations.

This short paper, which was presented at the third ASTM Symposium on Environmental Toxicology, and Risk Assessment, Atlanta, 1993, briefly reviews important recent developments and attempts to highlight critical issues which require further attention. The review covers five areas as follows:

1. Methodology Development
2. Standardisation
3. Data and Databases
4. Applications
5. Current Activities

METHODOLOGY DEVELOPMENT

Although much LCA methodology is founded on common and, overall, quite simple principles, differences in methodology, and opinions, between individual practitioners has on occasion resulted in some discrepancies between the results obtained. The need to resolve such differences by informed debate and to achieve a sensible, and acceptable, consensus was recognised by the Society of Environmental Toxicology and Chemistry (SETAC). SETAC has formed two LCA task groups, one in North America the other in Europe to specifically develop LCA science and methodology. Activities between the two groups are closely coordinated. A mechanism for generating debate and achieving consensus views on LCA which the groups have successfully used have been specialist workshops. These have brought together leading LCA experts and practitioners and also non-LCA experts from other disciplines whose expertise could be usefully applied to particular issues - for example, toxicologists, and decision theory experts.

The first two workshops covered generic issues, while later ones have addressed specific issues (Table 1).

TABLE 1 SETAC LCA Workshops

TOPIC	VENUE	DATE
Overall Methodology, Inventory	Smugglers Notch, Vermont, USA	Aug 1990
Overall Methodology	Leiden, Netherlands	Dec 1991
Impact Analysis	Sandestin, Florida, USA	Feb 1992
Data Quality	Wintergreen, Virginia, USA	Oct 1992
Code of Practice + Inventory Methodology	Sesimbra, Portugal	April 1993

The basic framework for conducting LCA's has been established comprising four basic components as follows (SETAC 1991; SETAC 1992):

1. Goal Definition and Scoping: Comprises defining the objective of the LCA, establishing the functional unit of the system being studied, setting boundaries for the LCA and establishing procedures for data accreditation, co-product allocation and energy accounting.

2. Inventory Compilation: Comprises assessing and quantifying all the inputs (energy, raw materials) and outputs (products, co-products, emissions, wastes) at each stage. The latter essentially cover raw material procurement, product manufacture, product use and disposal. The inventory is based on a process diagram characterising all relevant stages and operations involved.

3. Impact Assessment: This involves the translation of the quantitative inventory data (eg gaseous emissions) into actual environmental impacts (eg deforestation). Currently, impact assessment in LCA is at a very early stage of development due to many recognised difficulties, some of which are considered in further detail below.

4. Improvement Analysis: This constitutes the ultimate purpose of an LCA in which the Inventory and the environmental impacts are examined to ascertain items and issues most susceptible to remedial measures. Improvement Analysis should ideally be a continuous process conducted throughout all stages of the LCA.

A simple conceptual representation of the basic framework is depicted below (Figure 1).

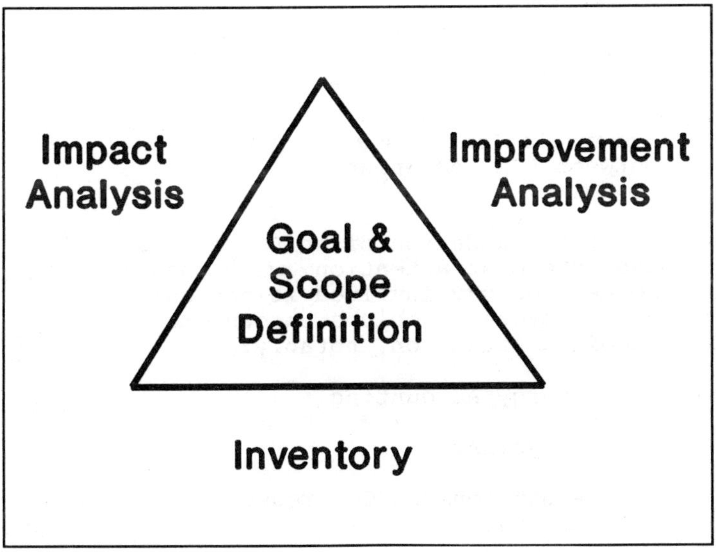

FIG. 1 Simple conceptual framework for LCA components.

This, of course, is oversimplified and in practice the LCA process is an iterative one (Fig. 2):

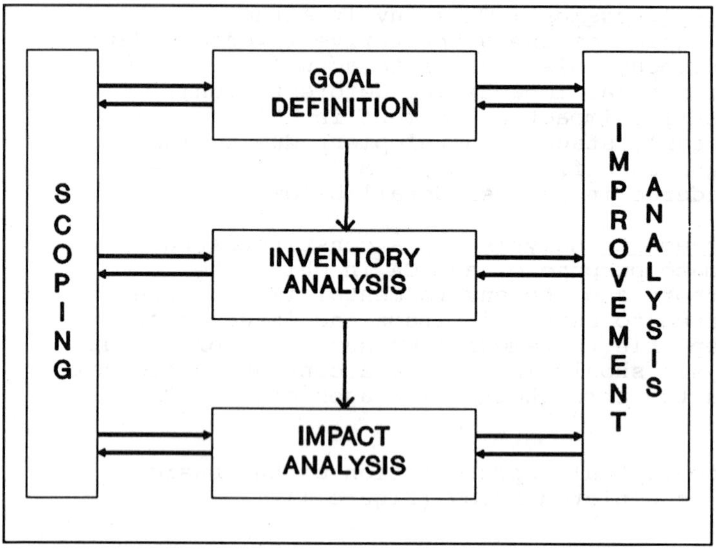

FIG. 2 Interrelationships and Interaction between LCA components.

The inventory is the foundation of an LCA and as such has received the most attention, with the result that the methodology involved is now quite well established. Several problems encountered earlier have received attention, notably:

- Energy Accounting
- Recycling
- Apportionment/Co-product Accounting

and the importance of proper functional unit and boundary definition has been emphasised.

Impact assessment, which relates the inventory inputs and outputs to actual environmental effects, is less well developed. Quantification and cross-comparison of impacts is notoriously difficult. Nevertheless, significant progress has been made, stemming from a recognition (SETAC 1993) that impact assessment itself comprises three stages, namely:

- Classification - in which emissions etc are grouped in terms of their environmental effect.

- Characterisation - in which the effects of these emissions are quantified.

- Valuation - in which relative effects and impacts are compared and, tentatively, aggregated.

Four ultimate environmental impact categories have been identified:

- Resource Depletion
- Human Health Effects
- Ecological Health Effects
- Social/Welfare Effects

The pathways to these from the inventory inputs and outputs have been characterised in terms of stressor chains. This is typically exemplified (Fig.3) by the pathway for sulphur dioxide outlined below:

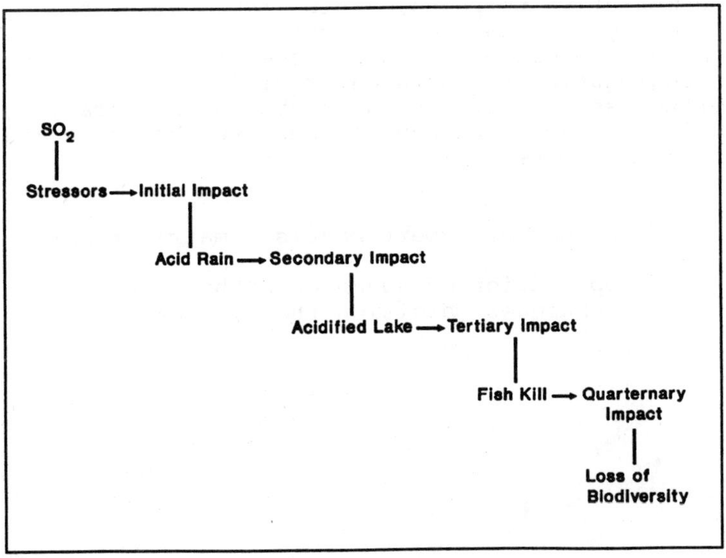

FIG 3. Example of Linkages Between Stressors and Impacts.

Quantification of impacts and stressors, and especially their combination or aggregation to give an "overall" environmental effect, is notoriously difficult and no satisfactory procedure has yet been developed. What has been recognised, is that several levels of data collection and treatment are possible and these have been categorised as follows:

- Loading Assessments
- Equivalency Assessments
- Toxicity, Persistence and Bioaccumulation Assessments
- Generic Exposure/Effects Assessment
- Site-Specific Exposure/Effects Assessment

A dilemma is that in going from the inventory to an actual environmental impact, the data involved becomes more diffuse, less precise - and thus more debatable.

A further dilemma is created by the need for an overall assessment to be given by an LCA, especially for comparative purposes. This itself creates a need for aggregated/combined data. Since fundamentally different parameters are involved, such aggregation presents major difficulties. Nevertheless, the pressures to obtain an overall result are severe and ways to resolve the issue are now being examined. These include:

- The use of expert panels - matrix ranking.
- Application of advanced mathematical techniques (decision theory etc).

STANDARDISATION

Differences between LCA studies, and the contention which has subsequently arisen, can in most cases be attributed to the use of different or, at least, badly specified methodologies and functional unit definitions. Such differences can, arguably, be resolved by the evolution, and adoption, of appropriate standards and operating procedures. Again, this has been recognised and there is now major activity directed at developing such standards. Bodies active include:

Global:

- International Standards Organisation (ISO)

International:

- Comité Europeen Standardisation (CEN)

National:

- Deutch Industrie Norm (DIN)
- American National Standards Institute (ANSI)
- British Standards Institute (BSI)
- Canadian Standards Association (CSA)
- Association Francois Normalisation (AFNOR)
- Environmental Protection Agency US (EPA)

Although initially fragmented, this activity is now being coordinated, with ISO taking the lead initiative. ISO, and also the others, have recognised the formative role which SETAC, as an independent organisation, can play in developing such standards, particularly through its evolution of an agreed and accepted Code of Practice.

Overall, there is no doubt that the establishment of transparent and ratified methodology and procedures, not only for LCA itself but attendant issues such as authentication (peer reviews etc) is necessary and would be of major benefit.

DATA AND DATABASES

The inventory is the heart of an LCA. Its compilation requires data and often such data is either not available or not accessible. This has imposed serious restrictions on the utility and application of LCA in practice. Again, the problem is a recognised one and efforts to resolve it are being made in earnest.

Much data is available concerning the grave-end of the cradle-to-grave spectrum. Thus, the fate and effect on the environment of many of the chemical species used today has been well documented and is available and applicable to LCA. The serious omissions and gaps occur at the cradle-end, principally involving raw material production, from base mineral or substrate procurement to manufacture. Production processes are in most cases proprietary and there is an understandable reluctance to release these data. Solutions to the problem, however, have been sought and developed. These have principally involved confidential averaging by third party institutes of data supplied to them by individual companies under appropriate secrecy agreements. These data, together with some generated or assembled by third party institutes themselves, are now increasingly becoming available in the public domain. At the present time these notably include:

<u>Industry Initiatives</u>:

Plastics Raw Materials:

> A major exercise on plastics raw materials is being conducted in Europe by the Plastics Waste Management Institute (PWMI). Data on the intermediate chemicals involved and on Polyethylene, Polypropylene, Polystyrene and has recently been published (PWMI 1993) and those for Polyvinyl Chloride (PVC) are currently being compiled. Other polymers, for example Polyurethane, Polyethylene Terephthalate (PET) will also be assessed in due course. PWMI itself is a sub-group of the Association of Plastic Manufacturers, Europe (APME).

Surfactants:

Surfactant sourcing (ie whether from petrochemicals or oleochemicals) is a critical issue. The European Centre of Studies on Linear Alkylbenzene (ECOSOL), a sector group of the European Chemical Manufacturers Association (Conseil Europeen Federation Industries Chimique - CEFIC) is currently preparing LCA inventories on the nine major surfactant types used commercially. These also include the preparation of intermediates and auxiliaries.

Independent Institutes etc:

These typically, but not exhaustively include:

- Open University, UK (I Boustead)
- Chalmers University, Goteborg, Sweden
- Franklin Associates, USA
- Eidgenossische Material Prufungs und Forschungsanstalt (EMPA)/Bundesamt fur Umwelt, Walt und Landschaft (BUWAL), Switzerland
- International Institute for Applied Systems Analysis (IIASA), Austria
- Centrum voor Milieukunde, Leiden (CML - Centre for Environmental Studies, Leiden)
- Fraunhofer Institut, Germany
- Umwelt Bundesamt (UBA, Federal Environmental Agency), Germany.

A related issue is data quality. Data quality standards are necessary in LCA to ensure confidence in the results and to enable subsequent validation. The issue has been addressed in a recent SETAC workshop where data quality assessment was confirmed to be an integral part of any LCA. A framework for data quality and its associated criteria, involving data quality indicators (DQI's), was formulated and the quality and characteristics of data from various sources was evaluated (SETAC, in press).

APPLICATIONS

LCA is a tool for assessing the overall environmental credentials of product manufacture and use and of service industry operations. Within industry, it is now being used to select products, ingredients and packaging having reduced environmental implications and to develop new ones. Externally, it is being applied by regulatory bodies to discriminate products for the purposes of ecolabel award and for selecting products for use in civic institutions etc.

The number and types of application has increased dramatically. Early subjects, comprise the by now familiar beverage containers, diapers and packaging. Now, LCA's are known to have been carried out on:

- Hairsprays
- Fabric Washing Detergents
- Cleaning Products
- Paints and Varnishes
- Window Frames
- Building Insulants
- Heating Boilers (combine heat and power units)
- Margarines and Spreads
- Motorcars
- Railway Vehicles
- Airboard Catering
- Auto-fuels (gasoline plus or minus MTBE)
- Rugs and Mats

and many more are being investigated (SETAC 1992b; Sustainability 1993).

As stated above, one of the main external applications, especially in Europe, has been for ecolabel award (MONITOR 1992). The European EC ecolabelling scheme is gaining pace: topics now well-advanced include:

- Lightbulbs
- Hairsprays
- Fabric Washing Detergents
- Washing Machines
- Paints and Varnishes
- Food Packaging

Many others are in the pipeline. A problem is that although LCA is stipulated as a main EC ecolabelling criterion, its proper application in practice has often, or nearly always, been hindered by lack of data. Because of this, many of the LCA's have necessarily been incomplete or, at best, streamlined. Not unexpectedly, this has created some contention (ENDS 1993). There is a need for a rational approach which reasonably embodies all LCA elements and for agreed and accepted impact assessment procedures, such that integration and cross-comparison are qualified and transparent.

OTHER ACTIVITIES

In addition to those covered above, other current LCA activities involve:

Globalisation - Interest in environmental matters and the application of LCA is growing in regions outside North America and Europe. Both the Organisation for Economic Cooperation and Development (OECD) and the United Nations Environmental programme (UNEP) are involved.

Wider Application - Some attention is being focussed on the use of LCA in technology assessments and in corporate decision making. The German parliamentary commission (Enquette) is assessing the use of LCA and related techniques in the political sphere and the International Chamber of Commerce (ICC) has established a working group, the World Industry Council on the Environment (WICE) to address the matter.

Methodology Development - Many bodies and institutes are active. The Society of Environmental Toxicology and Chemistry (SETAC) has taken a lead in developing LCA methodology and in coordinating activities worldwide. In Europe, a large number of institutes, organisations and companies are involved in LCA (Sustainability 1993), with major centres of activity in Scandinavia, the Netherlands and Germany. In North America, the US EPA has taken a leading role in LCA methodology development (EPA 1993a; EPA 1993b).

The most formative methodological development has been the production of a set of Guidelines for undertaking LCA's. These comprise a consensus from the world's leading practitioners and experts and emanated from the most recent SETAC workshop (SETAC 1993b).

Information Handling - As noted above, information accessibility and dissemination is vital to ensure a coordinated approach and avoid duplication and possible conflicts. The SETAC Newsletter is being developed and expanded to cater for this. The new version is a combined North American and European production and will, in future, incorporate semi-technical articles. A further information initiative is being undertaken by the Nordic group, in conjunction with the International Chamber of Commerce (ICC), in which a database of LCA's already undertaken is being compiled.

Databases - In Europe the Database position is being reviewed by the Society for the Promotion of Lifecycle Development (SPOLD). The European Chemical Manufacturers Association (CEFIC) are also examining the data situation, in particular the possibilities of extending the plastics (PWMI) and surfactants (ECOSOL) type of study to other raw materials.

SUMMARY AND CONCLUSIONS

Interest in Lifecycle Assessments (LCA's) has increased dramatically over the last few years. Activities have occurred across a broad front ranging from the development of methodology to applications in practice and use in the regulatory sphere. There has been criticism on the grounds of credibility and major efforts have been, and are being, expended to establish rational principles and develop unequivocal methodology which all practitioners can apply. The pace, and direction, of developments has been different between North American and Europe. In North America, the main emphasis has been on developing sound methodology. In Europe, the pressures for deploying the technique for regulatory or ecolabelling purposes, have led to a more urgent development of practical systems, notably involving streamlined approaches. Overall, the activity has involved a very broad spectrum of disciplines and affiliations. This has resulted in a major need for effective communication and linkages between all interested parties. The Society of Environmental Toxicology and Chemistry (SETAC) has played a major role in establishing these and, especially, in developing universally acceptable and deployable methodology. Data availability is still a fundamental problem hindering more widespread LCA deployment, especially in the public domain. Nevertheless, significant progress is being made toward establishing LCA as a reliable and credible technique and ensuring its proper use in practice.

REFERENCES*

Boustead, 1992, Eco-Balance Methodology for Commodity Thermoplastics, A Report for the European Centre for Plastics in the Environment (PWMI), Brussels, Belgium. Published by European Centre for Plastics in the Environment.

ECN, 1992, European Chemical News 30th November 1992, Report on Conference on Ecolabelling, Lifecycle Analysis and the Chemical Industry, 23-24 November 1992, Brussels.

ENDS, 1992, Environmental Data Services (ENDS) Report No 214 (November 1992), page 23.

ENDS, 1993, Environmental Data Services (ENDS) Report 222 (July 1993), p 27.

EPA, 1993, Lifecycle Design Manual: Environmental Requirements and the Product System (in conjunction with the University of Michigan), January 1993, Ref EPA/600R/R-92/226.

EPA, 1993b, Lifecycle Assessment: Inventory Guidelines and Principles (in conjunction with Battelle), February 1993, Ref EPA/600/R-92/245.

MONITOR, 1992, Update on Outlook on Eco-labelling and Environmental Claims, Monitor Bulletin 92-15 Global Business Relations Inc, New York.

SETAC 1991, A Technical Framework for Lifecycle Assessment, Workshop report from the Smugglers Notch, Vermont, USA, workshop held August 18-23, 1990.

SETAC 1992a, Workshop report from the SETAC-Europe workshop held Leiden, Netherlands, December 1991.

SETAC 1992b, Lifecycle Assessment: Workshop report 25-26 June 1992, Potsdam, Germany.

SETAC 1993a, Conceptual Framework for Impact Assessment, Workshop report from the Sandestin, Florida, USA workshop held February 1992.

SETAC 1993b, Guidelines for Lifecycle Assessment: A "Code of Practice", as drawn up at Sesimbra, Portugal workshop, 31 March-3 April 1993.

SETAC, In Press, A Practical Framework for LCA Data Quality, Workshop report from the Wintergreen, Virginia, USA, workshop held October 4-9, 1992.

SUSTAINABILITY 1993, The LCA Sourcebook: European Business Guide to Lifecycle Assessment, Sustainability/SPOLD, ISBN 0-9521904-0-0.

* The SETAC publications referred to can be obtained from the SETAC offices as follows:

NORTH AMERICA	EUROPE
1010 North 12th Avenue	Avenue E Mounier 83, Box 1
FL 32501 Pensacola	1200 Brussels
USA	Belgium
Tel: 904-469-9777	Tel: +32-2-772-7281
Fax: 904-469-9778	Fax: +32-2-770-5386

Methods Development

Marsha C. Black,[1] Katri Björkroth,[2] and Aimo Oikari[3]

PROBING THE ROUTES, RATES, AND MECHANISMS OF XENOBIOTIC ELIMINATION BY RAINBOW TROUT (*ONCORHYNCHUS MYKISS*) WITH A PHYSIOLOGICAL CHAMBER.

REFERENCE: Black, M. C., Björkroth, K., and Oikari, A., "Probing the Routes, Rates, and Mechanisms of Xenobiotic Elimination by Rainbow Trout (*Oncorhynchus mykiss*) with a Physiological Chamber," Environmental Toxicology and Risk Assessment - Third Volume, ASTM STP 1218, Jane S. Hughes, Gregory R. Biddinger, and Eugene Mones, Eds., American Society for Testing and Materials, Philadelphia, 1995.

ABSTRACT: The ability of aquatic organisms to efficiently biotransform and eliminate xenobiotics is an important strategy for reducing body burdens and thereby avoiding toxic effects of xenobiotic exposure. We have developed a plexiglass chamber that isolates the different xenobiotic elimination routes in fish, enabling the collection of biotransformation products over time from the gills, skin, urine, and feces of rainbow trout (*Oncorhynchus mykiss*). Trout were exposed to [^{14}C]-labeled pentachlorophenol (PCP) in the physiological chamber using two experimental treatments: (1) intraperitoneal (i.p.) injection of PCP into fish having no chemical or effluent preexposure (controls) and (2) i.p. injection of PCP into fish following preexposure to a complex pulp mill effluent for 2 weeks. Elimination of PCP residues was monitored from all routes for 24 to 48 h. Specific PCP biotransformation products were identified and quantified in urine, feces, and bile using high performance liquid chromatography (HPLC) to determine the effects of pulp mill effluent preexposure on the routes and rates of PCP elimination in exposed trout. This study demonstrates the utility of using the physiological chamber for studying the mechanisms of xenobiotic biotransformation and elimination.

KEYWORDS: elimination, biotransformation, pentachlorophenol, pulp mill effluents, preexposure, rainbow trout, *Oncorhynchus mykiss*

INTRODUCTION

Pollution inputs to the aquatic environment pose a significant threat to the health of aquatic biota and also to other organisms that depend on aquatic biota as a food source, including humans. Fish readily accumulate many hydrophobic organic pollutants by passive diffusion across the gills during respiratory processes or through the

---

[1]Assistant Professor, Environmental Health Science, 206 Dairy Science Bldg., The University of Georgia, Athens, GA 30602, USA

[2]Laboratory Technologist, Biology Department, University of Joensuu, FIN-80100 Joensuu, Finland

[3]Director, Laboratory of Environmental Protection, Helsinki University of Technology, FIN-02150 Espoo, Finland

food chain, and are especially susceptible to the effects of pollutants that can be bioaccumulated to toxic concentrations. The toxicity of some chemicals can be reduced through biotransformation processes, resulting in the formation of inactive or less active products, although biotransformation may result in the formation of a more toxic form (e.g. biotransformation of benzo[a]pyrene to the carcinogenic benzo[a]pyrene-7,8-dihydrodiol-9,10-epoxide) (Parke, 1981). Biotransformation products are usually eliminated more readily than their parent forms either because they are more hydrophilic or because they are able to utilize an active transport process, such as the organic anion transport system in the liver or tubular secretion processes in the kidney (Pritchard et al., 1991).

Fish biotransform many hydrophobic organic chemicals using Phase I reactions, primarily utilizing microsomal mixed function oxidase (MFO) enzymes, and Phase II conjugation reactions (reviewed by Binder et al., 1984). Many of the enzymes involved in these processes can be induced by recent or concomitant exposures of fish to a host of chemicals, including polycyclic aromatic hydrocarbons, polychlorinated biphenyls, DDT, polychlorinated dibenzodioxins and furans (reviewed by Lech et al., 1982; Melancon et al., 1988), and pulp mill effluents (Andersson et al., 1987; Lindström-Seppä and Oikari, 1989, 1990; Mather-Mihaich and Di Giulio, 1991). Induction of biotransformation enzymes may result in more rapid and/or more efficient biotransformation, which could then significantly reduce the residence time and toxicity of the accumulated xenobiotic (Melancon and Lech, 1979). Finally, elimination of the parent xenobiotic and biotransformed product(s) in fish can then occur by many different routes, depending on the physicochemical properties of the xenobiotic residue(s) and the physiological status of the fish. Potential elimination routes in fish include the gills, skin, kidney (urinary), and hepatobiliary (fecal) routes.

We hypothesize that the rates of xenobiotic elimination can be influenced by the biotransformation and elimination routes taken by the chemical, as well as by the circumstances of exposure, including physiologically or environmentally-induced changes in the organism (e.g., induction of biotransformation enzymes). Perhaps chemicals that only undergo either Phase I biotransformations or Phase II conjugations are eliminated more rapidly than those that undergo both Phase I transformations plus Phase II conjugation reactions. Elimination rates may also be faster for xenobiotics that are biotransformed and eliminated by the same tissue. Residence time and possibly toxicity of a xenobiotic would also be greater if a conjugated xenobiotic undergoes enterohepatic recirculation, in which the conjugated xenobiotic is deconjugated in the small intestine and reabsorbed as the parent form back into the systemic circulation. The xenobiotic can then be delivered to locations where toxic interactions with receptor tissues can occur and may be trapped in this enterohepatic circulation for extended periods of time. Finally, induction of Phase I and Phase II biotransformation enzymes could significantly increase the elimination rates of xenobiotics using these pathways, thus reducing their residence times. Clearly, potential differences in elimination rates exist, given these alternatives for biotransformation and elimination.

In order to test this hypothesis we designed and fabricated a physiological chamber that would separate xenobiotic elimination routes in fish. We present results of an initial study with this chamber, in which we characterized and quantified the elimination of pentachlorophenol by adult rainbow trout, with and without preexposure to pulp mill effluents.

MATERIALS AND METHODS

Fish

Adult rainbow trout (*Oncorhynchus mykiss*) were obtained from the Kontiolahti and Keskijärvi fish farms (eastern Finland). Trout were acclimated at 15 °C in flowing, nonchlorinated tap water for two weeks prior to experimentation and were fed daily *ad libitum* with trout chow (Ewos-Vaasa ST40, Suomen Rehu Oy, Finland) until 24 h prior to experimentation. Mean trout weights (± SD) were 456 (± 58) g for control trout (n = 4) and 580 (± 80) g (n = 3) for trout preexposed to diluted pulp mill effluents.

Chemicals

Radiolabeled pentachlorophenol (PCP) ([U-^{14}C]PCP) with a specific activity of 1.37 GBq/mmol and ≥ 98% purity was purchased from CEA/Cen Saclay Molécules Marquées (Gif-sur-Yvette, France). Working solutions of PCP (approximately 100 μg/kg) were prepared just prior to i.p. injection by evaporating the carrier solvent (toluene) under a gentle stream of nitrogen and reconstituting the residue with a small volume of absolute ethanol (50 - 100 μl). The ethanol solutions were diluted with saline (0.9% NaCl), so that the final solution to be injected into the fish contained ≤ 10% ethanol.

Untreated bleached kraft mill effluent (BKME) from processes using both hardwood (60%) and softwood (40%) was acquired from Kaukas Oy, Lappeenranta, Finland. A three-day composite sample was collected in plastic containers and stored in the dark at 4 °C until needed. This single collection provided sufficient effluent for the entire experiment, including preexposures and chamber exposures.

Effluent Preexposure

Trout were preexposed to diluted BKME in a 530-liter stainless steel tank for 2 weeks under flow-through conditions. Effluent was mixed with nonchlorinated tap water just before exposure to yield a 3.4% (± 0.4) solution of BKME. During the preexposure period, flow rates of diluted BKME to the exposure tank averaged 112 ml/min, with an average exposure temperature of 13.8 °C. Oxygen concentrations were maintained at 80 - 90% saturation and the pH of the preexposure water with BKME was 7.1. The primary toxic components of BKME, resin acids and chlorophenolics, were quantified by gas chromatography in composite samples of the diluted effluent (Table 1).

TABLE 1--Toxic Components of Diluted Pulp Mill Effluent (3.4%)

Component	μg/l
Resin Acids	
Neoabietic acid	3.7
Pimaric acid	5.7
Abietic acid	9.2
Isopimaric acid	9.5
Dehydroabietic acid	15.4
Chlorophenolics	
2,4,6-Trichlorophenol	0.08
Tetrachlorocatechol	0.12
Pentachlorophenol	0.15
3,4,5-Trichloroguaiacol	0.26
Tetrachloroguaiacol	0.26

Surgical procedures

Trout were anaesthesized with 100 mg/L MS-222 (3-aminobenzoic acid, ethyl ester, Sigma Chemical Corp., St. Louis, MO) and placed on a dry surgical table. The dorsal aorta was cannulated following the method of Soivio and Nynolm (1975). The cannula was filled with heparinized saline (1 mg/mL ammonium heparin, Sigma Chemical Corp.) and plugged with a hedgehog quill. An i.p. cannula was then inserted into the peritoneal cavity, secured with sutures, filled with saline, and similarly plugged. Cannulated trout were transferred to a recovery cage in nonchlorinated tap water (controls) or 3.4% BKME (effluent preexposed trout) for 12 to 18 hours. On the following day these trout were anaesthesized in a surgical bath with a more dilute solution of MS-222 (20 - 30 mg/L) and transected by severing the spinal cord just posterior to the operculae. Following transection urinary and fecal catheters were inserted and secured with sutures. Trout were then transferred to the physiological chamber to recover from the surgical manipulations and acclimate to the chamber for 12 to 18 hours before i.p. injection of PCP.

Physiological Chamber

A physiological chamber designed to enable the collection of xenobiotic elimination products was constructed of plexiglass with the following dimensions: 12 x 14 x 38.5 cm (Fig. 1). The chamber is divided into two sections, A and B, by a latex partition that is attached to the bottom and sides of the chamber and fits snugly around the trout's midsection just posterior to the operculae. Aerated water is continuously recirculated to sections A and B by a peristaltic pump. The approximate total volume of recirculating water in section A was 6700 ml and in section B, 6300 ml. An experimental temperature (± SD) of 11.1 (± 1.4) °C was maintained in the physiological chamber throughout the exposures.

The integrity of the latex barriers was tested (with and without trout present in the chamber) by adding methyl orange to the rear chamber (B) and analyzing the water in chamber A by UV-Visible spectroscopy for the presence of methyl orange after 8 - 12 h. No leakage was ever observed in random tests of the chamber.

After overnight acclimation in the chamber, trout were injected with radiolabeled PCP dissolved in saline via the i.p. cannula at the following calculated dosages: 121 ± 3 μg/kg for control trout and 124 ± 19 μg/kg for effluent-preexposed trout. The PCP was injected manually over 10 to 15 minutes, followed by a 0.5 ml saline rinse. The total injected volume was ≤ 2.0 ml.

Although BKME-preexposed trout were exposed to 0.15 μg/L PCP for 2 weeks prior to the experiment (Table 1), very little PCP is expected to be accumulated by these fish during the preexposure period. At the pH of the preexposure water PCP is 99.4% ionized; therefore, only 0.6% is available for gill uptake. Calculations of potential PCP uptake by BKME-preexposed trout over the 14-d preexposure period were made based on PCP uptake efficiencies for trout (McKim et al., 1986) and average trout respiratory volumes (Black and McCarthy, 1990; Black et al., 1991). Additional PCP uptake by BKME-preexposed trout was estimated to be 0.9 μg, less than 2% of the total amount of PCP injected into each fish.

Trout elimination routes were separated by the following barriers: urine and feces were collected by catheters; skin elimination products were measured in water samples collected from section B; and gill elimination products were measured in water samples collected from section A, which was corrected for skin elimination based on body surface area measurements. Water was sampled from sections A and B of the chamber at 4, 8, 12, 24, 36 (n = 4 controls) and 48 h (n = 2 controls) after the radiolabeled compounds were injected. The volume of feces in the fecal catheter was recorded at each sampling times. Urine was collected automatically by a fraction collector at 4-h intervals during the experimental period. All elimination products from control and BKME-preexposed trout were monitored for 36 and 24 h, respectively. Fecal and biliary elimination of PCP was also monitored in two control fish for 48 h. The experimental duration for BKME-exposed trout was shorter than for controls due to their reduced viability after 28 to 30 hours in the physiological chamber.

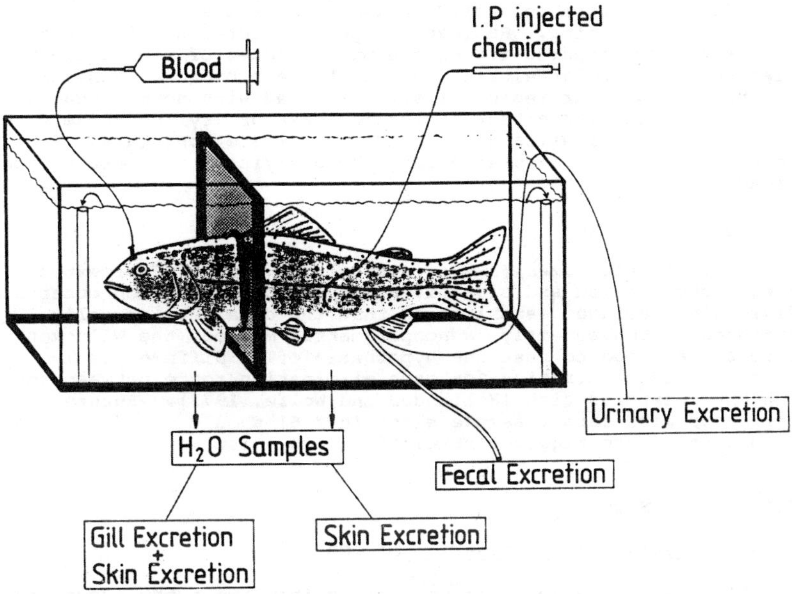

FIG. 1--The physiological chamber.

Compound Analyses

The total amounts of radiolabeled PCP and PCP biotransformation products in water, urine, and fecal samples were measured by liquid scintillation counting. Ten ml of scintillation cocktail (Luma Gel, Lumac Inc., Olen, Belgium) were added to water samples (5 ml), urine samples (0.1 to 1 ml), or fecal samples dissolved in 1 N NaOH (0.01 to 1 ml) and the ^{14}C activity was measured with a liquid scintillation counter (LKB-Wallac Rackbeta, Model 1217, Turku, Finland). Additional water and diluted urine samples (5 ml, in duplicate) were adjusted to pH 3.0 to 3.5 with phosphoric acid and extracted with toluene to separate and quantify the polar metabolites of PCP. The ^{14}C activities of the toluene (PCP) and aqueous layers (polar metabolites of PCP) were determined by liquid scintillation counting as previously described.

Conjugated biotransformation products of PCP in urine, bile, and feces were identified and quantified by enzyme hydrolysis followed by high performance liquid chromatography (HPLC) (Hewlett Packard Model 1050 HPLC, HP 1040A diode array detector, HP Hypersil ODS column) and scintillation counting of HPLC fractions collected at 1-minute intervals. Glucuronide conjugates (PCP-GA) were hydrolyzed by incubating a 20-μl sample, buffered to Ph 6.8 with 170 μl of 0.1 M phosphate buffer, with β-glucuronidase (isolated from *Escherichia coli*, Mannheim Boeringer) for 2 h at 37 °C (modified from Oikari and Ånäs, 1985). Sulfate conjugates (PCP-SO_3H) were hydrolyzed by incubating 20-μl samples buffered to Ph 5.0 with 170 μl of 0.2 M acetate buffer with arylsulfatase (isolated from *Aerobacter aerogenes*, Mannheim Boeringer) for 2 h at 37 °C (modified from Kukkonen and Oikari, 1988). Untreated and hydrolyzed samples were adjusted to pH 3 with concentrated phosphoric acid and were analyzed by HPLC. Pentachlorophenol and PCP conjugates were detected at 214 nm using a gradient mobile phase of acetonitrile (10 to 80% over 20 minutes) and phosphoric acid (pH 3). Eluent fractions were collected at 1-min intervals for 25 min for liquid scintillation counting. Radioactive peaks before and after enzyme hydrolysis were compared for each sample. Zones of radioactivity collected from a polar elution region that exhibited a quantitative shift to a less polar region (i.e., co-eluted with nonconjugated PCP) after hydrolysis with either β-glucuronidase or arylsulfatase were assumed to be the cleaved glucuronide or sulfate conjugate. Conjugate concentrations were calculated from the activities of these shifted radioactive peaks.

Statistical Analyses

Small sample sizes (n = 4, controls; n = 3, BKME-preexposed trout) for each observation and significant biological variation observed among individuals precluded establishing that the data were normally distributed. Consequently, a nonparametric method, the Wilcoxon rank sum test, was used to test the hypothesis of no differences in cumulative PCP elimination for each elimination route between control and BKME-preexposed fish (Hollander and Wolfe, 1973). Future experiments with larger sample sizes (n ≥ 6) should yield results amenable to a more rigorous statistical analysis.

RESULTS AND DISCUSSION

Biotransformation and elimination of PCP

Elimination routes--For control rainbow trout the predominant elimination route for PCP residues (nonbiotransformed PCP plus biotransformation products of PCP) during the first 24 h after injection was the gill, accounting for 40 to 60% of the total amount of PCP residues eliminated by all routes (Fig. 2a). Elimination via the skin was a minor route for the first 12 h; but became more predominant by 24 h and surpassed gill elimination of PCP at 36 h to become the major elimination route, along with fecal elimination. Urinary elimination of PCP by control trout was a fairly consistent, but minor route at all sampling times, accounting for 10 to 20% of the total elimination of PCP residues. Fecal elimination of PCP residues increased from 20 to nearly 40% of the total elimination during the 36-h experimental period and was one of the major routes of elimination by 36 h. At the end of the experiment, both feces removed from the anterior colon and bile contained large quantities of radiolabeled PCP residues (up to 2.6 μg PCP residues/g feces and 50 ng PCP residues/μL bile), indicating that fecal elimination should continue to be a major elimination route.

All elimination routes for PCP residues were also utilized by BKME-preexposed trout, but different patterns for elimination were detected compared with control trout (Fig. 2b). No single route of elimination predominated in BKME-preexposed trout during the initial 8 hours of exposure; although by 8 h and throughout the duration of the experiment, skin elimination was consistently the least utilized route, dropping to 10% of the total elimination by 24 h. By 12 h urinary and fecal routes were the major routes of elimination, with 34 and 28% of the total elimination, respectively. Fecal elimination continued to increase in prevalence and accounted for nearly half of the total

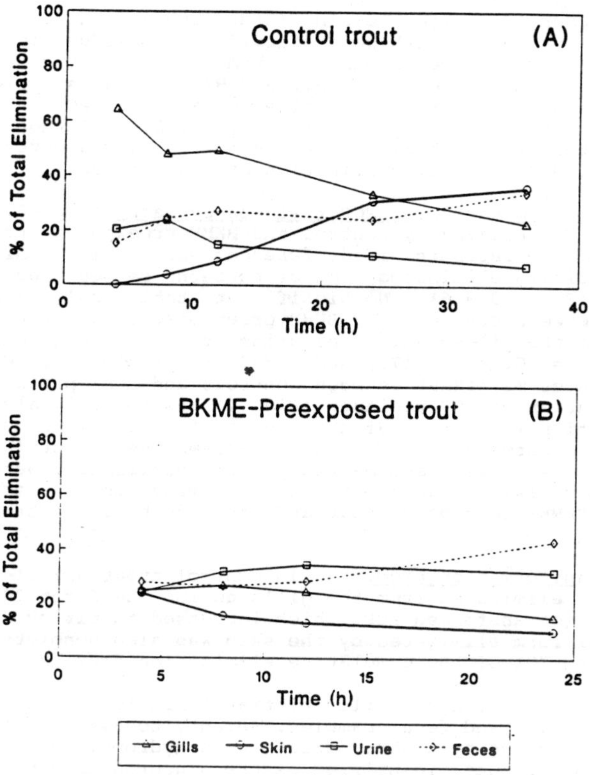

FIG. 2--Percentage elimination of PCP residues by all routes for control and BKME-preexposed trout at each elimination time.

elimination of PCP residues by 24 h, whereas urinary elimination appeared to have reached a plateau of approximately 32% of total elimination by 12 h, which continued for the duration of the experiment.

This study may be the first to isolate all possible four elimination routes for PCP or any other xenobiotic in fish. McKim and colleagues (1986) used a similar chamber combined with urinary and fecal catheters to separate the routes of elimination of PCP residues in trout; but did not measure skin elimination of PCP. In fact, skin is the most often ignored route in elimination studies; yet, as our results reveal, it may not always be a minor route, especially before significant hepatobiliary elimination begins. Naphthalene is also eliminated in significant quantities by the skin (Varanasi et al.,1978). Further elimination studies of additional compounds with the physiological chamber will enable a more accurate determination of the role of skin in the elimination of xenobiotics by fish.

Other studies have measured the appearance of xenobiotic residues in water and have hypothesized differential elimination due to physiological constraints. For example, Stehly and Hayton (1989a) assumed that fecal elimination of PCP residues was minor after a 64-h exposure because of evidence in some fish species that bile secretion (plus secretion of xenobiotic residues in the bile) into the small intestine may occur only after feeding (Eadsforth and Hutson, 1984). Because their experimental fish were starved, PCP residues measured in the water were assumed to be eliminated from the gills or kidneys (urine), and not from the feces (Stehly and Hayton, 1989a). In contrast, we measured significant fecal elimination of PCP in our study, even after 72 h without feeding. Clearly, physical isolation of elimination routes by our physiological chamber allows a more direct determination of differential elimination of xenobiotics.

Cumulative elimination of PCP residues by each route--Cumulative elimination of PCP residues by control and BKME-preexposed trout were compared by route to determine if differences existed in elimination rates, net quantities eliminated, and/or patterns between the two groups for each route (Figs. 3 - 6). No significant statistical differences were observed between controls and BKME-preexposed fish for PCP residue elimination from the gills, skin, and urine from 0 to 24 h (Wilcoxon rank sum test; $\alpha =$ 0.443, 0.171, and 0.343, respectively). However, pattern differences may exist between controls and BKME-preexposed fish for skin elimination of PCP residues (Fig. 4) and possibly also for urinary elimination (Fig. 5). Significant differences in cumulative fecal elimination between control and BKME-preexposed trout (Wilcoxon rank sums test, $\alpha = 0.022$), and marked pattern differences were also evident, with a striking increase in fecal elimination rate occurring after 12 h for BKME-preexposed trout and after 36 h for controls (Fig. 6).

PCP biotransformation products--In control trout 52% of the radiolabeled PCP eliminated from the gills during the first 24 h was composed of nonbiotransformed PCP, which increased to 61% by 36 h. The primary chemical form eliminated by the skin was also nonbiotransformed PCP, contributing 70% of the cumulative elimination from skin measured at 36 h.

On the other hand, hydrophilic biotransformation products predominated in urine and fecal samples. Seventy to 84% of the PCP eliminated in the urine by control trout was a hydrophilic biotransformation product, identified as the glucuronide conjugate of PCP (PCP-GA) in a limited number of samples. BKME-preexposed trout also primarily eliminated PCP via the urine as PCP-GA (avg = 91% eliminated as PCP-GA; 9% eliminated as PCP). Fecal samples from BKME-preexposed trout also contained mostly conjugated PCP, identified as the sulfate conjugate (PCP-SO_3H). No conjugate identifications were made in control fecal material, due to the addition of 1 N NaOH to dissolve the solids in the samples for scintillation counting. Because NaOH was determined to break conjugate bonds, neither extractions nor HPLC analyses could be successfully performed on control feces to determine the percentages of PCP and PCP conjugates.

Sulfate conjugates of PCP were also detected in the bile of control trout, along with PCP-GA and nonconjugated PCP. An interesting pattern was detected in the relative amounts of these three products analyzed in bile collected after two different elimination times in control fish (Fig. 7). In trout sampled at 36 h, significant quantities of nonconjugated PCP were detected in the bile, which constituted an average of 42% of the total PCP residues analyzed in the bile. Average percentages of PCP-GA and PCP-SO_3H in these trout were nearly equivalent, at 31 and 27% of the total PCP residues measured. Trout sampled at 48 h had markedly less nonconjugated PCP (avg = 4%), similar percentages for PCP-GA (avg = 32%), and much higher percentages of PCP-SO_3H (avg = 64%) in bile samples than found in trout sampled earlier. In comparison, conjugate concentrations in bile sampled from BKME-preexposed fish after 24 h were strikingly similar to the 48 h values for control fish, with averages of 5% PCP, 27% PCP-GA, and 68% PCP-SO_3H (Fig. 7).

The observations of distinct conjugation patterns in bile from all trout and the coincidence of an apparent accelerated elimination

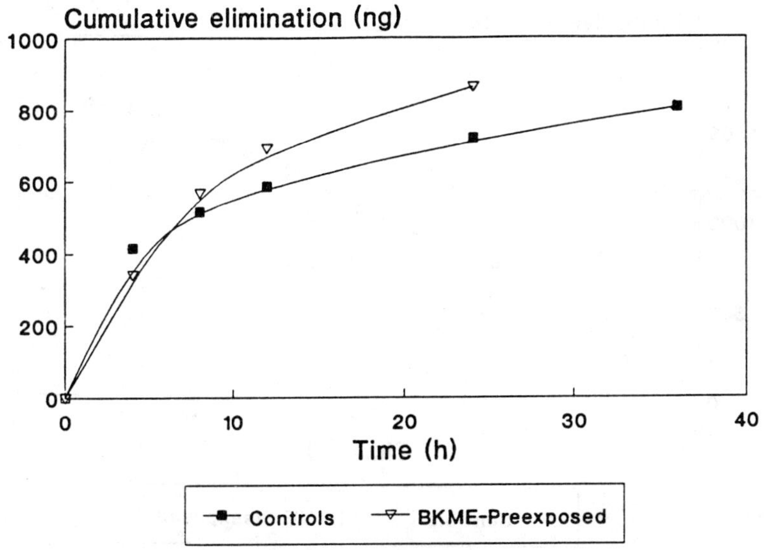

FIG. 3--Elimination of PCP residues by the gills of control and BKME-preexposed trout.

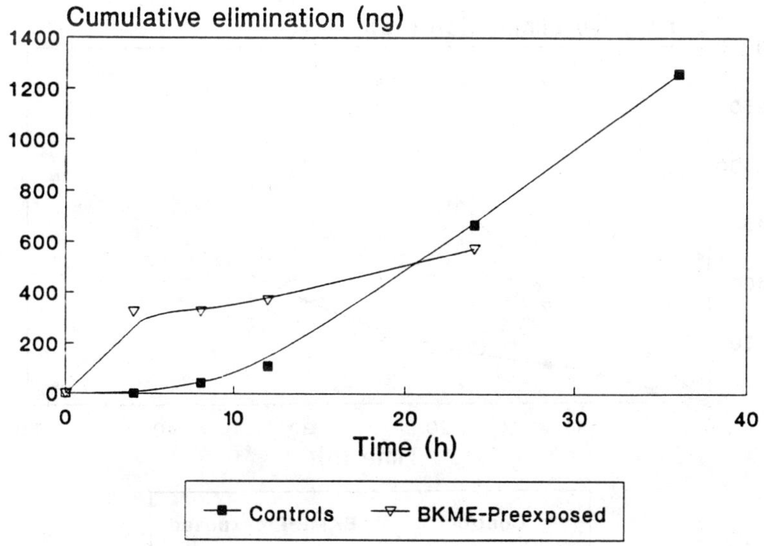

FIG. 4--Elimination of PCP residues by the skin of control and BKME-preexposed trout.

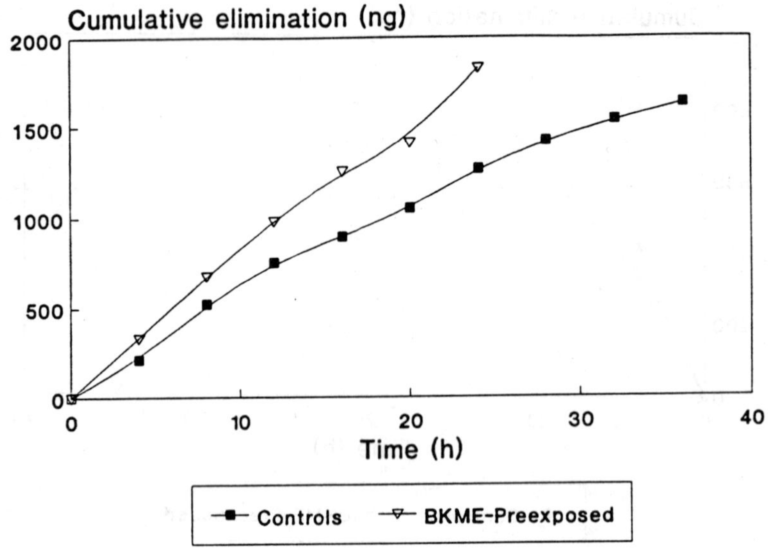

FIG. 5--Elimination of PCP residues via the urine of control and BKME-preexposed trout.

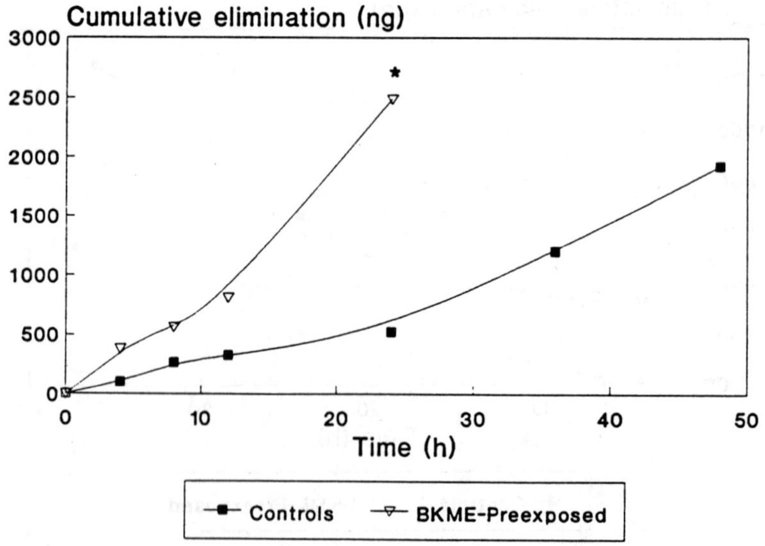

FIG. 6--Elimination of PCP residues via the feces of control and BKME-preexposed trout.

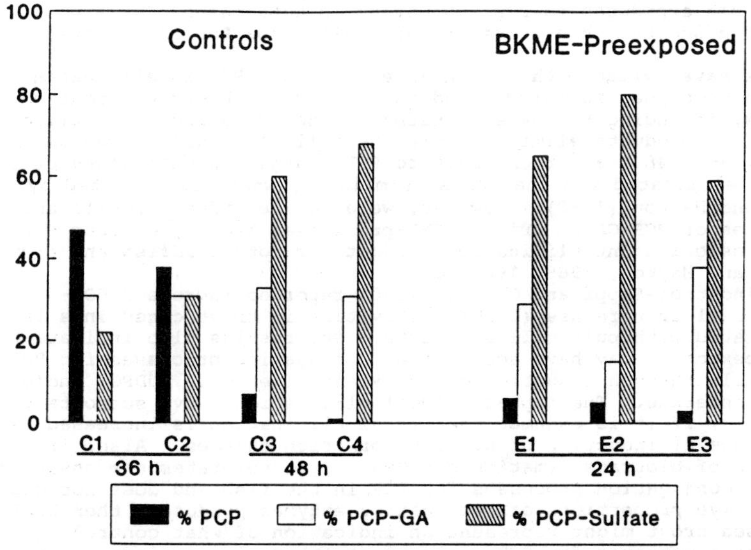

FIG. 7--Percentages of PCP, PCP-GA, and PCP-SO_3H identified in the bile of control and BKME-preexposed trout.

response in BKME-preexposed trout merit some speculation about possible biotransformation mechanisms for PCP in trout. Differences in the relative amounts of nonconjugated PCP, PCP-GA, and PCP-SO_3H measured in bile samples of control and BKME-preexposed trout may be due to reabsorption and enterohepatic cycling of nonconjugated PCP and hydrolyzed PCP-GA. Ultimately the reabsorbed PCP may be reconjugated to PCP-SO_3H, which would appear in bile prior to its elimination in the feces. The indication of a biphasic elimination curve for fecal elimination observed in BKME-preexposed fish also appears to support this hypothesis. From 0 to 12 hours the cumulative elimination curve for PCP residues is similar in slope to the control curve (Fig. 6). However, the slope (≈ elimination rate) from 12 to 24 hours in BKME-preexposed trout is three times that of the earlier time period (0 to 12 h for BKME-preexposed trout) and for the 0 to 36 h elimination in control trout. We also have limited data indicating that control fish exhibit a similar increase in elimination rate; however, in control fish this rate increase is not evident until 48 h, rather than at 24 h as seen in BKME-preexposed trout. Based on this data, the increased elimination rates appear to coincide with the increased appearance of sulfate conjugates in the bile. Furthermore, only the sulfate conjugate and parent PCP was detected in the feces of BKME-preexposed trout.

Others have reported detecting three forms of PCP residues (PCP, PCP-GA and PCP-SO_3H) in the bile of goldfish (*Carassius auratus*) (Stehly and Hayton, 1988) and rainbow trout (*Oncorhynchus mykiss*) (Stehly and Hayton, 1989a, 1989b) after exposure to PCP in water for 64 to 96 h. The sulfate conjugate was identified as the major elimination product released to water by goldfish, accounting for 81% of total PCP residues eliminated (Stehly and Hayton, 1988), and was the only metabolite released by trout (Stehly and Hayton, 1989a). No attempts were made to separate elimination routes, thus appearance of PCP residues in the water included elimination from the gills, urinary, and fecal routes. Kobayashi (1978) and Lech and colleagues (1978) report detecting only the PCP-GA and nonconjugated PCP in the bile of goldfish and trout after

48- and 8-h exposures to PCP. However, in both cases, PCP exposure times were shorter than those in which all three PCP forms were detected.

We have evidence that soon after exposure PCP is eliminated in both the unchanged form (PCP) and as hydrophilic biotransformation products, including PCP-GA eliminated in the urine and unidentified hydrophilic products eliminated via the gills and skin. Eventually (e.g., > 36 - 48 h after exposure to PCP) large concentrations of PCP-SO_3H are eliminated via the feces, similar to what was reported by Stehly and Hayton (1988). However, we also identified significant quantities of PCP-GA in urine (BKME-preexposed trout), whereas PCP-GA was an insignificant elimination product for both goldfish and trout (Stehly and Hayton, 1988, 1989a).

Lindström-Seppä and Oikari (1990) reported increased UDP-glucuronosyl transferase (UDPGT) activities in trout caged in a lake contaminated with pulp mill effluents. Our results also indicate that BKME-preexposure may have accelerated conjugation processes for PCP, most likely through induction of the Phase II enzymes, UDPGT and/or sulfotransferase. The biphasic fecal elimination curve supports this hypothesis, if it is assumed that fecal elimination is increased as a consequence of induction of biotransformation enzymes. Also, if induction of biotransformation enzymes only accelerates the onset of "normal" conjugation processes for PCP in the fish and does not change the relative proportions of conjugating enzymes produced, then BKME-preexposed trout might represent an indication of what control elimination patterns for PCP would be at later time periods. The similarity in the net proportions of PCP and PCP conjugates and the specific ratios of conjugates in bile collected at 48 h in controls and at 24 h in BKME-preexposed trout further suggest that this may be the case. Oikari and Ånäs (1985) found that bile collected from yearling rainbow trout exposed to 2% BKME for 30 days also contained similar ratios of PCP and PCP conjugates (4% PCP; 96% conjugates) as the 48 h controls and 24 h BKME-preexposed trout in our experiment. On the other hand, McKim and colleagues (1986) found a ratio of PCP:biotransformation products in rainbow trout bile after a 48-h PCP exposure that is more similar to values for our 36-h controls (45% PCP: 55% biotransformation products), than our BKME-preexposed trout. This would be expected because in McKim's study trout were exposed to waterborne PCP, which would result in a more gradual accumulation than would result from i.p. injection, due to the increased absorption and distribution times following the waterborne exposure.

This hypothesis could be tested further in future physiological chamber experiments by extending control elimination times to 72 or 96 h and measuring specific conjugate formation at those later times. Then conjugate formation by controls at 72 or 96 h could be compared to the conjugation pattern of additional BKME-preexposed trout at 24 h. Furthermore, analysis of UDP-glucuronosyl transferase and sulfotransferase activities in liver microsomes of fish exposed to BKME would also verify whether or not induction of these enzymes is occurring.

SUMMARY AND CONCLUSIONS

A physiological chamber was used to measure elimination of pentachlorophenol via the gills, skin, urinary, and fecal routes in control trout (PCP injected without preexposure) and BKME-preexposed trout (PCP injected after a 2-week preexposure to pulp mill effluents). Effluent preexposure significantly accelerated fecal elimination of PCP residues, and potential differences in urinary and skin elimination patterns were observed. Specific conjugated biotransformation products were identified in bile samples, and a consistent temporal pattern was observed in both control and effluent-preexposed fish, but was delayed in control trout. Our results suggest that effluent preexposure may affect PCP elimination rates by accelerating the formation of the sulfate conjugate in the liver. Our evidence for enterohepatic cycling of PCP residues may explain the delayed onset of significant fecal elimination of PCP. The results from this study demonstrate the utility of using the metabolism chamber for studying the mechanisms of xenobiotic biotransformation and elimination.

ACKNOWLEDGMENTS

We wish to thank Tiina Petänen and Riita Pietarinen for expert technical assistance and Jussi Kukkonen, John F. McCarthy, S. L. Burks and Margaret S. Ewing for valuable suggestions for the project and/or manuscript. This research was sponsored by the National Science Foundation Program for Long and Medium-Term Research at Foreign Centers of Excellence (# INT-8907738) and the Academy of Finland/Research Council for the Environmental Sciences.

REFERENCES

Andersson, T., Bengtsson, B.-E., Förlin, L., Härdig, J., and Larsson, Å., 1987, "Long-term effects of bleached kraft mill effluents on carbohydrate metabolism and hepatic biotransformation enzymes in fish," Ecotoxicology and Environmental Safety, Vol. 13, pp. 53-60.

Binder, R. L., Melancon, M. J., Lech, J.. J., 1984, "Factors influencing the persistence and metabolism of chemicals in fish," Drug Metabolism Reviews, Vol. 15, pp. 697-724.

Black, M. C. and McCarthy, J. F., 1990, "Effects of sublethal exposure to chlorine on the uptake of polychlorinated biphenyl congeners by rainbow trout, *Salmo gairdneri* (Richardson)," Aquatic Toxicology, Vol. 17, pp. 275-290.

Black, M. C., Millsap, D. S., and McCarthy, J. F., 1991, "Effects of acute temperature change on respiration and toxicant uptake by rainbow trout, *Salmo gairdneri* (Richardson)," Physiological Zoology, Vol. 64, pp. 145-168.

Eadeforth, C. V. and Hutson, D. H., 1984, "Formation of carbohydrate, sulphate, and other xenobiotic conjugates," Foreign Compound Metabolism, J. Caldwell and G. D. Paulson (eds.), Taylor and Francis Ltd., London, pp. 171-184.

Hollander, M. and Wolfe, D. A., 1973, Nonparametric Statistical Methods, John Wiley and Sons, New York.

Kobayashi, K. 1978, "Metabolism of pentachlorophenol in fishes," Pentachlorophenol: Chemistry, Pharmacology, and Environmental Toxicology, K. R. Rao (ed.), Plenum Press, New York, pp. 89-105.

Kukkonen, J. and Oikari, A., 1988, "Sulphate conjugation is the main route of pentachlorophenol metabolism in *Daphnia magna*," Comparative Biochemistry and Physiology, Vol. 91C, pp. 465-468.

Lech, J. J., Glickman, A. H., and Statham, C. N., 1978, "Studies on the uptake, disposition, and metabolism of pentachlorophenol and pentachloroanisole in rainbow trout (*Salmo gairdneri*)," Pentachlorophenol: Chemistry, Pharmacology, and Environmental Toxicology, K. R. Rao (ed.), Plenum Press, New York, pp. 107-113.

Lech, J. J., Vodicnik, M. J., and Elcombe, C. R., 1982, "Induction of monooxygenase activity in fish," Aquatic Toxicology, L. J. Weber (ed.), Raven Press, New York, pp. 107-148.

Lindström-Seppä, P. and Oikari, A., 1989, "Biotransformation and other physiological responses in whitefish caged in a lake receiving pulp and paper mill effluents," Ecotoxicology and Environmental Safety, Vol. 18, pp. 191-203.

Lindström-Seppä, P. and Oikari, A., 1990, "Biotransformation and other physiological responses in rainbow trout (*Salmo gairdneri* Richardson) caged in a lake receiving effluents of pulp and paper industry," Aquatic Toxicology, Vol. 16, pp. 187-204.

Mather-Mihaich, E. and Di Giulio, R. T., 1991, "Oxidant, mixed-function oxidase and peroxisomal responses in channel catfish exposed to a bleached kraft mill effluent," Archives of Environmental Contamination and Toxicology, Vol. 20, pp. 391-397.

McKim, J. M., Schmieder, P. K., and Erickson, R. J., 1986, "Toxicokinetic modeling of [^{14}C]pentachlorophenol in the rainbow trout (*Salmo gairdneri*)," Aquatic Toxicology, Vol. 9, pp. 59-80.

Melancon, M. J., Binder, R.. L., and Lech, J. J., 1988, "Environmental induction of monooxygenase activity in fish," Toxic Contaminants and Ecosystem Health: A Great Lakes Focus, M. S. Evans (ed.), John Wiley and Sons, New York, NY, pp. 215-236.

Melancon, M. J. and Lech, J. J., 1979, "Uptake, biotransformation, disposition, and elimination of 2-methyl naphthalene in several fish species," Aquatic Toxicology, L. L. Marking and R. A. Kimmerle (eds.), American Society for Testing and Materials STP 677, ASTM, Philadelphia, pp. 5-22.

Oikari, A. and Ånäs, E., 1985, "Chlorinated phenolics and their conjugates in the bile of trout (*Salmo gairdneri*) exposed to contaminated waters," Bulletin of Environmental Contamination and Toxicology, Vol. 35, pp. 802-809.

Parke, D. V., 1981, "Cytochrome P-450 and the detoxification of environmental chemicals," Aquatic Toxicology, Vol. 1, pp. 367-376.

Pritchard, J. B., Walden; R., and Oikari, A., 1991, "Dehydroabietic acid, a major anionic contaminant of pulp mill effluent, reduces both active *p*-aminohippurate transport and passive membrane permeability in isolated renal membranes," Journal of Pharmacology and Experimental Therapeutics, Vol. 259, pp. 156-163.

Soivio, A. and Nynolm, K., 1975, " A technique for repeated sampling of the blood of individual resting fish," Journal of Applied Biology, Vol. 62, pp. 207-217.

Stehly, G. R. and W. L. Hayton, 1988, "Detection of pentachlorophenol and its glucuronide and sulfate conjugates in fish bile and exposure water," Journal of Environmental Science and Health, Vol. B24, pp. 355-366.

Stehly, G. R. and W. L. Hayton, 1989a, "Metabolism of pentachlorophenol by fish," Xenobiotica, Vol. 19, pp. 75-81.

Stehly, G. R. and W. L. Hayton, 1989b, "Disposition of pentachlorophenol in rainbow trout (*Salmo gairdneri*): effect of inhibition of metabolism," Aquatic Toxicology, Vol. 14, pp. 131-147.

Varanasi, U., Uhler, M., and Stranahan, S. I., 1978, "Uptake and release of naphthalene and its metabolites in skin and epidermal mucous of salmonids," Toxicology and Applied Pharmacology, Vol. 44, pp. 277-289.

David Gruber[1] and Cathia Frago[2]

METHODS TO IMPROVE THE SENSITIVITY OF AN AUTOMATED BIOMONITORING SYSTEM

REFERENCE: Gruber, D., and Frago, C., **"Methods to Improve the Sensitivity of an Automated Biomonitoring System,"** Environmental Toxicology and Risk Assessment - Third Volume, ASTM STP 1218, Jane S. Hughes, Gregory R. Biddinger, and Eugene Mones, Eds., American Society for Testing and Materials, Philadelphia, 1995.

ABSTRACT: The biomonitoring system was designed to assess changes in toxicity of wastewater or surface water on a real-time basis using fish as the sensors. Previous research indicated that there were other responses in addition to the breathing rate which might be equally or more sensitive to changes in toxicity. These included fish activity (turns and episodes) and changes in the shape of the waveform generated as the fish breathes. To investigate the usefulness of these responses, four methods were used: strip-chart recordings, split-screen video techniques, Fast Fourier Transformation techniques, and a data replay software program. As a result of this research, the software of the biomonitoring system has been modified to include the additional responses which showed promise to increase the sensitivity of the system. Field testing of the system will be the next step.

KEYWORDS: biomonitoring, toxicity, fish, wastewater, coughs, turns, sensitivity, Fast Fourier Transformation

BACKGROUND

Biomonitoring systems use living organisms as sensors to assess water quality. Several automated biomonitors exist, but only few have evolved into models that can be used on-site and continuously. The main characteristic distinguishing these systems is the species of organism used as the sensors, which can be bacteria, algae, invertebrates, and fish. Of these systems, those monitoring fish behavior have been researched the most and have the greatest number of commercial applications (Gruber et al. In press). A fairly comprehensive review of the various automated biomonitors developed to date has been presented by Gruber et al. (In press), and Gruber and Diamond (1988).

The biomonitor used in the current research uses fish as the living sensors. Although much research has been conducted using waste water effluents, in the field, these biomonitors have successfully been

[1]President, Senior Scientist, Biological Monitoring, Inc., P.O. Box 184, Blacksburg, VA 24063.

[2]Environmental Engineer, Biological Monitoring, Inc., P.O. Box 184, Blacksburg, VA 24063.

used to monitor water quality at water treatment plant intakes. Our biomonitoring system has been used to rapidly detect toxicity problems in both water and wastewater. In addition, our research indicates that this system has the potential for being used as a predictor of the type of compound causing toxicity. However, problems such as clogging of the water distribution system due to the high turbidities typically found in wastewater, have occurred, in particular, when used on a continuous basis. To address this shortcoming, modifications to the system's valves and pipes are currently in progress. These include increasing the pipe diameter and/or replacing the presently used needle valves with ball or plug valves.

SYSTEM DESCRIPTION

Basically the system receives a continuous water source which flows through 8 to 12 tanks, each of which holds one fish. Figure 1 shows the basic set up of the biomonitor except that 12 tanks, instead of 8, were used. This entire set up is housed in a cabinet which is 61 cm long, 61 cm wide, and 183 cm high. The flow rate of the water into

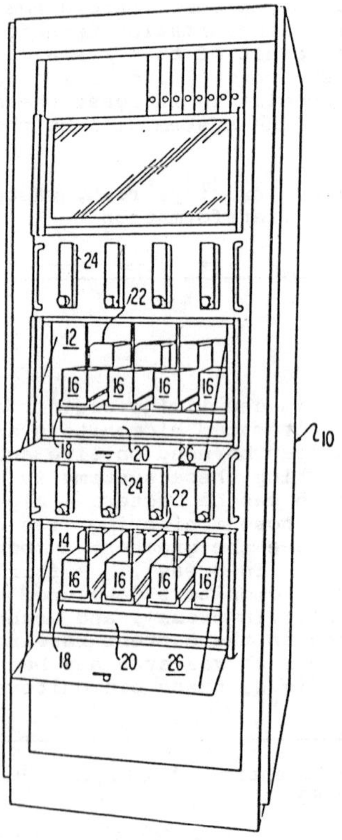

FIG. 1 - Physical layout of the biomonitor used in the experiments [reprinted from Gruber, 1992]. 10 biomonitoring housing; 12 & 14 monitoring modules; 16 exposure tank; 18 rack for four exposure tanks; 20 drain tray; 22 automatic fish feeder; 24 flow meter; 26 hinged door.

each tank is controlled by a flow metering valve. The tanks are arranged in groups of 4 in a module that has a hinged door so that the fish are kept in darkness during monitoring. Each fish is fed daily, except during experimentation, by means of an automatic feeder which sits on top of the tank.

Figure 2 shows a diagram of an individual fish tank. The glass tank is approximately 5 cm wide and 23 cm long. Water enters into the far right portion of the tank and then flows through the tank from right to left exiting through the standpipe on the far left end of the tank.

Each tank has 2 parallel stainless steel electrodes (labelled as # 52 and 54 in the Figure) which are about 9 cm apart, with the first electrode placed 3.5 cm from the front end of the chamber. The electrodes pick up the signal generated by the fish's bioelectric field. This signal, generated by the fish during breathing and other movements, is then filtered and amplified to make it more prominent. From the amplifier the signal is carried to either a strip-chart recorder or to the computer where it is continuously displayed on the monitor.

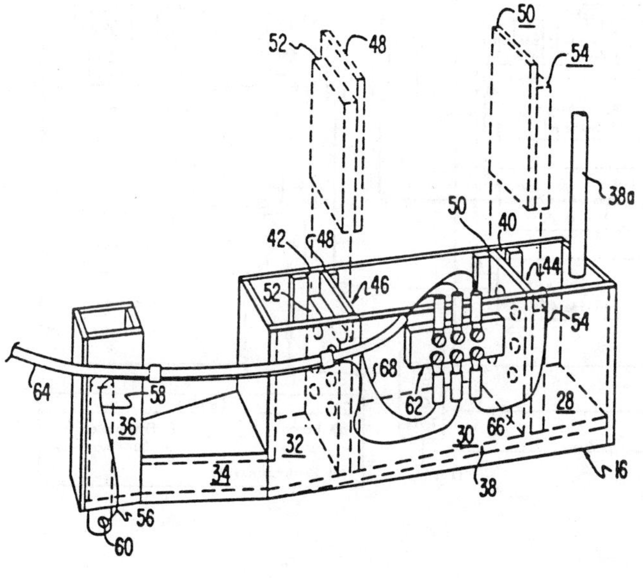

FIG. 2 - Fish (exposure) tank which houses one fish [reprinted from Gruber, 1992]. 16 exposure tank; 28 water inlet section; 30 area occupied by fish; 32 water outlet section; 34 tapered outlet; 36 water overflow section; 38 sloping floor of tank; 38a Teflon® tubing for water inlet; 40 & 42 slots for electrode assemblies; 44 & 46 electrode assemblies; 48 & 50 barrier plates of electrodes; 52 & 54 electrode plates; 56 standpipe; 58 grounding wire; 60 stainless steel screw; 62 terminal block; 64 cable to amplifier; 66 & 68 electrode wires.

conductivity, pH, dissolved oxygen, and temperature of water from one of the modules was continuously monitored and recorded.

Figure 3 shows the flow of water through the system as well as the pathway of the electrical signal from the fish to the computer and strip-chart recorder. In the experiment conducted as part of the current research, 4 fish received control water, 4 fish received a high dose of pollutants, and 4 fish received a low dose of pollutants. In addition, the conductivity, pH, dissolved oxygen, and temperature of water from one of the modules was continuously monitored and recorded. The organisms used in this experiment were Juvenile Bluegill sunfish, Lepomis macrochirus, less than 4.5 cm in length.

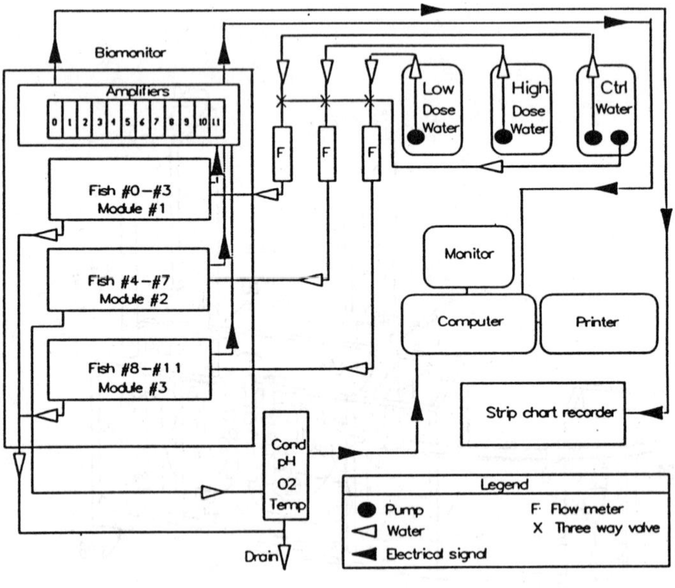

FIG. 3 - The biomonitoring system. Solid lines with white arrows depict water flow through the system. Dotted lines with black arrows depict the signal and data flow.

Figure 4 shows the typical signal which is seen on the strip-chart recorder or computer monitor during monitoring or experimentation. Each complete cycle represents one breath of the fish. Nineteen complete cycles or breaths are shown here. Prior to the current research, the software program was designed to assess the breathing or ventilatory rate of the fish to detect changes in water quality as follows.

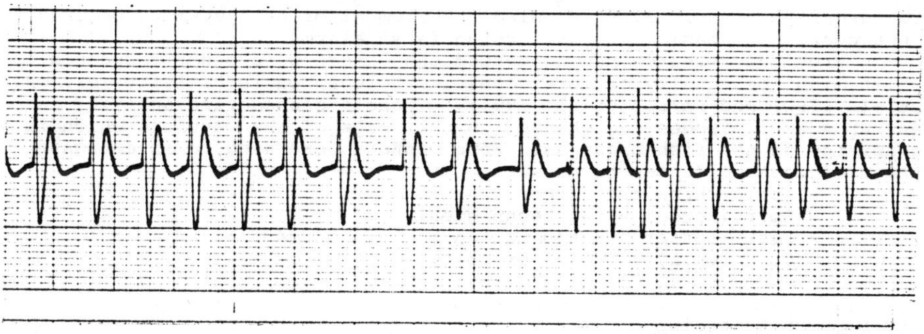

FIG. 4 - Waveform generated by fish under control water conditions.

First the user selects the number of minutes that will be used to estimate the ventilatory rate. This is called the assessment interval. The program is set up so that one minute is the shortest interval that can be selected. That is, data sampled at 30 times per second are averaged at intervals of at least one minute. These data, averaged at every minute are believed to give intervals small enough to give a good assessment of the fish's behavior while rendering a database which is manageable in size.

Second, the user selects the numbers of assessment intervals that will be used to determine the mean ventilatory frequency (or breathing rate). This is the sample size for statistical analyses.

Third, the user selects how many standard deviations will be used to define "the acceptable range" of the mean frequency.

Fourth, the user selects the number of fish that must be 'out-of-range' for an alarm to be generated.

For example, using an assessment interval of 10 minutes, a sample size of 6, and an acceptable range of 3 standard deviations, the following data here were generated during monitoring:

FISH #1 VENTILATORY RATE IN HERTZ (cycles per second)

@	1:50 PM	0.85
@	2:00 PM	0.97
@	2:10 PM	0.82
@	2:20 PM	1.14
@	2:30 PM	0.77
@	2:40 PM	0.95

For these data, the mean frequency is 0.91 hertz (Hz) and the standard deviation is 0.133. Thus, the acceptable range for the mean frequency is 0.511 to 1.309 Hz. If at 2:50 PM, the ventilatory frequency is 1.51 Hz, this value is 'out-of-range', and Fish #1 is designated as being in a "warning" state. If the number of fish in 'warning' is equal to the number selected for the out-of-range, then an alarm is generated.

Thus, prior to the current research only mean ventilatory frequency was used during monitoring.

MAJOR RESEARCH OBJECTIVES AND METHODS

The purpose of the current research was to: (1) improve the sensitivity of the biomonitoring system, so that it is sensitive enough to detect changes in water quality that might adversely affect the biota in a receiving stream or the safety of a drinking water supply, and (2), to assess the feasibility of using the biomonitoring system to be used on a continuous basis without causing false alarms.

Previous research had suggested that there were other responses which might be equally or more sensitive to changes in toxicity (Diamond et al. 1990, and Parson et al. 1991). These included fish activity such as turns and episodes and changes in the shape of the waveform which is generated as the fish breathes. Four methods were used to investigate the usefulness of these responses:

1 - Strip-chart recordings;
2 - Split-screen video techniques;
3 - Fast Fourier Transformation techniques; and
4 - Data replay software program.

Strip-chart Recordings

A total of 7 experiments were performed as part of this research effort. The experimental design was set up so that 4 fish received control water, 4 fish received a high dose effluent, and four received a low dose effluent. Four experiments utilized an industrial effluent containing various heavy metals. Table 1 shows the chemical analysis results for cyanide, hexavalent chromium, aluminum, cadmium, lead, nickel and zinc. These heavy metals were selected for analyses because they are part of the industrial discharger's National Pollutant Discharge Elimination Permit. Table 2 shows the concentrations and time to response of experiments A - D. Three experiments used a municipal waste water effluent, spiked with diazinon which is a commonly used insecticide, at a final concentration of 37.5 mg/L for the high dose, and at 18.75 mg/L for the low dose. Initially, all chambers had control water in them, causing the incoming effluent concentration to be diluted until enough time had been allowed for the control water to be completely replaced.

TABLE 1: CHEMICAL ANALYSIS OF EFFLUENT FOR EXPERIMENTS A, B, C, AND D

Sample	CN mg/L	Cr^{+6} mg/L	Al mg/L	Cd mg/L	Cr mg/L	Pb mg/L	Ni mg/L	Zn mg/L
A	<DL*	<DL	1.1	0.0026	0.058	0.079	0.048	0.130
B	<DL	<DL	0.5	0.0019	0.069	0.054	<DL	0.212
C	<DL	<DL	2.3	<DL	<DL	0.041	<DL	0.108
D	<DL	<DL	1.0	<DL	<DL	<DL	<DL	0.095
Detection Limit	0.02	0.05	0.1	0.0001	0.001	0.001	0.001	0.005

*<DL = Less than the detection limit

In all of these experiments, significant changes in the ventilatory frequency occurred within 1/2 hour after exposure to the effluents. As shown in table 2, the time to a response to heavy metals ranged from 3 to 11 minutes for fish exposed to the high dose, and from 3 to 29 minutes for fish exposed to the low dose. For the diazinon experiments, the time to a response ranged from 3 - 10 minutes for the high dose and from 4 - 6 minutes for the low dose (table 3). These results imply that the biomonitoring system can respond to toxic compounds in the water in a relatively short period of time, especially when compared with traditional toxicity tests that require a minimum of 24 hours to produce an answer.

TABLE 2: TIME TO RESPONSE USING VENTILATORY FREQUENCY - HEAVY METALS

Experiment	Time to Response in Minutes (Concentration at Response)	
	High Dose	Low Dose
A	9 (37% effluent)	3 (12.5% effluent)
B	7 (32% effluent)	7 (16% effluent)
C	3 (25% effluent)	4 (12.5% effluent)
D	11 (38% effluent)	29 (47% effluent)

TABLE 3: TIME TO RESPONSE USING VENTILATORY FREQUENCY - DIAZINON

Experiment	Time to Response in Minutes (Concentration at Response)	
	High Dose	Low Dose
E	3 (18.8 mg/L)	4 (9.4 mg/L)
F	10 (30 mg/L)	5 (7.5 mg/L)
G	6 (22 mg/L)	6 (11 mg/L)

Split-screen Video Techniques

The split-screen set-up is shown in Figure 5. It allows the researcher to simultaneously view and record the fish within the monitoring chamber and the strip-chart recording of the waveform generated as the fish breathes. This methodology has been very important because it allows the researcher to correlate behavior with changes or patterns seen on the strip chart. In turn, this enables the computer programmer to devise ways in which these changes in behavior can be automatically detected, counted, and assessed statistically. For example, when a fish lines up and faces the flow of water through the tank, the first part of the waveform is deflected upward. If the fish turns 180° and faces the opposite direction, the first part of the waveform is deflected downward. Electronically, this change in direction is detected by a change in polarity which is easily programmable. Once these changes were incorporated into the software, the split-screen video set up was again used, but this time the computer screen was observed simultaneously with the fish. This allowed the programmers to ascertain if the software was counting fish turns correctly, and if not, to modify the software accordingly.

In a similar manner, episodes were identified. An episode was defined as a series of very rapid movements by the fish which was characterized on the strip chart as a high amplitude, high frequency event. With the use of the split screen video setup, these episodes were documented as one or more coughs during which the fish reversed the flow of water over the gills. After seeing this pattern over and over again as the fish were exposed to pollutants (at subacute levels), software was written to detect and count them, and will be further investigated.

One of the observations that was noted during the experiments with

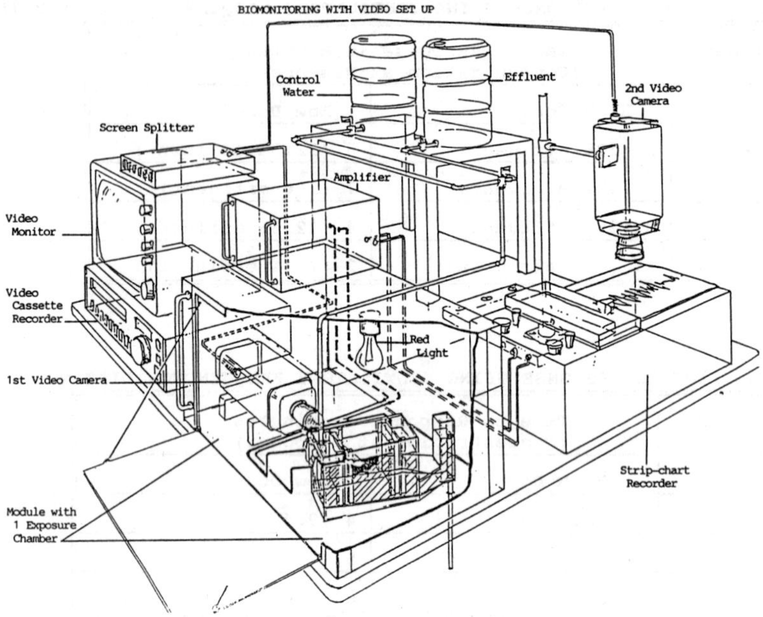

FIG. 5 - Setup of the biomonitoring split-screen video monitoring experiments.

the effluent containing several heavy metals was a double-peak on one half of the waveform. In Figure 6, the top strip chart shows the waveform of a fish receiving control water prior to exposure to about 25% wastewater effluent. The lower one shows the waveform after 37 minutes of exposure. This waveform is very regular, but the shape of one-half of the waveform has a double-peak unlike the waveform under control water conditions. This pattern was seen in every fish that was exposed to the effluent with heavy metals.

Other consistent patterns were seen during exposure to a municipal effluent which was spiked with diazinon. In Figure 7, the top portion shows the pattern after about 4 hours of exposure. The bottom portion shows the pattern after about 2.5 hours of exposure in a separate experiment but also with the diazinon-spiked effluent. In this instance double peaks were consistently seen on both halves of the waveform for all the experiments.

The question that was raised was "How could these changes be detected?" The method that was tried was Fast Fourier Transformation (FFT) Techniques.

Fast Fourier Transformation Techniques

FFT allows the transformation of spectrum data from the time domain to the frequency domain. A computer program was written so that 1-minute sequences of ventilatory data could be transformed as requeste

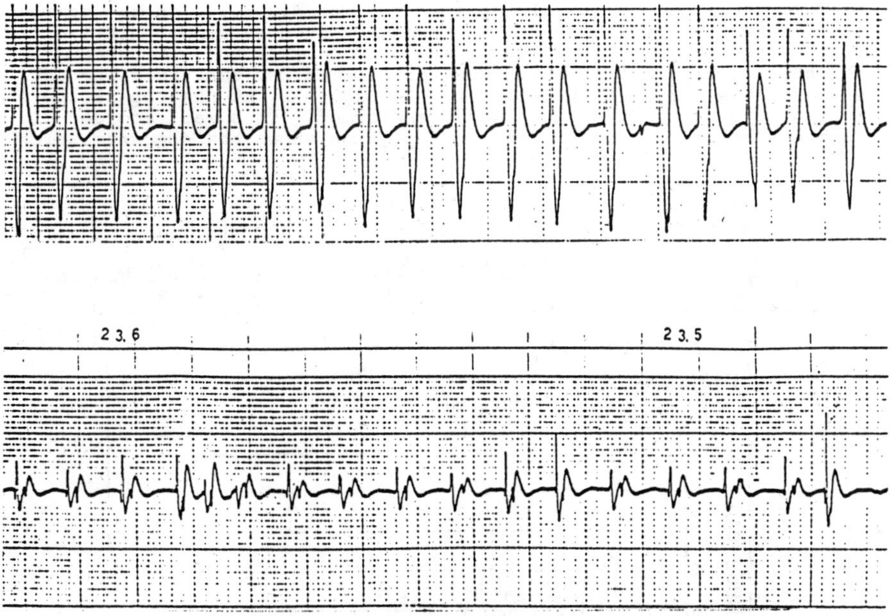

FIG. 6 - Top: Fish ventilatory waveform one minute prior to exposure to heavy metals. Bottom: fish ventilatory waveform 37 minutes into the exposure period. Note the consistency of the double-peak pattern.

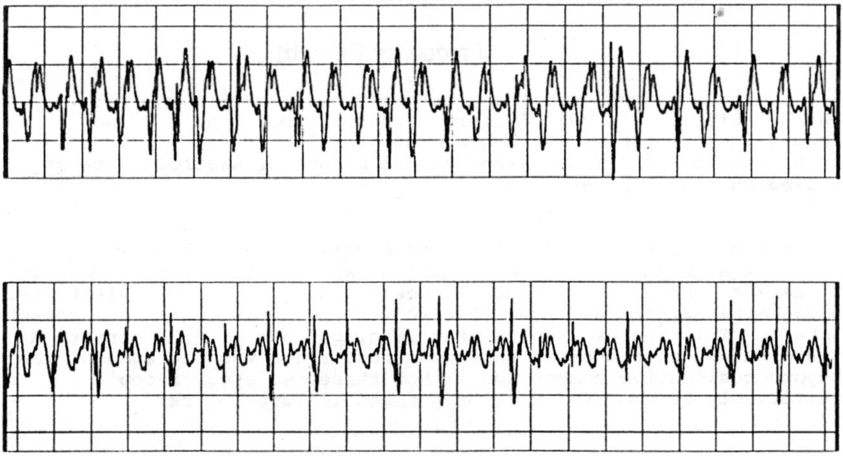

FIG. 7 - Fish ventilatory waveforms during diazinon-spiked effluent exposure experiments. Top: approximately 4 hours into the exposure period during April 30, 1992, experiment. Bottom: approximately 2.5 hours into the exposure period on May 8, 1992.

during monitoring. The resulting spectrum was displayed on the computer screen. A hard copy of the spectrum was obtained by simply hitting the 'print screen' key on the computer. A hard copy of the 1-minute ventilatory waveform data which was transformed was available through the use of the strip-chart recorder. In Figure 8, at the top is the one minute of frequency data which was transformed. This was recorded during control conditions. The lower portion shows the spectrum which

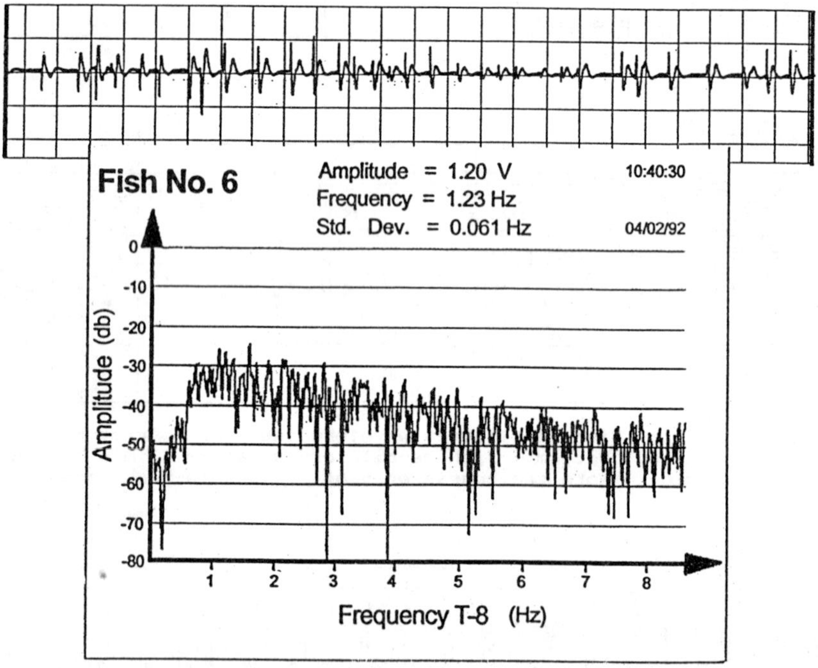

FIG. 8 - FFT of a normal waveform pattern. Top: the FFT was performed on this one-minute segment of ventilatory data. Bottom: spectral display of FFT performed on one minute of waveform data as displayed on the computer monitor.

was produced as a result of the FFT procedure. Figure 9 shows a spectrum of a one-minute sequence during exposure to the effluent with heavy metals. Note that the double-peaked waveform was prevalent during this one-minute interval. Qualitatively these two spectra look somewhat different. This approach looks promising, but due to time constraints of the grant which supported this research, there was not enough time to go beyond qualitative comparisons. How these two spectra could quantitatively be compared will be pursued in future work.

Data Replay Software Program

This software program was written so that fish response data (ventilatory frequency, turn frequency, episode frequency, and waveform amplitude) could be saved during monitoring and then replayed after the experiment was finished. In this way the parameters used to generate alarms could be varied, and the results (time to an alarm) compared.

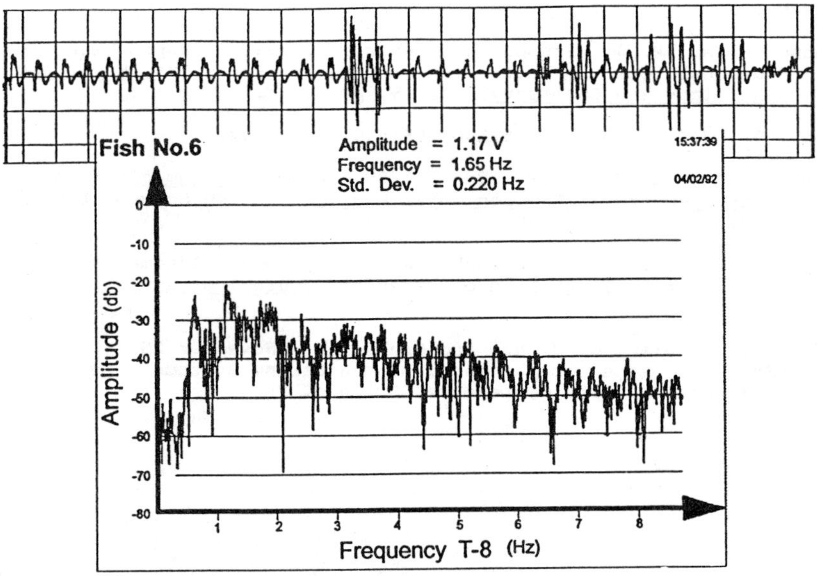

FIG. 9 - FFT of a double-peak waveform pattern. Top: FFT was performed on this one-minute segment of ventilatory data. Bottom: spectral display of FFT performed on one minute of waveform data as displayed on the computer monitor.

The data for each response type was "replayed" many times varying the assessment interval, sample size, acceptable range of the mean, and number of fish out-of-range or in warning for an alarm. In this way, the combination of parameters which made the system more sensitive were identified. Sensitivity was defined by the time to an alarm (want a rapid response) and number of false alarms (don't want alarms generated if there isn't any change in water quality or toxicity.)

CONCLUSIONS

The four methods described here have provided support to the original premise that there are fish responses, in addition to ventilatory frequency, which can be continuously monitored in order to assess changes in water quality. The next step will be to conduct field tests using the automated monitor to validate the usefulness of these additional responses under on-site monitoring conditions.

ACKNOWLEDGEMENTS

The authors wish to express their gratitude to the National Science Foundation's Small Business Innovative Research (SBIR) grant program (Grant No. III-9223109). Without this support, this present research effort would not have been possible.

REFERENCES

Diamond, J. M., M. J. Parson, and Gruber, D., 1990, "Rapid Detection of Sublethal Toxicity Using Fish Ventilatory Behavior", Environmental Toxicology and Chemistry, Vol. 9, pp. 3-11.

Gruber, D., U.S. Patent No. 5,140,855, 25 Aug. 1992.

Gruber, D. and Diamond, J.M., Eds., 1988, Automated Biomonitoring - Living Sensors as Environmental Monitors, Ellis Horwood Ltd., London.

Gruber, D., Frago, C., and Rasnake, W.J., In press, "Automated Biomonitors - First Line of Defense", Journal of Aquatic Ecosystem Health.

Parson, M. J., Diamond, J. M., and Gruber, D., November 10-14, 1991, "Research needs for Automated Biomonitoring Systems," Proceedings, AWWA Water Quality Conference, Orlando, FL.

Joseph W. Gorsuch,[1] Merrilee Ritter,[2] E. Raymond Anderson[3]

COMPARATIVE TOXICITIES OF SIX HEAVY METALS USING ROOT ELONGATION AND SHOOT GROWTH IN THREE PLANT SPECIES

REFERENCE: Gorsuch, J. W., Ritter, M. L., and Anderson, E. R., "**Comparative Toxicities of Six Heavy Metals Using Root Elongation and Shoot Growth of Three Plant Species,**" Environmental Toxicology and Risk Assessment - Third Volume, ASTM STP 1218, Jane S. Hughes, Gregory R. Biddinger, and Eugene Mones, Eds., American Society for Testing and Materials, Philadelphia, 1995.

ABSTRACT: Cucumber (*Cucumis sativus* L. var. Chicago Pickler), lettuce (*Lactuca sativa* L. var. Buttercrunch), and millet (*Panicum miliaceum*) seeds were exposed for seven days to six or more concentrations of cadmium (Cd), chromium (Cr VI), copper (Cu), manganese (Mn), nickel (Ni), and zinc (Zn). The responses of the germinating seeds, root lengths, and plant heights were compared. The procedure employs seeds exposed in pouches which are held in a vertical position to aqueous solutions of the six test metals at 22 ± 2°C in the dark.

Cucumber and lettuce are test species recommended by the U.S. EPA (FIFRA), U.S. FDA, and OECD for environmental assessments. Millet, a riverine species of the Midwest, has been used by the Illinois State Water Survey to evaluate environmental effects of chemicals and waste water effluents.

---

[1]Senior Environmental Toxicologist and Group Leader, Eastman Kodak Company, Environmental Sciences Section, Corporate Health and Environment Laboratories, B-306, Kodak Park, Rochester, NY, 14652-3617.

[2]Biostatistician, Eastman Kodak Company, Manufacturing Quality Assurance Organization, B-320, Kodak Park, Rochester, NY, 14652-3615.

[3]Chemist, Eastman Kodak Company, Environmental Sciences Section, Corporate Health and Environment Laboratories, B-65, Kodak Park, Rochester, NY, 14650-1818.

The endpoints chosen were the IC_{50} (concentration causing 50% inhibition of root elongation or of plant heights, in comparison to the control) value and the NOEC (No-Observed-Effect Concentration) value. Both endpoints were determined after 5 and 7 days exposure. Root elongation was the most sensitive measure of inhibition. Lettuce was the most sensitive species to chromium and cadmium and equally sensitive as cucumber and millet to the other four metals. Inhibitory effects were usually greater after 7 days exposure than at 5 days.

The results from this study are compared with those obtained by the Illinois State Water Survey, which used test solutions prepared from the same stock and exposed seeds from the same lot as those used in our trials in 10 cm disposable petri dishes containing Whatman No. 1 filter paper. IC_{50} values obtained in our study differed significantly from those obtained by the Illinois State Water Survey study. The reasons for these differences will be discussed in the paper.

KEYWORDS: phytotoxicity (bioassay), root elongation, lettuce, cucumber, millet, cadmium, chromium VI, copper, manganese, nickel, zinc

---

Several seed germination and root elongation methods have been used over the past three decades to evaluate the effects of chemicals, effluents, and contaminated soil elutriates on plants (Horowitz 1965; Kuboi and Fujii 1984; Ratsch and Johndro 1986; Myhill and Konzak 1967; Gorsuch et al. 1990; Linder et al. 1990; Wang and Keturi 1990). Cucumber and lettuce are test species recommended the the U.S. EPA (Holst and Ellwanger 1982), U.S. FDA (U.S. Food and Drug Administration 1987), and OECD (Organization for Economic Cooperation and Development 1984) for ecological hazard assessment. Millet has been used primarily by the Illinois State Water Survey (ISWS) (Wang 1985a, 1985b) since it has wide distribution in the midwest and is a major food source for waterfowl.

A comparative root elongation and early growth study was conducted between ISWS and Eastman Kodak Company (Kodak) involving three species of plants and their responses to six heavy metals to evaluate any differences between two methods of exposure of the plants. The six heavy metals were cadmium (Cd), chromium VI (Cr), copper (Cu), manganese (Mn), nickel (Ni), and zinc (Zn).

The pouch method (Gorsuch, et al. 1990) used in our laboratory, involved germinating seeds in vertically oriented pouches. The ISWS used a petri dish method (Wang 1987; Wang and Williams 1988), which involved germinating seeds in petri dishes horizontally oriented. In the Kodak study, the IC_{50} and NOEC values were determined after 5 and 7 days of exposure for both plant height and root elongation. The ISWS measured only root elongation after 5 days of exposure to test solutions.

The results of the Kodak and ISWS studies were compared to determine any differences due to methodology. The endpoints chosen for comparison were the IC_{50} (the concentration causing 50% inhibition of root elongation or plant height) value and the NOEC (No-Observed-Effect Concentration) value.

MATERIALS AND METHODS

Test Species

The species studied were cucumber (Cucumis sativus L. var. Chicago Pickler), lettuce (Lactuca sativa L. var. Buttercrunch), and millet (Panicum miliaceum). The two laboratories used seeds from the same lots. The seeds used in our studies, which were received from ISWS in plastic containers, were stored at -10°C when not being used. The seeds were treated with Chlorox™ at a 1:10 dilution ratio for 20 minutes, thoroughly rinsed with water, and air-dried. Cucumber root elongation from this seed lot was observed to decrease by 50% after 6 months of storage. No other abnormal findings from these seeds were observed.

Preparation of Test Solutions

Six metal stock solutions were prepared by ISWS from the following metal salts: $CdCl_2{\bullet}2H_2O$, K_2CrO_4, $CuCl_2{\bullet}2H_2O$, $MnCl_2{\bullet}4H_2O$, $NiCl_2{\bullet}6H_2O$, and $ZnCl_2$. Aliquots of the metal stock solutions were shipped to Kodak in plastic bottles and refrigerated until used. Some stock solutions were more than 6 months old before they were used. The pH of the test solutions was not altered. Diluent solutions were made at Kodak using distilled water and at ISWS using deionized water. Distilled water was used as the control solution in the growth pouch method. Seeds from the three plant species were exposed at Kodak to varying concentrations of heavy metals according to the following schedule:

Cd	Cr	Cu	Mn	Ni	Zn
		(mg of metal ion/L)			
643	100	462	600	170	500
386	60	278	360	102	300
232	36	167	216	61	180
139	22	100	130	37	108
83	13	60	78	22	65
50	8		46	13	39
30	5		28	8	23

The six metal stock solutions were analyzed on receipt by Kodak for the metal ions using Inductively Coupled Plasma (ICP) Atomic Absorption Spectroscopy. Test solutions were not analyzed. Test concentrations were based on stock solution concentrations.

Test Design

The root elongation and early growth effects tests were performed in seed-pack growth pouches (manufactured by Northrup, King, and Company) with the following conditions:

Plant Species:	Lettuce	Cucumber	Millet
Number of Replicates:	6 pouches	6 pouches	6 pouches
Number of Seeds/Replicate:	10 seeds/pouch	8 seeds/pouch	10 seeds/pouch
Light Conditions:	darkness	darkness	darkness
Temperature Conditions:	22 ± 2°C	22 ± 2°C	22 ± 2°C
Orientation:	vertical	vertical	vertical
Measurements Taken:	5 and 7 days	5 and 7 days	5 and 7 days

Seeds were equally distributed in the trough of the growth pouch and 20 mL of test solution or diluent water were added down the back side of the paper toweling, which served to moisten the seeds. The bottom of the pouch was gently raised to thoroughly immerse the paper in the solution. During an exploratory trial using the copper solution, chromatographic effects (a gradient of copper was observed on the paper, decreasing from top to bottom) were shown to occur unless the solutions were dispersed at the top of the pouch. Growth pouches were placed vertically in racks which were then placed in light-free chambers where they were incubated at 22 ± 2°C and 60 ± 10% relative humidity.

Measurements and Endpoint Calculations

After 5 days and 7 days exposure to the test and control solutions, plant height and root length were measured (to the nearest mm). At Day 5, pouches were removed from the growth chamber only long enough to obtain these measurements and then were returned to the dark until Day 7. Morphological changes and percent germination (radicle length = 0.5mm) were recorded. The IC_{50} values were determined by comparing the values of the treated plants with the mean of control plants. The NOEC value was determined to be the highest exposure level that was not significantly different from the control mean.

Statistical Methods

The data for each observation day were examined for outliers in each exposure group using Z scores and an alpha risk of 0.01. Outliers were removed from the data, and the remaining values for each replicate were averaged, yielding six responses for each exposure group. For each replicate, the mean of each exposure group was divided by the respective mean of the control group. This variable was analyzed by analysis of variance (ANOVA). If a difference was detected among the exposure means (alpha = 0.05), Scheffe's test was done to detect which means were different. ANOVA and Scheffe's test were also applied to the raw data to detect mean differences among the exposure and control groups.

If the control means were different from the exposure means (alpha = 0.05), the exposure means were plotted against the metal concentrations. Both linear and quadratic regression models were fit to the data. The IC_{50} values were derived from the better fitting model, which was determined by the R-squared value, parsimony, and analysis of residuals. Confidence bands which included the variation in the control means were calculated and plotted around the curves. The confidence limits for the IC_{50} values were read from the graphs of these curves. The NOEC values were determined using Scheffe's test.

RESULTS

Germination Response

No statistical differences were noted in percent germination among the three plant species for any metal concentrations.

Five Days of Exposure

Plant Height--The three plant species *(Table 1)* were most severely affected by chromium (lowest IC_{50} values) in both plant heights and root lengths. Plant height was generally less sensitive to exposure than was root length. IC_{50} values for cadmium and copper were above the exposure range for cucumber and lettuce. Millet height was enhanced (taller than millet control height) after exposure to manganese and zinc. IC_{50} values for copper were not estimable in this study for any plant. IC_{50} values for nickel using millet heights were not estimable. Millet, however, had the lowest cadmium IC_{50} value of the three plant species for plant height.

Root Lengths--Across the three species, chromium was most toxic, followed by nickel. The sensitivity to cadmium, copper, and zinc were approximately equal. Manganese had the least toxic effect of any metal on root lengths of all plant species. Toxicity was observed to decrease in the order **Cr > Ni > Zn = Cd = Cu > Mn.**

With regard to plant height among the species, cucumber and lettuce were generally more sensitive to heavy metals than was millet, except for cadmium. For root length, relative sensitivity among plant species was metal dependent, although some metals were equally toxic to all three plant species.

TABLE 1--Day 5 IC_{50} Values (mg/L) and [95% Confidence Ranges].

Plant Heights

Metal	Cucumber		Lettuce		Millet	
Cadmium	>800	[710-n.e.]	>800	[n.e.-n.e.]	190	[150-250]
Chromium	56	[49- 65]	55	[47- 65]	98	[83-123]
Copper	>600	[590->600]	>600	[595->600]	>600	[540-n.e.]
Manganese	635	[575-785]	750	[670-920]	enhancement	
Nickel	200	[164-n.e.]	175	[167-187]	>200	[n.e.-n.e.]
Zinc	530	[490-600]	820	[630-n.e.]	enhancement	

n.e. = not estimable from graph

TABLE 1 (contd)--Day 5 IC_{50} Values (mg/L) and [95% Confidence Ranges].

Root Lengths

Metal	Cucumber		Lettuce		Millet	
Cadmium	400	[350-460]	215	[175-275]	425	[380-485]
Chromium	57	[53- 62]	20	[18- 23]	39	[34- 44]
Copper	400	[342-500]	545	[435->600]	395	[310-580]
Manganese	630	[535-810]	643	[612-805]	783	[600-n.e.]
Nickel	124	[112-138]	101	[90-116]	127	[112-151]
Zinc	287	[275-315]	277	[218-n.e.]	525	[445-655]

n.e. = not estimable from graph

Seven Days of Exposure

Plant Height--The toxicity of copper to cucumber, lettuce, and millet increased from Day 5 to Day 7 ***(Table 2)***. Chromium remained the most toxic metal for the three plant species at Day 7, but no substantial increase in toxicity was detected when compared to Day-5 results. Millet continued to show enhanced growth from manganese and zinc exposures.

Root Lengths--Chromium was the most toxic metal for all plants, with a slight increase in toxicity from Day 5. Copper and zinc were more toxic to millet roots at Day 7 than at Day 5.

No consistent pattern of relative sensitivity to the six metals was observed among the three plant species for either plant heights or root lengths, although cucumber and lettuce were generally more sensitive than millet. Responses (percent inhibition) for plant heights and root lengths exposed to the six metals for 5 days and 7 days are presented in Figures 1-12.

TABLE 2--Day 7 IC_{50} Values (mg/L) and [95% Confidence Ranges].

Plant Heights

Metal	Cucumber		Lettuce		Millet	
Cadmium	700	[600->800]	>800	[750-n.e.]	330	[260-500]
Chromium	52	[47- 59]	57	[46-n.e.]	105	[85-142]
Copper	445	[390-530]]	560	[509->600]	565	[485-n.e.]
Manganese	666	[605-800]	995	[800-n.e.]	enhancement	
Nickel	not estimable		174	[164-198]	>200	[n.e.-n.e.]
Zinc	555	[450-745]	590	[490->720]	enhancement	

n.e. = not estimable from graph

TABLE 2 (contd)--Day 7 IC_{50} Values (mg/L) and [95% Confidence Ranges].

Root Lengths

Metal	Cucumber		Lettuce		Millet	
Cadmium	370	[320-430]	185	[155-235]	290	[245-350]
Chromium	34	[31- 38]	18	[15- 20]	29	[26- 33]
Copper	140	[122-160]	295	[210-n.e.]	280	[220-380]
Manganese	530	[480-610]	580	[505-682]	683	[575-895]
Nickel	116	[106-130]	91	[80-103]	132	[113-161]
Zinc	160	[145-180]	192	[157-252]	450	[392->500]

n.e. = not estimable from graph

DISCUSSION

Results from the ISWS study are compared to Kodak results in Table 3.

TABLE 3--Comparison of Day 5 Root Elongation Endpoints. Pouch Method Versus Petri Dish Method*

IC_{50} Values (mg metal ion/L)

Metal	Cucumber		Lettuce		Millet	
	Pouch	Petri Dish	Pouch	Petri Dish	Pouch	Petri Dish
Cadmium	400	15.0	215	2.4	425	11.0
Chromium	57	44.0	20	3.7	39	17.0
Copper	400	2.8	545	2.4	395	2.8
Manganese	630	65.0	643	35.0	783	140.0
Nickel	124	11.0	101	0.83	127	3.0
Zinc	287	30	277	11	525	64

NOEC Values (mg metal ion/L)

Metal	Cucumber		Lettuce		Millet	
	Pouch	Petri Dish	Pouch	Petri Dish	Pouch	Petri Dish
Cadmium	83	n.a.	83	n.a.	232	3.9
Chromium	22	n.a.	8	n.a.	13	4.7
Copper	167	n.a.	100	n.a.	100	0.7
Manganese	216	n.a.	360	n.a.	600	28
Nickel	61	n.a.	37	n.a.	61	1.4
Zinc	108	n.a.	108	n.a.	108	12

* Petri dish values according to Wang, 1987.
n.a. = not available

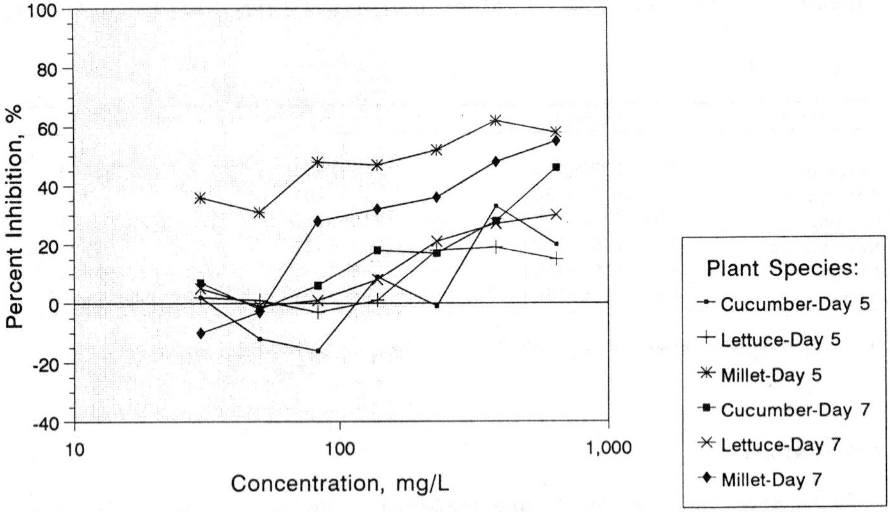

Fig. 1--Plant height responses of cucumber, lettuce, and millet to *cadmium* exposures at Day 5 and Day 7

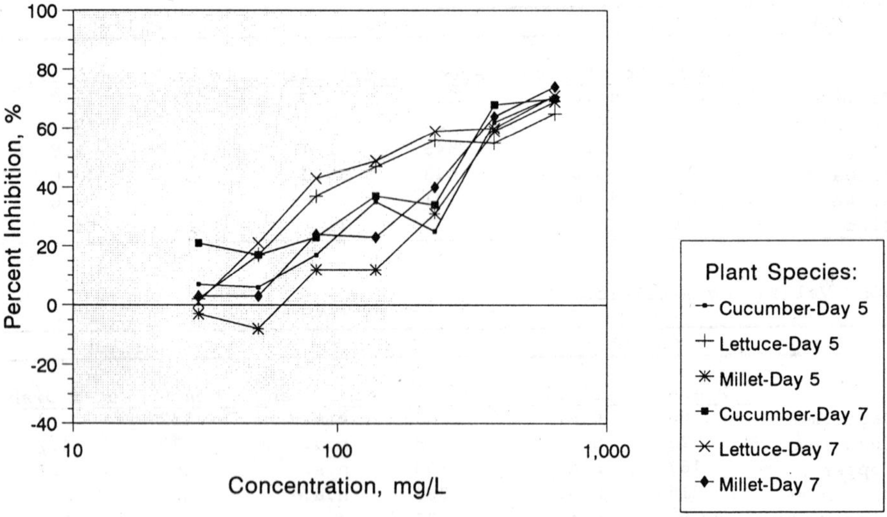

Fig. 2--Root length responses of cucumber, lettuce, and millet to *cadmium* at Day 5 and Day 7

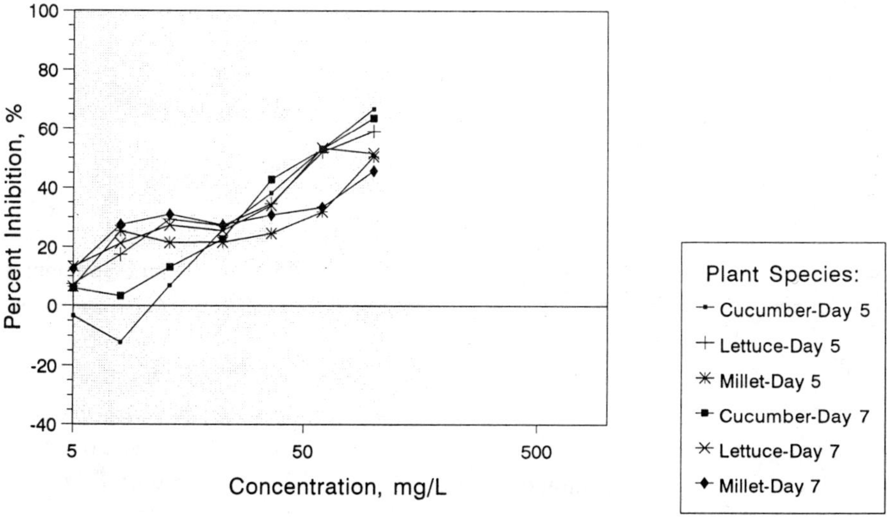

Fig. 3--Plant height responses of cucumber, lettuce, and millet to ***chromium*** exposures at Day 5 and Day 7

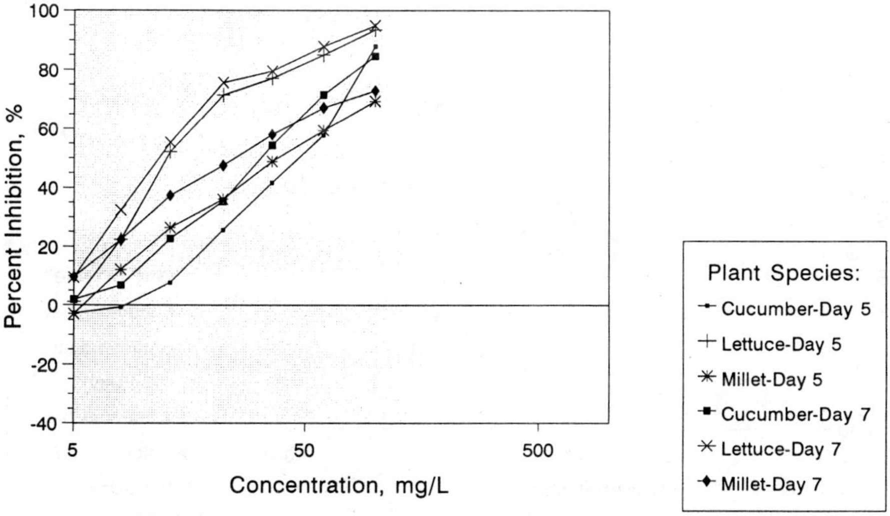

Fig. 4--Root length responses of cucumber, lettuce, and millet to ***chromium*** at Day 5 and Day 7

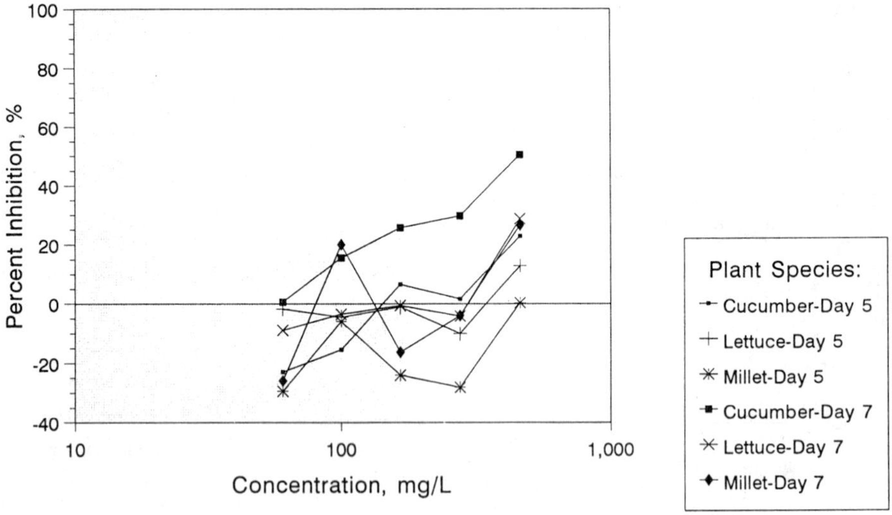

Fig. 5--Plant height responses of cucumber, lettuce, and millet to ***copper*** exposures at Day 5 and Day 7

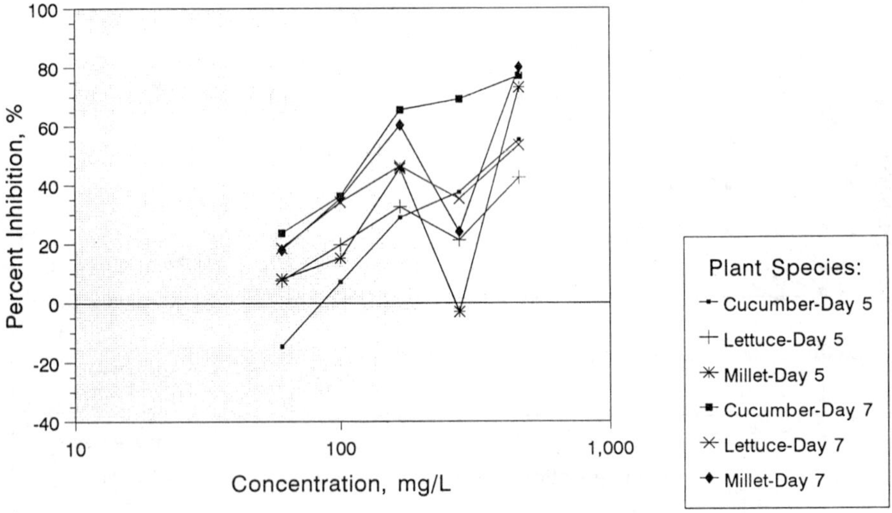

Fig. 6--Root length responses of cucumber, lettuce, and millet to ***copper*** at Day 5 and Day 7

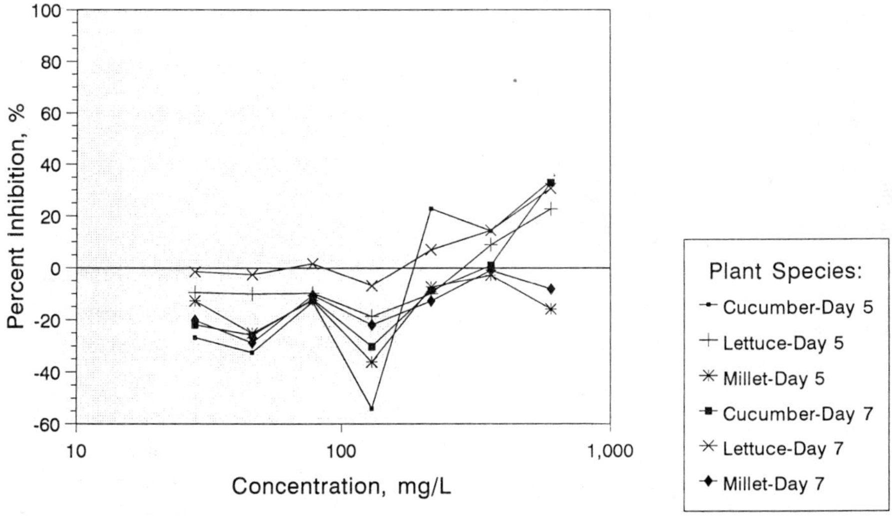

Fig. 7--Plant height responses of cucumber, lettuce, and millet to ***nickel*** exposures at Day 5 and Day 7

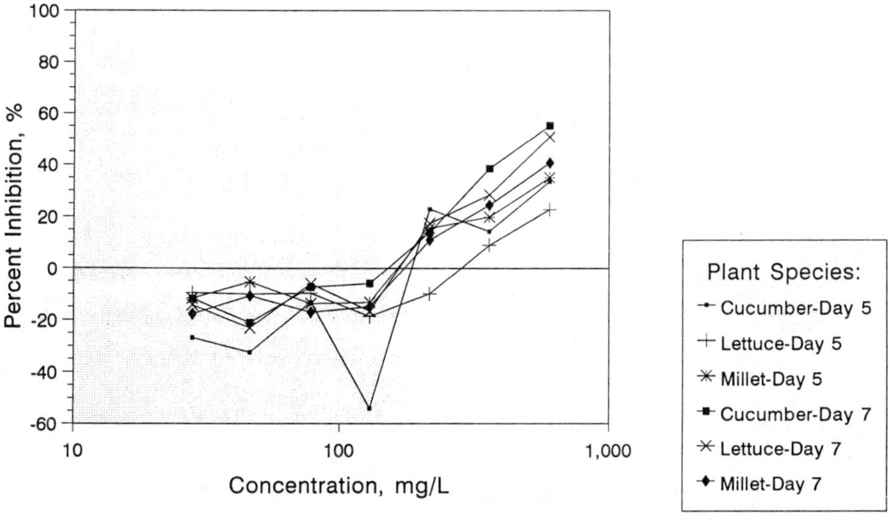

Fig. 8--Root length responses of cucumber, lettuce, and millet to ***nickel*** at Day 5 and Day 7

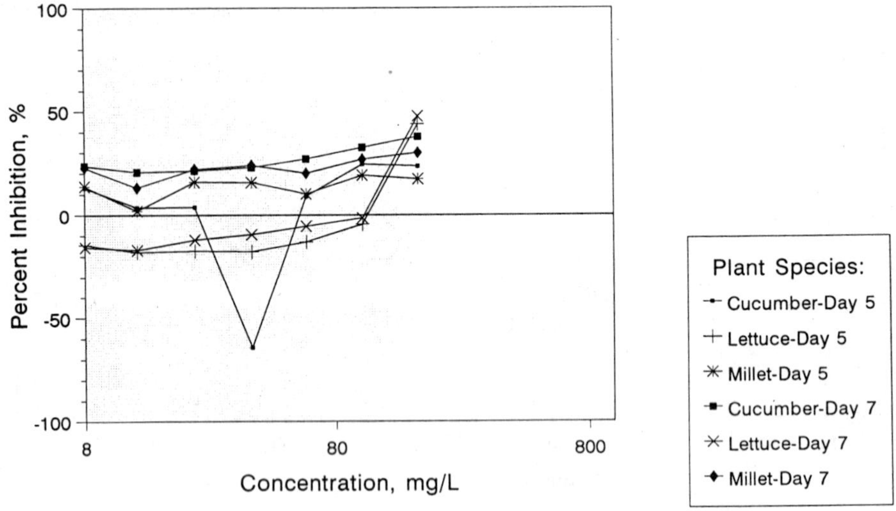

Fig. 9--Plant height responses of cucumber, lettuce, and millet to ***manganese*** exposures at Day 5 and Day 7

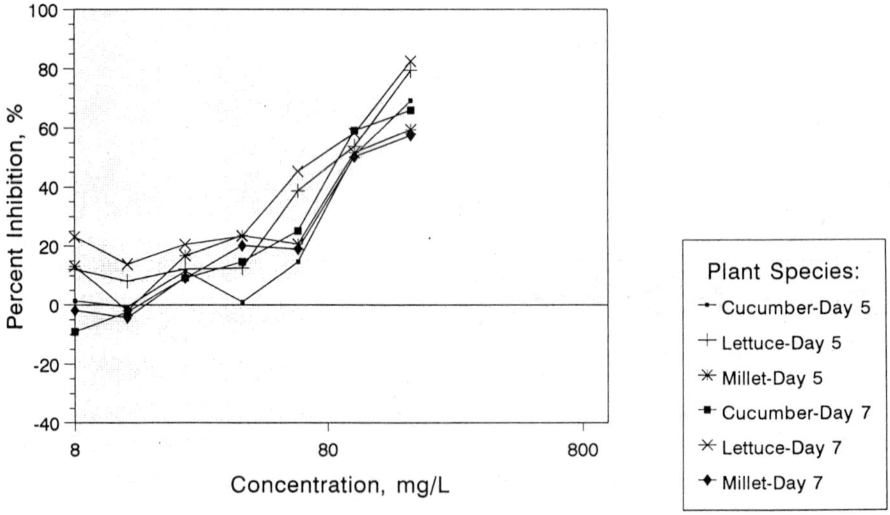

Fig. 10--Root length responses of cucumber, lettuce, and millet to ***manganese*** at Day 5 and Day 7

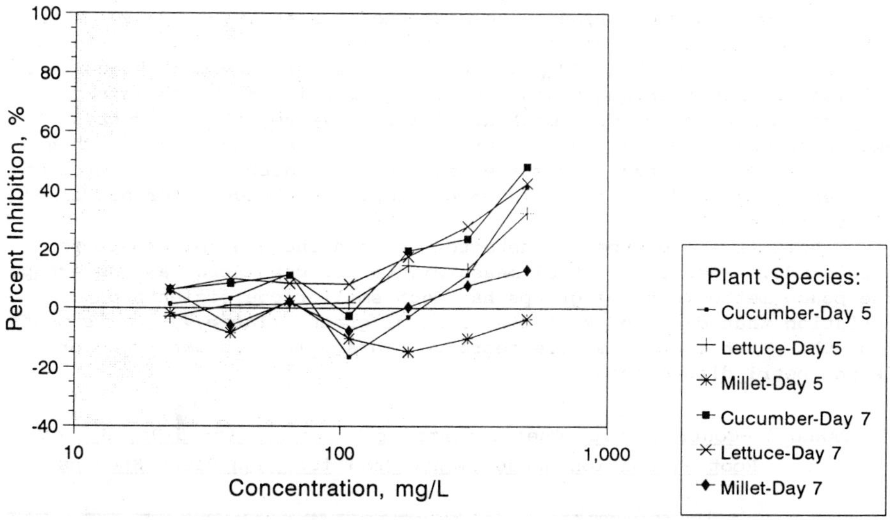

Fig. 11--Plant height responses of cucumber, lettuce, and millet to ***zinc*** exposures at Day 5 and Day 7

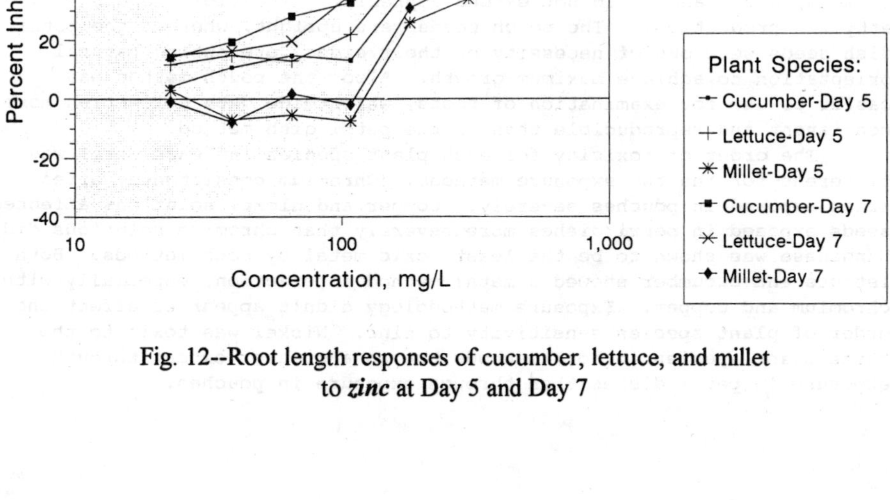

Fig. 12--Root length responses of cucumber, lettuce, and millet to ***zinc*** at Day 5 and Day 7

The most notable finding between the ISWS and Kodak data was the order of magnitude or greater differences in toxicity shown by the two methods. Both the 5-Day IC_{50} and the NOEC values were much higher for all metals except chromium and for all species in the pouch method compared to the petri dish method. The IC_{50} values for all metals except chromium were at least 1 or 2 orders of magnitude larger when using the pouch method as compared to the petri dish method. Chromium, however, responded similarly in both exposure techniques for all three plant species.

Another difference was detected between the control groups for each study. When the control measurements are considered as one group, the pouch method control groups had much smaller coefficients of variation than did the petri dish control groups ***(Table 4)***. This means that the pouch method is more reproducible and more robust to error than is the petri dish method.

TABLE 4--Control Group Coefficients of Variation for 5-Day Millet Root Elongation Measurements (mm) for Each Plant Species.

Plant	Pouch Method			Petri Dish Method*		
	mean	std	cv	mean	std	cv
Cucumber	75.4	14.8	20.1	55	30	55
Lettuce	44.1	11.1	25.1	42	15	36
Millet	66.2	20.8	31.5	45	28	62

* Petri dish values according to Wang, 1987.
std = standard deviation
cv = coefficient of variation

Generally, roots grew 37, 5, and 47% longer in the pouch method ***(Table 4)***, presumably because they had the room to grow along with assistance from gravity (geotropism), whereas the petri dish roots were crowded, bent, and could not extend appreciably (possibly leading to ethylene production). The pouch seeds were upright, whereas the petri dish seeds were out of necessity on their sides, preventing natural orientation to achieve maximum growth. Also, the pouch method was easier to use for examination of roots, which made data collection more consistent and reproducible than in the petri dish method.

The order of toxicity for each plant species and each metal was different for the two exposure methods. Chromium consistently affected seeds exposed in pouches severely. Copper and nickel solutions affected seeds exposed in petri dishes more severely than chromium solutions did. Manganese was shown to be the least toxic metal by both methods. Both lettuce and cucumber showed a metal-method interaction, especially with chromium and copper. Exposure methodology didn't appear to affect the order of plant species sensitivity to zinc. Nickel was toxic to the three plant species in both methods but to a greater extent through exposure in petri dishes than through exposure in pouches.

CONCLUSIONS

With the exception of chromium VI, the pouch method resulted in less toxicity to lettuce, cucumber, and millet from exposure to heavy metal solutions than did the petri dish method of exposure. Chromium was the most toxic metal tested by both exposure methods. There is an assay method-heavy metal interaction in toxicity, implying that it is very important to choose the best assay for the species or investigator bias will be introduced. The pouch method is more suitable for assay purposes than the petri dish method because of its ease of use and consistency of data. The pouch method is statistically more reproducible and is more robust to error than the petri dish method. The pouch method provides a more natural environment and is less constrictive to plant growth and development than is the petri dish method. The vertical growth allows for easy measurement of the roots.

The findings from the pouch method demonstrated that reduction in root length was the most sensitive plant response, followed by reduction in plant height. Germination response was not a sensitive measure of metal toxicity. Longer exposure (7 days vs 5 days) to metal solutions resulted in increased effects from some of the metals.

REFERENCES

Gorsuch, J.W., Kringle, R.O., and Robillard, K.A., 1990. "Chemical Effects on the Germination and Early Growth of Terrestrial Plants," Plants for Toxicity Assessment, ASTM STP 1091. W. Wang, J.W. Gorsuch, and W.R. Lower, Eds. American Society for Testing and Materials, Philadelphia, PA, pp. 49-58.

Holst, R.W. and Ellwanger, T.C., 1982. Pesticide Assessment Guidelines, Subdivision J, "Hazard Evaluation: Non-Target Plants," Office of Pesticide and Toxic Substances, United States Environmental Protection Agency, Washington, D.C.

Horowitz, M., 1965. "A Rapid Bioassay for PEBC and its Application in Volatilization and Adsorption Studies," Weed Research, Vol. 6, pp. 22-36.

Kuboi, T. and Fujii, K., 1984. "A New Method for Seedling Assay of Phytotoxic Substances: Liquid Shaking Culture," Soil Science and Plant Nutrition, Vol. 30, pp. 209-218.

Linder, G., Greene, J.C., Ratsch, H., Nwosu. J., Smith, S. and Wilborn, D., 1990. "Seed Germination and Root Elongation Toxicity Tests in Hazardous Waste Site Evaluation: Method Development and Application," Plants for Toxicity Assessment, ASTM STP 1091, W. Wang, J.W. Gorsuch, and W.R. Lower, Eds., Americam Society for Testing and Materials, Philadelphia, PA., pp. 177-187.

Myhill, R.R. and Konzak, C.E., 1967. "A New Technique for Culturing and Measuring Barley Seedlings," Crop Science, Vol. 7, pp. 275-276.

Organization for Economic Cooperation and Development, "Terrestrial Plants: Growth Test," OECD Guideline for Testing of Chemicals, No. 208, Paris, 1984.

Ratsch, H. and Johndro, D., 1986. "Comparative Toxicity of Six Test Chemicals to Lettuce Using Two Root Elongation Test Methods," Journal of Environment Monitoring Assessment, Vol. 6, pp. 267-276.

U.S. Food and Drug Administration, "Seed Germination and Root Elongation," FDA Environmental Assessment Technical Guide No. 4.06, Center for Food Safety and Applied Nutrition and Center for Veterinary Medicine, U.S. Department of Health and Human Services, Washington, D.C.

Wang, W., 1985a. "The Use of Plant Seeds in Toxicity Tests of Phenolic Compounds," Environment International, Vol. 11, pp. 49-55.

Wang, W., 1985b. "Use of Millet Root Elongation for Toxicity Tests of Phenolic Compounds," Environment International Vol. 11:49-55.

Wang. W., 1987. "Root Elongation Method for Toxicity Testing of Organic and Inorganic Pollutants," Environmental Toxicology and Chemistry, Vol. 6, pp. 409-414.

Wang, W., and Williams, J.M., 1988. "Screening and Biomonitoring of Industrial Effluents Using Phytotoxicity Tests," Environmental Toxicology and Chemistry, Vol. 7:(8), pp. 645-652.

Wang, W., and Keturi, P.H., 1990. "Comparative Seed Germination Tests Using Ten Plant Species for Toxicity Assessment of a Metal Engraving Effluent Sample," Water, Air, and Soil Pollution, Vol. 52, pp. 369-376.

Allen M. Nielsen,[1] Paul A. Filler,[1] John E. Heinze,[1] and Thomas M. Lachocki[1]

A MODIFIED ASTM SEMI-CONTINUOUS ACTIVATED SLUDGE TEST TO COMPARE NONIONIC SURFACTANT BIOLOGICAL REMOVAL

REFERENCE: Nielsen, A. M., Filler, P.A., Heinze, J.E., and Lachocki, T.M. **"A Modified ASTM Semi-Continuous Activated Sludge Test to Compare Nonionic Surfactant Biological Removal,"** Environmental Toxicology and Risk Assessment-Third Volume, ASTM STP 1218, Jane S.Hughes, Gregory R. Biddinger, and Eugene Mones, Eds., American Society for Testing and Materials, Philadelphia, 1995.

ABSTRACT: The Semi-Continuous Activated Sludge (SCAS) test of the ASTM "Standard Test Method for Biodegradability of Alkylbenzene Sulfonates" (D2667-89) was modified and used to compare the biological removal of new carbohydrate-based surfactants (CBS). The SCAS test was modified in three ways: the units were miniaturized, natural sewage replaced synthetic sewage, and analysis for dissolved organic carbon (DOC) replaced methylene blue active substance as the analytical method. The modified test distinguished between compounds that underwent minimal to complete biological removal by establishing a percent removal at a "steady state" (typically reached within two weeks). The method is inexpensive, easy, and efficiently compares biological removal of surfactants or other water-soluble compounds. This study shows that random substitution of hydroxyl hydrogens on glucose inhibits biological removal. In contrast specific regio-substitution at the 3-O or 1-O positions did not inhibit biological removal.

KEYWORDS: carbohydrate-based surfactants, SCAS test, biological removal, biodegradation, substituted glucose, acclimation

The SCAS test was initially developed by The Soap and Detergent Association (1965) for evaluating the biodegradation of surfactants by using analytical methods capable of detecting anionic and nonionic surfactants (The Soap and Detergent Association 1969). The ASTM slightly modified the SCAS test and adopted it as ASTM D2667-89. Several years later the Organization for Economic Cooperation and Development (OECD) significantly altered the SCAS test by utilizing a natural sewage background feed and using a nonspecific analytical method (DOC) to follow removal. It was adopted as "OECD Guidelines for Testing of Chemicals - Inherent Biodegradability: Modified SCAS Test". Guideline 302A, 12 May 1981. The OECD 302A guideline was adopted virtually

[1]Senior Research Scientist, Chemist, Research Manager and Senior Research Chemist, respectively, Research and Development Department, Vista Chemical Company, P.O. Box 200135, Austin, Texas 78720-0135.

unchanged by the United States Environmental Protection Agency in the Toxic Substances Control Act Test Guidelines as §796.3340 "Inherent biodegradability: Modified SCAS test", September 27, 1985.

The SCAS methodology has been used extensively to evaluate the fate of many chemicals upon exposure to sewage sludge. Examples from the literature include studies which determined the fate in the SCAS test of surfactants (Larson 1979; Naylor et al. 1988; Nielsen 1991); detergent builders (Vashon et al. 1982; King et al. 1980); commercial phthalate esters (Saeger and Tucker 1973; O'Grady et al. 1985) and hair care rinse conditioners (Waters et al. 1991). The SCAS methodology is also commonly used to develop acclimated microbial populations for other biodegradability studies (Larson 1979; Struijs and Stoltenkamp 1986).

Vista Chemical Company recently implemented a development program to investigate carbohydrate-based surfactants (CBS). It was anticipated that the overall fate in sewage sludge of numerous compounds would need to be estimated, and in response to this need the modified SCAS test described in this paper was conceived and implemented. The modifications were based on the concepts presented in the OECD 302A guidelines of using a natural sewage background feed and a nonspecific analytical method (DOC). The DOC removal characteristics of over fifty water-soluble compounds were determined with this methodology which proved to be inexpensive and easy to execute. Using this method it was noted that substitution patterns of the hydroxyl hydrogens on glucose did affect their DOC removal and apparent biodegradation characteristics.

EXPERIMENTAL METHOD

Test Compounds

The test compounds were synthesized or purchased commercially. All of the commercially obtained materials were high purity >99%. The compounds synthesized were generally 40 to 50 percent active; the organic portion of all the materials was > 80 percent active with many >95%. The nonactive portion was generally water, trace salts and unreacted sugar.

Biological Test System

A modification of the SCAS test of ASTM Standard Test Method for Biodegradability of Alkylbenzene Sulfonates (D2667-89), was used to screen the apparent biodegradability of over fifty carbohydrate-based surfactants. The test method was modified in three ways: (1) the units were miniaturized and built of glass rather than methyl methacrylate (Fig.1), (2) synthetic sewage was replaced by a domestic waste water, and (3) the methylene blue active substance analysis for anionic surfactants was replaced by the DOC analysis (EPA test method 415.1, Organics-Combustion or Oxidation Products, Environmental Monitoring and Support Laboratory, in Methods for Chemical

Analysis of Water and Wastes, EPA-600/4-79-020) a generalized analytical method for determining the loss of water-soluble organic compounds.

The modifications made it possible to operate twenty miniaturized SCAS units in a standard 5 foot laboratory ventilated hood over an extended period of time (approximately one year).

Since in our experience the use of synthetic sewage background feed (ASTM D 2667-89) has caused sludge settling problems, it was replaced with wastewater influent to the Anderson Mill MUD Wastewater Treatment Plant of Austin, Texas. The plant is an activated sludge system which treats about four million kg of residential and restaurant wastewater per day. Each day at approximately 10:00 a.m. the influent was collected, filtered through glass wool and used as background feed.

The activated sludge for the test was obtained from the aeration unit of the Anderson Mill plant and was sieved through a Number 200 ASTM E11 sieve (75 μm pore size) before use . The concentration of activated sludge in the SCAS units was maintained between 2000 and 3000 mg/L volatile suspended solids (VSS).

The daily protocol consisted of: (1) aerating the units for twenty three hours, (2) turning off the air and allowing the sludge to settle for thirty minutes, (3) removing the supernatant (effluent) for DOC analysis, and (4) replacing the supernatant with background feed containing the surfactant. The pH in the units ranged from 6.5 to 7.5. Dissolved oxygen (DO) levels sagged to 0.2 mg/L after addition of feed. DO levels recovered after 6 - 8 hours of aeration and were maintained at >4.5 mg/L for at least 16 hours of the 23-hour cycle.

DOC Analysis

Compounds were generally tested at 20 mg/L (active) which corresponded to 10 - 15 mg/L DOC, but concentrations were also increased two to three fold at various times during the test. Samples of the effluents (supernatants) were collected each day after the sludge has settled for thirty minutes. The samples were filtered through MILLEX®-HV[1] (0.45 μm) Durapore membrane filters, preserved with concentrated sulfuric acid (H_2SO_4) to <pH 1, and analyzed for DOC in a Model 700 Total Organic Carbon Analyzer manufactured by O.I. Corporation, College Station, Texas. The MILLEX®-HV filters do not contribute appreciable DOC (< 0.25 mg/L). The Model 700 analyzer removes the inorganic carbon by acidification and purging; it then treats the sample with sodium persulfate ($Na_2S_2O_8$) at 100 °C, purges, traps, desorbs and analyzes the released carbon dioxide (CO_2) as per EPA method 415.1.

---

[1]Millipore Corporation, Bedford, MA.

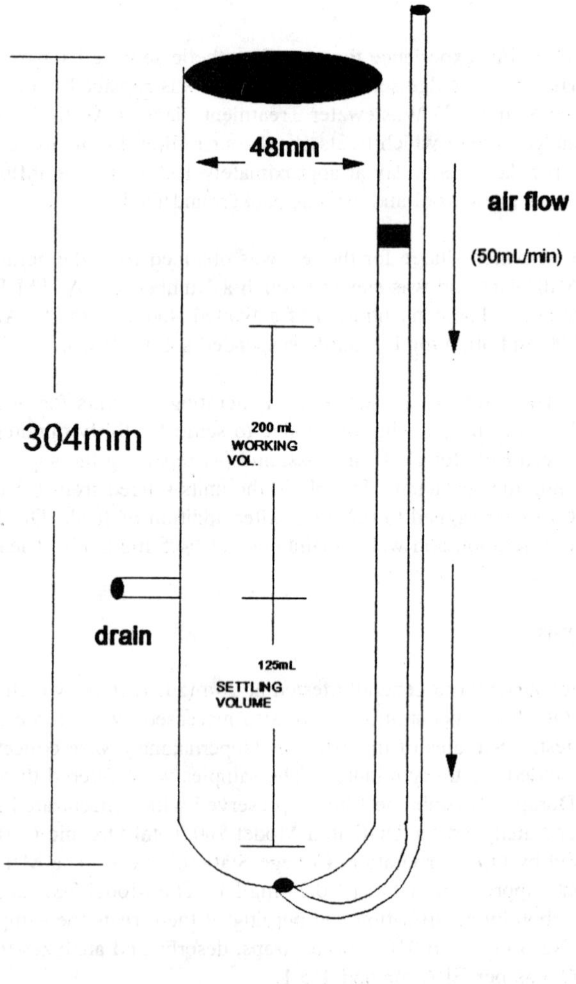

Fig.--1. Semi-continuous activated sludge aeration chamber

Percent Biological Removal

The daily percentage biological removal for a test compound was calculated according to the following equation:

$$\text{Removal (day x), \%} = [\,S_i - S_e)/S_i] \times 100 \qquad (1)$$

where:

S_i = the average DOC analyses of three distilled water solutions containing at least 20 mg/L (active) of the test compound and

S_e = DOC analysis of the effluent minus the average DOC values for the blanks (background feed only, no test chemical) .

Adsorption

Both biodegradation and adsorption contribute to the removal of soluble compounds in the Modified SCAS test. However, the amount of adsorption which occurred was not measured in this study.

RESULTS

Using a natural sewage background feed rather than a synthetic sewage feed maintained the excellent settling characteristics of the activated sludge unit (ASU) microbial populations over the 276 day testing period. The operation of the SCAS units was relatively trouble free and allowed for long-term exposure of over fifty water soluble surfactants to the natural population of sewage sludge microorganisms. It was, however, necessary to occasionally amend the units with fresh ASU sludge to maintain sludge VSS levels at 2000-3000 mg/L since the organic carbon levels in the background feed were low (30-70 mg/L DOC).

As further evidence that the units were functioning well, it was noted that a C_{12} LAS (linear alkylbenzene sulfonate) showed a 95.2% average DOC removal, and a standard deviation of 4.1% over the test period. This value compared well with the 92-93% DOC removal values reported for two commercial LAS samples in a SCAS test (Larson 1979).

The modified SCAS methodology appeared to separate the test compounds into three classes according to percent dissolved organic carbon removal (Table 1). A visual inspection of the data (Fig. 2) suggested that the average percent DOC removal values were clustered in three groups for test materials which showed high (≥ 87%), intermediate (≤ 87% - ≥ 10%), and low (≤ 10%) DOC removals in the modified SCAS

TABLE 1--Classification of Compounds by Modified SCAS Methodology.

Group	# Compounds	"Steady State" DOC LOSS, % (Average)	STD. DEV. % (Average)	Data Points (N) (Average)	% Rel. Error (Average)
Class I	16	97.4	3.92	17	4.07
Class II	30	33.2	8.99	16	30.6
Class III	6	4.75	11.75	29	817

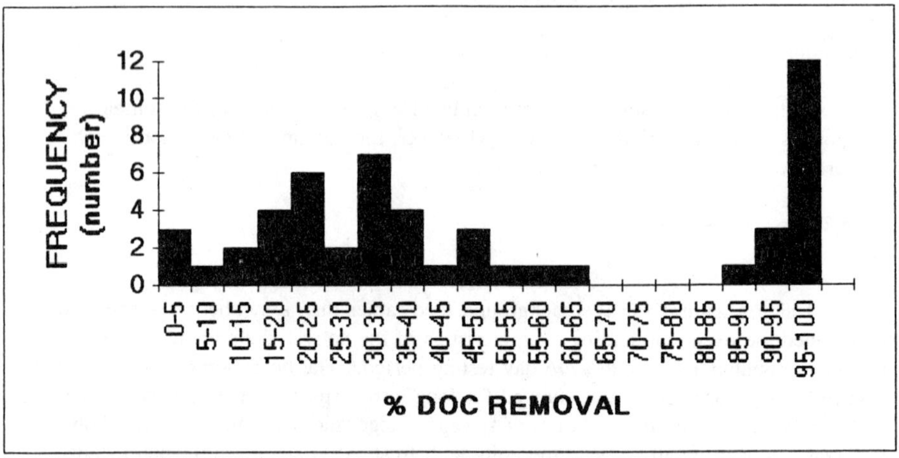

FIG. 2.--Distribution of % removal values.

test. Analysis of variance (Box et al. 1978) confirmed that the three classes were statistically significantly different from each other.

Those compounds in the first class showed a ≥87% average DOC removal during the "steady state" (the period after acclimation was completed). This high level of removal was usually noted immediately (Fig. 3 and Fig. 4), but three of the fourteen compounds in class I required an acclimation period from one to twenty days to reach this consistently high level of DOC removal as illustrated in Fig. 5 and Fig. 6 . Once "steady state" was reached, the class I compounds showed a consistently high daily DOC removal with a low level of variability (average standard deviation of < 5%).

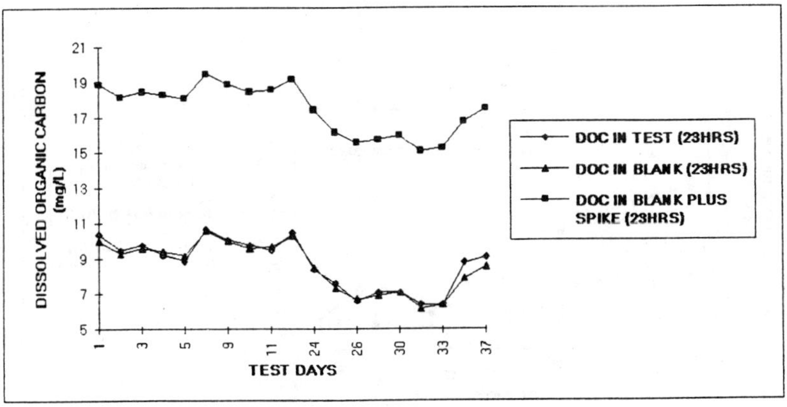

Fig. 3--A comparison of 23hr 3-O-methyl-alpha-D-glucopyranose DOC levels to 23hr blank and blank plus spike DOC values.

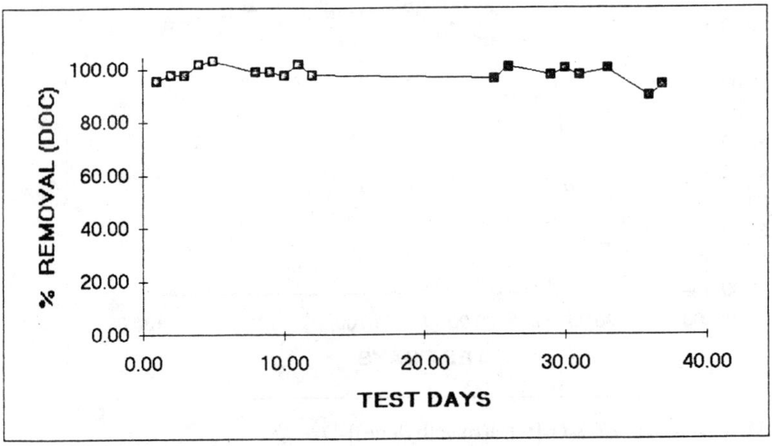

FIG. 4--DOC removal of 3-O-methyl-alpha-D-glucopyranose in modified SCAS test (by daily % removal).

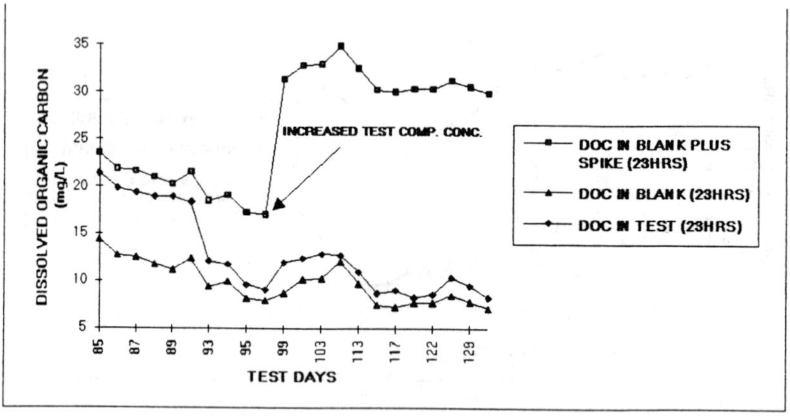

Fig. 5--A comparison of 23hr 3-O-[tetra(oxyethylene)]-D-glucopyranose DOC levels to 23hr blank and blank plus spike DOC values.

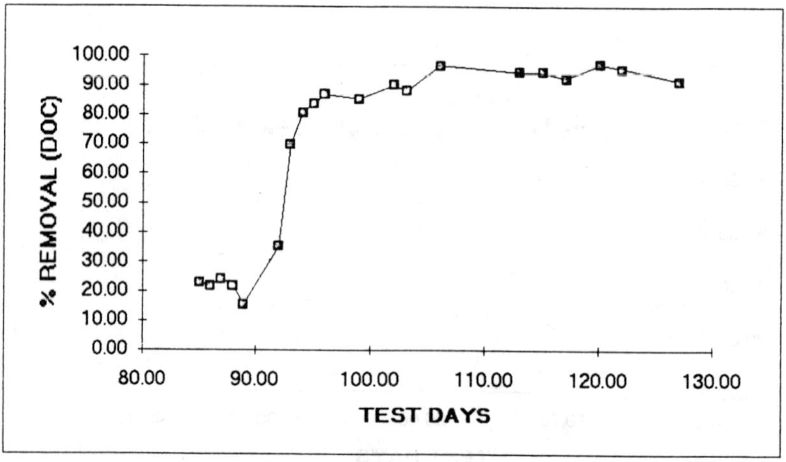

Fig. 6--DOC removal of 3-O-[tetra(oxyethylene)]-D-glucopyranose in modified SCAS test (by daily % removal).

The second class of compounds showed an intermediate range of DOC removals (≤ 87% - ≥ 10%). Acclimation to high average percent removals never occurred even if a class II material were tested for several months (Fig. 7 and Fig. 8). High variability was noted (9% average standard deviation).

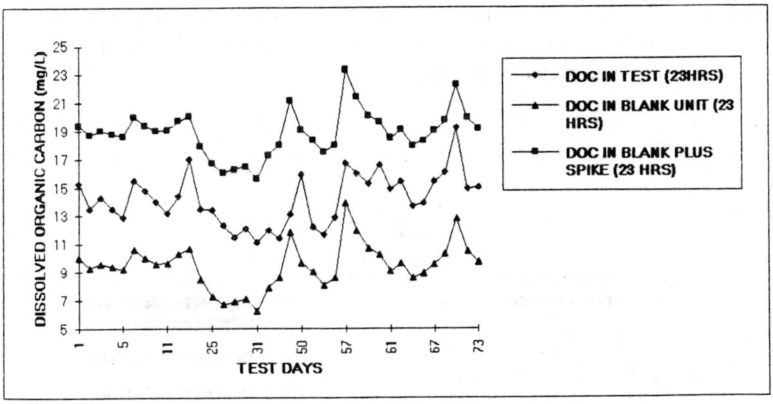

Fig. 7--A comparison of 23hr 2,3,4,6-ethoxylated (1.5 eq.)-methyl-D-glucopyranoside DOC levels to 23hr blank and blank plus spike DOC values.

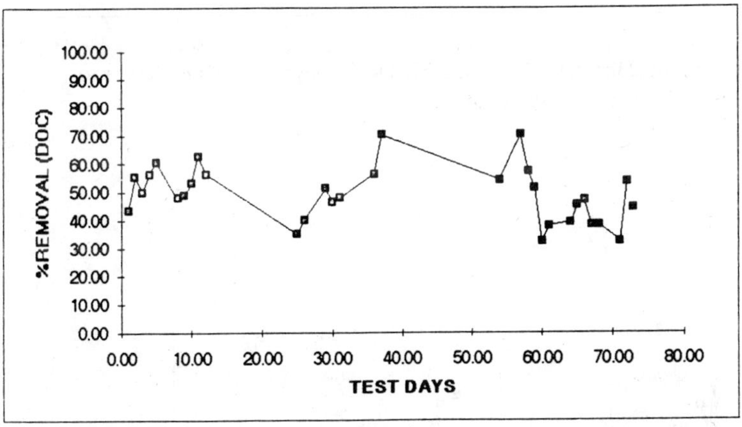

Fig. 8--DOC removal of 2,3,4,6-ethoxylated (1.5 eq.)-methyl-D-glucopyranoside in modified SCAS test (by daily % removal).

The third group of chemicals underwent very little if any DOC removal in the modified SCAS test (<10%). The example shown in Fig. 9 and Fig. 10 illustrated that no acclimation occurred and reproducibility was poor.

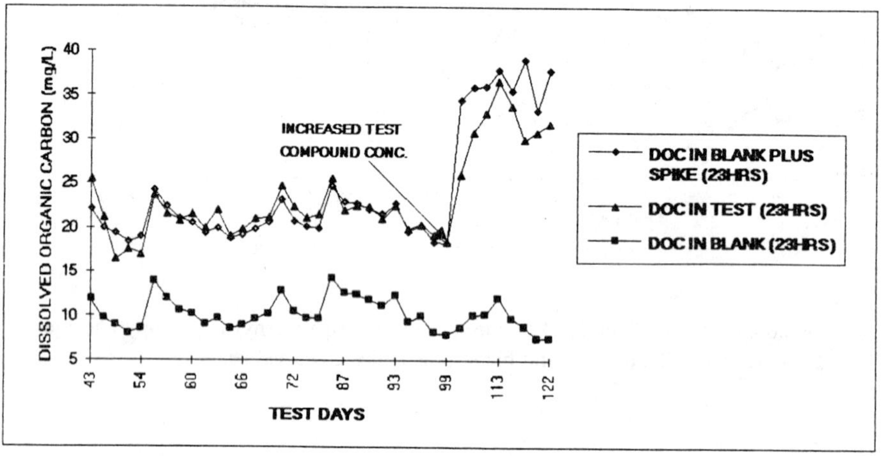

Fig. 9--A comparison of 23hr 2,3,4,6-tetramethyl-D-glucopyranose DOC levels to 23hr blank and blank plus spike DOC values.

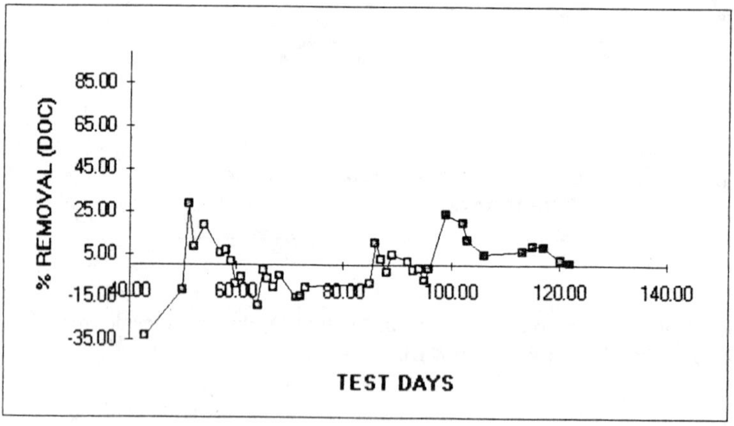

Fig. 10 --DOC removal of 2,3,4,6-tetramethyl-D-glucopyranose in modified SCAS test (by daily % removal).

The use of a natural sewage feed resulted in high and variable DOC values in the blank units (background feed, no test chemical) after the 23 hour aeration period. Therefore, in order to evaluate the relationships between the DOC concentrations in the test units and blanks, these data were plotted in figures 3,5,7 and 9 for typical compounds of classes I, II and III. Also shown in these figures are the calculated values for DOC which would theoretically be present in the effluents of the test units if no removal of the test compound occurred over the 23 hour aeration period (blank + test compound spike).

Comparisons of the DOC values in the effluents of the test units, blanks and blanks + spikes, which were graphically displayed in figures 3,5,7, and 9 were summarized in Table 2. It is clear that the effluent DOC values from the class I compounds were very close to the blank DOC concentrations but different than the blank + spike levels (signal to noise ratios of 2-3). In contrast, the effluent DOC values for the class III compound were very close to the blank + spike DOC concentrations and different from the blank DOC concentrations. The effluent DOC values of the class II test chemical were clearly different from the blank or blank + spike DOC levels.

In addition to providing an evaluation of the modified SCAS methodology, this study revealed information concerning the effects on DOC removal of hydroxyl hydrogen substitutions of glucose (Table 3). Unsubstituted glucose showed nearly complete (100% ± 8.3%) DOC removal in the SCAS test. Further more, regio-specific substitutions at the 3-O or 1-O positions resulted in apparently easily biodegradable compounds (class I), even though some required an acclimation period. Additional random substitutions in the 2-O, 4-O and 6-O positions inhibited DOC removal which resulted in compounds which would likely be characterized as partially or non-biodegradable (class II or III) chemicals. This example illustrated how the modified SCAS test could be used as an initial screening tool for evaluating the apparent biodegradability of water-soluble chemicals. However, extensive additional confirmatory testing would be required before a judgement could be reached concerning the environmental acceptability of these compounds.

TABLE 2. Examples of DOC concentrations in effluents from modified SCAS units

Compound	Class	"Steady State" Effluent DOC Concentrations (Mg/L)				Average "Steady State" DOC Removal			
		Mean	Std. Dev.	N	% Rel. Error	Mean	Std. Dev.	N	% Rel. Error
3-O-methyl-alpha-D-glucopyranose	I								
Test Unit		8.73	±1.45	19	16.60	98.5	± 3.2	19	3.25
Blank Unit		8.60	±1.43	19	16.62				
[1] Blank + Spike		17.50	±1.43	19	8.17				
3-O-[tetra(oxyethylene)]-D-glucopyranose	I								
[2] Test Unit		9.62	±1.52	9	15.80	94.6	± 2.0	9	2.11
Blank Unit		8.40	±1.60	9	19.04				
Blank + Spike		31.10	±1.60	9	5.14				
2,3,4,6-ethoxylated(1.5eg.)-methyl-D-glucopyranoside	II								
Test Unit		14.18	±1.82	37	12.83	50.1	±12.0	37	23.9
Blank Unit		9.49	±1.62	37	17.07				
Blank + Spike		18.89	±1.62	37	8.58				
2,3,4,6-tetramethyl-D-glucopyranose	III								
Test Unit		21.09	±2.23	29	10.57	-3.2	±11.9	29	372
Blank Unit		10.46	±1.77	29	16.92				
Blank + Spike		20.76	±1.77	29	8.53				

[1] Calculated DOC values which would be present in test unit effluent if NO loss of test compound occurred.
[2] Data for days 106-131 (Fig. 6)

TABLE 3--Effect of positional substitution on apparent biodegradation of glucose

Substituted Glucose		"Steady State" DOC Loss, %			Acclimation to "Steady State"
Position	Substituent	Mean	Std. Dev.	Days	Days
1	CH_3	99.6	2.8	3	0
3	CH_3	99.4	5.0	20	0
3	C_{10}	92.0	6.1	6	9
3	$(EO)_4$	92.5	3.7	13	13
3	$(EO)_2C_8$ [a]	91.1	3.5	11	0
3	$(EO)_6C_{12}$	91.7	2.0	7	0
1,2,3	CH_3	14.0	8.4	15	0
2,3,4,6	CH_3	0.5	12.6	37	0
1 2,3,4,6	CH_3 $(EO)_{1.5}$	48.5	9.8	35	0
1 2,3,4,6	CH_3 [b] $(EO)_6$-C_8-C_{10}	35.2	12.5	38	0

[a] This structure signifies that D-glucopyranose has been regio-specifically substituted at the hydroxyl group corresponding to carbon 3 in the glucose molecule with an average of two equivalents of ethylene oxide. The ethylene oxide residue is subsequently capped with a normal alkyl group with eight carbons (C_8H_{17}).

[b] This structure signifies that methyl-D-glucopyranoside has six equivalents of ethylene oxide residues randomly substituted at hydroxyl groups that correspond to carbons 2,3,4, and 6 in the glucose molecule. Subsequently, the ethylene oxide residues are capped with one equivalent of an alkyl group that are added randomly to either the 2,3,4, or 6 positions. The alkyl groups is a mixture of octyl (C_8H_{17}, 42.5%) and decyl ($C_{10}H_{19}$, 57.5%) alkyl groups.

DISCUSSION

The purpose in modifying the SCAS test was to develop an inexpensive, relatively trouble-free and effective method for screening the fate of a large number of water - soluble compounds upon exposure to sewage sludge. The experience of this study suggests that this methodology will satisfy these three criteria.

The cost for operating the modified SCAS methodology was minimal. It required about 50% of a technican's time to operate twenty SCAS units which included maintenance, sampling and analyses. The use of a nonspecific analytical method (DOC analysis) reduced costs by eliminating the need for new analytical methods or the requirement for syntheses of radiolabeled test compounds.

The use of natural sewage as background feed allowed for long-term, trouble-free operations. In our experience, the use of synthetic sewage background feed as in ASTM D2667-89 apparently caused population changes in the natural sludge. This change was manifested by color shifts and poorer settling. After ten to fifteen days of use, the sludge would usually disperse, stop settling and had to be replaced. On the other hand, if settled domestic sewage were used as the background feed, SCAS sludges maintained the orginal color and excellent settling properties of the starting ASU sludge, and SCAS units could be successfully operated for at least eighteen months.

The negative aspect of using a sewage background feed in conjunction with a nonspecific analysis is that it introduced a high (8-10 mg/L DOC) and variable (17-19 % relative error) background (blank unit effluent) DOC value in the percent DOC removal calculation. The OECD 302A guideline recognized that high levels of DOC would be present in the blank and stated that about "...10 mg/litre of dissolved organic carbon remain in the supernatant liquor of the control experiment." The authors of the OECD guideline also predicted that the extent of DOC removal should be within 6% for the range of 80 -100% removal if at least 20 mg/L DOC of test compound is used and the DOC determination is ± 5%. These predictions agreed well with the results for LAS and the other class I compounds (Table 1).

Despite the high and variable background DOC values, it was possible with the modified SCAS test to discriminate between those compounds which underwent high, intermediate, and low or no DOC removal (Table 2 and Figures 3, 5, 7 and 9). Since compounds known to undergo moderate or poor biodegradation in the SCAS test were not included as controls, it was not possible to determine the accuracy of removal for class II and III compounds.

The biochemical rationale is not known for the negative effect on apparent biodegradability and DOC removal of random substitutions in the 2-O, 4-O and 6-O positions of glucose. It is reasonable to speculate that the geometries of the randomly substituted molecules are altered sufficiently to no longer fit into the active sites of the enzymes utilized to biodegrade the molecules with regio-specific substitutions at the 3-

O and 1-O positions.

CONCLUSIONS

The modified SCAS test is a cost effective method for determining the overall fate of water-soluble compounds in the presence of sewage sludge.

This methodology separated the test compounds into three classes based on high (≥87%), intermediate (≤87% - ≥10%) and low or no (≤10%) average DOC removals.

By using this test it was possible to demonstrate that specific regio-substitutions at the 3-O and 1-O positions of glucose do not inhibit apparent biodegradability, but random substitutions at the other positions adversely affect the DOC removal characteristics of these compounds.

REFERENCES

Box, G., Hunter, W.G., and Hunter, J.S., 1978, Statistics for Experimenters: An Introduction to Design, Data Analysis and Model Building, John Wiley and Sons, New York.

King, J. E., Hopping, W. D., and Holman, W. F., 1980, "Treatability of Type A Zeolite in Waste Water 1," Journal of Water Pollution Control Federation, Vol. 52, No. 12, pp. 2875-2886.

Larson, R. J., Dec. 1979, "Estimation of Biodegradation Potential of Xenobiotic Organic Chemicals," Applied And Environmental Microbiology, Vol. 38, No. 6, pp. 1153-1161.

Naylor, C. G., Castaldi, F. J., and Hayes, B. J., 1988, "Biodegradation of Nonionic Surfactants Containing Propylene Oxide," Journal of the American Oil Chemists' Society, Vol. 65, No. 10, pp. 1669-1676.

Nielsen, A. M., 1991. "Primary and Ultimate Biodegradation of Linear Alkylbenzene Sulfonate(LAS) and Aquatic Toxicity of LAS Biodegradation Intermediates," Biodeterioration & Biodegradation 8: Proceedings of the 8th International Symposium 26-31 August 1990, Windsor, Ontario, Canada, Edited by Rossmoore, H.W., Elsevier Science Publishers Ltd., New York, pp. 377-379.

O'Grady, D. P., Howard, P.H., and Werner, A. F., 1985, "Activated Sludge Biodegradation of Twelve Commercial Phthalate Esters," Applied and Environmental Microbiology, Vol. 49, No. 2, pp. 443-445.

Saeger, V. W. and Tucker, E. S., August 1973, "Phthalate Esters Under Ready Biodegradation," Plastics Engineering, Vol. 29, No. 8, pp. 46-49.

Struijs, J. and Stoltenkamp, J., 1986, "Ultimate Biodegradation of 2,3 and 4 Nitrotoluene," Science of the Total Environment, Vol. 57, No. 0, pp. 161-170.

The Soap and Detergent Association Subcommittee on Biodegradation Test Methods, 1965, "A Procedure and Standards For the Determination of the Biodegradability of Alkyl Benzene Sulfonate and Linear Alkylate Sulfonate," Journal of the American Oil Chemists' Society, Vol. 42, pp. 986-993.

The Soap and Detergent Association Subcommittee on Biodegradation Test Methods, 1969, "The Status of Biodegradability Testing of Nonionic Surfactants," Journal of the American Oil Chemists' Society, Vol. 46, pp. 432-438.

Vashon, R. D., Jones, W. J., and Payne, A. G., 1982. " The Effect of Water Hardness of Nitrilo Tri Acetate Removal and Microbial Acclimation in Activated Sludge," Water Research, Vol. 16, No. 9, pp. 1429-1432.

Waters, J., Kleiser, H. H., How, M. J., Barratt, M. D., Birch, R. R., Fletcher, R. J., Haigh, S. D., Hales, S. G., Marshall S. J., Pestell, T. C., 1991. " A New Rinse Conditioner With Improved Environmental Properties," Tenside Surfactant Detergents, Vol. 28, No. 6, pp. 460-468.

Author Index

A

Allstock, M. S., 303
Anderson, E. R., 377

B

Bartell, S. M., 3
Biddinger, G. R., 3
Björkroth, K., 351
Black, M. C., 351
Bollman, M., 61

C

Cece, A., 318
Costlow, Jr., J. D., 267
Cunningham, P. A., 267

D

Darrow, T., 61
Dillon, T. M., 201
Duncan, P. B., 242

E

Evans, D. W., 267

F

Ferson, S., 97
Filler, P. A., 393
Fleming, W. J., 303
Frago, C., 365

G

Gillett, C., 61
Gorsuch, J. W., 377
Gruber, D., 365

H

Hallam, T. G., 157
Heinze, J. E., 393
Henderson, G., 61
Henson, S. M., 157
Hovatter, P. S., 288
Hunter, R. S., 172

J

Jaworska, J. S., 157, 172
Johnson, J. K., 29

K

King, R., 61

L

Lachocki, T. M., 393
Landis, W. G., 79, 133
Lassiter, R. R., 157
Lightfoot, D., 61
Linder, G., 61
Long, T. F., 97

K

Kross, B. C., 29

M

MacGregor, M. A., 187
Markiewicz, A. J., 133
Matthews, G. B., 79, 133
Matthews, R. A., 79, 133
McKinney, W. R., 157
Momot, J. J., 303
Moore, D. W., 201
Moschner, K. F., 318

N

Nielsen, A. M., 393
Nwosu, J., 61

O

Oikari, A., 351
Ott, S., 61

P

Pfleeger, T., 61
Postlethwaite, D., 332

R

Reish, D. J., 201
Ritter, M., 377
Rose, K. A., 242
Ross, R. H., 288

S

Salazar, M. H., 216, 242
Salazar, S. M., 216, 242
Schultz, T. W., 172
Scott, P. K., 111

T

Trowbridge, K. R., 111

V

Vigna, J. R., 29

W

Walsh, G. E., 187
Weber, D. E., 187
Wilborn, D., 61
Wilson, J. E. H., 267

Subject Index

A

Agricultural conservation and management practices, 29
Alachlor, 303
Alkylbenzene sulfonates biodegradability, 393
Amphibians, freshwater, 288
Artificial intelligence, nonmetric clustering, 79
Assessment endpoints, 3
Assessment process, risk, 61
Assessment protocol, rapid, 29
Assessment tools, 3
Association analysis, 133
ASTM standards
  D 2667: 393
Automated biomonitoring system, 365

B

Bioaccumulation, 111, 216, 242
Boric acid, 288

C

Cadmium, 377
Chemical analyses, 61
CHEMICALC2, 318
Chromatography, high performance liquid, 267, 351
Chromium, 377
Clay minerals, 187
CLOGP, 318
Clustering, nonmetric, 79
Copper, 242, 377
Co-product allocation, 332
Correlation structure, 97
Cucumber, 377
Cucumis sativus, 377

D

Daphnia magna, 157, 288
Dependency bounds, 97
Diflubenzuron, 267
Dose-response data, 3, 216, 242

E

Echinochloa crusgalli, 187
Embryotoxicity, shrimp, sediment effect on, 267
Endpoints
  assessment, 3
  mortality, 172, 288, 377
  toxicity testing, 79
Energy accounting, 332
Escherichia coli, 157
Expert systems, 79
Exposure-response assays, 3

F

Fast Fourier transformation, 365
Fate modeling, 111
Field monitoring, 79
Field screening, 61
Field tests, 216, 242
Fish, 157, 172, 288, 351, 365
Freshwater versus saltwater, boron toxicity, 288

G

Gambusia affinis, 288
Geographic information systems, 3
Glovers Creek Watershed Protection Project, 29
Glucose, substituted, 393
Growth rate/inhibition, 172, 187, 201, 351
  grass shrimp, 267
  mussels, 216, 242
  plant, 377

H

Herbicides, 303
Hydrophobicity, 172, 318

I

Impact assessment, 332
Individual-based models, 157
International Organization for Standardization, 332
Invertebrates, 288

J

Jet fuel, 133

L

Lactuca sativa, 377
Lake Ontario, 111
Lettuce, 377
Lifecycle assessment, 332
Limanda limanda, 288
Limnoria lignorum, 288

M

Macroinvertebrates, 29
Manganese, 377
Metals, 377
Methylene blue, 393
Microcosm, multivariate analysis in, 133
Millet, 377
Milltown Reservoir wetlands, 61
Minnow, 172, 288
Modeling, 318
  capabilities, 3
  fate, 111
  individual-based, 157
  predator-prey community, 157
  transport, 111
  upwardly scaled, 3
Monte Carlo simulation, 97
Multispecies tests, 79
Multivariate analysis, 133
Mussel transplants, 216, 242
Mytilus galloprovincialis, 216
Mytilus trossulus, 242

N

Narcosis, 172
Nereis (Neanthes) arenaceodentata, 201
Nickel, 377
Nonlinear oscillations, 133
Nonmetric clustering, 79, 133
Nonpoint source pollution, 29

O

Octanol-water partition coefficients, 318
Oncorhynchus mykiss, 157, 351

P

Palaemonetes pugio, 267
Panicum miliaceum, 377
Pentachlorophenol, 351
Photosynthesis, pondweed, 303
Pimephales promelas, 172, 288
Plastics, 332
Polychaetes, 201
Polychlorinated biphenyls, 111
Pondweed, 303
Potamogeton pectinatus, 303
Predator-prey communities, 157
Probabilistic arithmetic, 97
Puget Sound, 242
Pulp mill effluents, 351

Q

Quantitative structure activity relationships, 157, 318

R

RBP II, 29
Respiration, pondweed, 303
Respiratory uncoupling, 172
Rhizosphere microorganisms, 187
Root elongation, 377
Root nodulation, 187

S

Sago pondweed, 303
Salmonids, 111
San Diego Bay, 216
SCAS, semicontinuous activated sludge test, 393
Screening methods
  field, 61
  laboratory, 61

Sediments, 61, 201, 216, 242, 267
simulated, 187
Sesbania macrocarpa, 187
SETAC, 332
Shelter Island Yacht Basin, 216
Shrimp, grass, 267
Sludge test, 393
Sodium borate, 288
Spartina alterniflora, 187
Split screen video techniques, wastewater toxicity, 365
Standard Aquatic Microcosm, 133
Strip-chart readings, wastewater toxicity, 365
Surfactants, 318, 332, 393

T

TBT, 242
Tetrahymena pyriformis, 157, 172
Tissue accumulation, 242
Transplant mussels, bioassays with, 216, 242
Transport modeling, 111
Trout, 157, 351

V

Volume fraction analyses, 172

W

Wastewater toxicity, 365, 377
Water food webs, 111, 157
Water plants, 187
Water flea, 157, 288
Water sediments, 187, 201, 242, 267
Watershed protection project, 29
Water soluble fraction, 133
Waveform, 365
Wetlands, 187
risk assessment, 61
Worms, 201
Worst case analysis, 97

X

Xenobiotic transformation, 351

Z

Zinc, 377